D1761256

Neuro-Ophthalmology Illustrated

2nd Edition

Valérie Biousse, MD
Cyrus H. Stoner Professor of Ophthalmology
Professor of Ophthalmology and Neurology
Emory University School of Medicine
Neuro-ophthalmology Unit
Emory Eye Center
Atlanta, Georgia

Nancy J. Newman, MD
Leo Delle Jolley Professor of Ophthalmology
Professor of Ophthalmology, Neurology, and Neurological Surgery
Emory University School of Medicine
Neuro-ophthalmology Unit
Emory Eye Center
Atlanta, Georgia

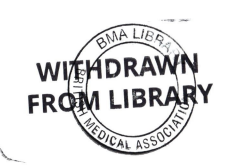
Thieme
New York • Stuttgart • Delhi • Rio de Janeiro

Executive Editor: William Lamsback
Managing Editor: Elizabeth Palumbo
Director, Editorial Services: Mary Jo Casey
Editorial Assistant: Mohammad Ibrar
Production Editor: Sean Woznicki
International Production Director: Andreas Schabert
Vice President, Editorial and E-Product Development:
Vera Spiller
International Marketing Director: Fiona Henderson
International Sales Director: Louisa Turrell
Director of Sales, North America: Mike Roseman
Senior Vice President and Chief Operating Officer:
Sarah Vanderbilt
President: Brian D. Scanlan
Printer: Asia Pacific Offset

Library of Congress Cataloging-in-Publication Data

Biousse, Valérie, author.
Neuro-ophthalmology illustrated / Valérie Biousse,
Nancy J. Newman. – Second edition
p. ; cm.
ISBN 978-1-62623-149-8 (softcover) –
ISBN 978-1-62623-150-4 (eISBN)
I. Newman, Nancy J., author. II. Title.
[DNLM: 1. Eye Diseases–diagnosis–Atlases. 2. Eye Diseases–
therapy–Atlases. 3. Eye Manifestations–Atlases. 4. Nervous
System Diseases–complications–Atlases. WW 17]
RE46
617.7–dc23   2014032080

Important note: Medicine is an ever-changing science undergoing continual development. Research and clinical experience are continually expanding our knowledge, in particular our knowledge of proper treatment and drug therapy. Insofar as this book mentions any dosage or application, readers may rest assured that the authors, editors, and publishers have made every effort to ensure that such references are in accordance with **the state of knowledge at the time of production of the book.**

Nevertheless, this does not involve, imply, or express any guarantee or responsibility on the part of the publishers in respect to any dosage instructions and forms of applications stated in the book. **Every user is requested to examine carefully** the manufacturers' leaflets accompanying each drug and to check, if necessary in consultation with a physician or specialist, whether the dosage schedules mentioned therein or the contraindications stated by the manufacturers differ from the statements made in the present book. Such examination is particularly important with drugs that are either rarely used or have been newly released on the market. Every dosage schedule or every form of application used is entirely at the user's own risk and responsibility. The authors and publishers request every user to report to the publishers any discrepancies or inaccuracies noticed. If errors in this work are found after publication, errata will be posted at www.thieme.com on the product description page.

Some of the product names, patents, and registered designs referred to in this book are in fact registered trademarks or proprietary names even though specific reference to this fact is not always made in the text. Therefore, the appearance of a name without designation as proprietary is not to be construed as a representation by the publisher that it is in the public domain.

© 2016 Thieme Medical Publishers, Inc.

Thieme Publishers New York
333 Seventh Avenue, New York, NY 10001 USA,
1-800-782-3488
customerservice@thieme.com

Thieme Publishers Stuttgart
Rüdigerstrasse 14, 70469 Stuttgart, Germany,
+49 [0]711 8931 421
customerservice@thieme.de

Thieme Publishers Delhi
A-12, Second Floor, Sector -2, NOIDA -201301,
Uttar Pradesh, India, +91 120 45 566 00
customerservice@thieme.in

Thieme Publishers Rio de Janeiro, Thieme Publicações Ltda.
Argentina Building 16th floor, Ala A, 228 Praia do Botafogo
Rio de Janeiro 22250-040 Brazil, +55 21 3736-3631

Printed in China

5 4 3 2 1

ISBN 978-1-62623-149-8

Also available as an e-book:
eISBN978-1-62623-150-4

MIX
Paper from
responsible sources
FSC® C012521
www.fsc.org

We dedicate this book to our students.

Contents

Contents

Preface to the 1st edition

Neuro-ophthalmology is the "overlap" specialty between ophthalmology and neurology. It covers all the disorders that may affect those parts of the central nervous system devoted to vision: the afferent visual system (the pathways for visual input and processing), which encompasses more than one third of the supratentorial brain mass, and the efferent system (the pathways for ocular motor control and pupillary function), which crisscrosses throughout the brainstem and cerebellum. Indeed, it is hard to imagine a neurologic disorder that could not have neuro-ophthalmic manifestations. Hence, neuro-ophthalmology has also been referred to as "applied neuroanatomy."

Neuro-ophthalmology is also that part of ophthalmology that most scares ophthalmologists and that most confuses neurologists. Ophthalmologists, skilled in the direct inspection of the eye, are accustomed to seeing the pathology, rather than inferring it. Brain tumors, ischemic events, and inflammation can present with the same patient complaints such as refractive error, dry eye, or cataract, but the implications for management and prognosis are dramatically different, and correct diagnosis is essential. Neurologists, although perhaps more comfortable with the diagnosis and management of life-threatening neurologic processes, are often challenged by the techniques of the examination of the visual system-skills frequently neglected in their training and relegated to "eye doctors." Diagnosing brain disease using the eye examination is not easy if the components of the eye examination include skills and techniques unfamiliar to the neurologist.

Perhaps most importantly, neuro-ophthalmology is deeply rooted in a certain way of thinking. It begins first and foremost with neuroanatomy, moves next to the mechanisms of disease, then generates a differential diagnosis of which specific disorders to consider, and finally addresses the appropriate management for diagnosis and treatment: (1) Where? (2) How? (3) What? (4) Now what? For example, in a patient presenting with visual loss, the first step is to localize the lesion along the pathways of vision (Where?). Let's say that the localization is the optic nerve. The second step, then, is to review all those categories of disease that can affect the optic nerve (inflammatory, vascular, compressive, toxic, etc.) and decide which one best fits the clinical profile of the case

(How?). Once the likely mechanisms have been identified, specific disorders can be considered (What?). Ultimately, the appropriate diagnostic tests and further management will depend on the preceding process of logical thinking (Now what?).

Welcome to *Neuro-Ophthalmology Illustrated*. It is hard to imagine a more "visual" subspecialty than neuro-ophthalmology. All the layers of the eye are available for direct inspection using the techniques and tools of the ophthalmologist, and all the features of the brain are exposed by today's exquisite advances in neuroimaging. Over the course of 20 years of teaching medical students, residents, fellows, and practitioners, we have personally acquired over 20,000 unique clinical images. We have used more than 1000 of these images in this book to illustrate the phenomenal richness of clinical neuro-ophthalmology. More than an atlas, *Neuro-Ophthalmology Illustrated* aims to provide the essential information on basic clinical neuro-ophthalmology and to simplify the perceived complexity of neuro-ophthalmology, without sacrificing comprehensiveness.

This book began with the idea of a small, practical, and portable manual for medical students and residents, especially residents preparing for board examinations in ophthalmology, neurology, and neurosurgery, as well as those pursuing careers in neuroradiology, otolaryngology, and even primary care. We have attempted to compensate for the diversity of our audience by providing the necessary basic information on the two primary specialties that overlap to become neuro-ophthalmology. For the ophthalmology-naive student of neurology, we provide a basic introduction into the anatomy, physiology, and examination of the eye. For the ophthalmologist, we reciprocate with practical examples of brain anatomy and circuitry, as well as the fundamentals of neuroimaging. The book is structured to include sections on the essential components of the neuro-ophthalmic examination and evaluation; disorders of the visual afferent system, pupil, ocular motor efferent systems, orbit, and lid; evaluation of the nonorganic patient; and common or classic neurologic and systemic disorders with important neuro-ophthalmic manifestations. A more comprehensive index appears at the end of the book. The emphasis is on how to think about these disorders, from symptoms and signs, to localization, differential diagnosis, and management.

Neuro-ophthalmologists are teachers. We teach ophthalmologists about the brain and neurologists and neurosurgeons about the eye. We facilitate communication between specialties and among physicians. Although we believe our book is still the practical manual it was meant to be, we hope that the richness of the illustrations will serve as a reference for practitioners in all the related fields and for our fellow teachers of neuro-ophthalmology. We hope that *Neuro-Ophthalmology Illustrated* facilitates your learning and your teaching.

Preface to the 2nd edition

Over the 6 years since the publication of the first edition, *Neuro-Ophthalmology Illustrated* has sold by the thousands. Reviews have been spectacular and we are overwhelmed by the positive response worldwide, from both trainees and mentors. It has been lauded as "the best soft-cover training manual in neuro-ophthalmology", "a tour de force", and even "a great stocking stuffer for every neurology and ophthalmology resident". We are very proud and humbled by its success.

We hope now to have made it better. This second edition has been fully updated. Although the overall structure of the book remains the same, new sections have been added and space used more efficiently. Illustrations have been enlarged and clarified, the inevitable errors identified by our eagle-eyed trainees have been corrected, and feedback from our readers has been incorporated. We hope you enjoy!

Acknowledgements

We wish to thank those who have helped us with this second edition. Specifically, we are grateful to William Lamsback, Thieme's Executive Editor for Ophthalmology Publications, and to our Managing Editor, Liz Palumbo, who shepherded this book and us through the trials of publication. Finally, we thank Philip S. Garza ("almost M.D.") for his exquisitely careful proofreading.

Valérie Biousse
Nancy J. Newman

1 The Neuro-ophthalmic Examination

A detailed neuro-ophthalmic examination is part of routine neurologic and ophthalmic examinations. It is a powerful means to detect and localize lesions that involve the visual system. Documentation of the extent of damage within the visual system is also an invaluable method to assess the effect of various therapies and often guides the management of numerous neurologic and neurosurgical disorders.

The extent of the neuro-ophthalmic examination varies depending on the patient's complaints, but parts of it should always be performed in detail in selected neurologic disorders, and some parts of the neuro-ophthalmic examination should be systematically performed in most neurologic and systemic diseases. For example, in a patient with an occipital infarction, evaluations of visual acuity, color vision, and formal visual fields are the most important. A patient with known multiple sclerosis needs a thorough examination, because all functions involved in the visual system may be affected. In a patient complaining of diplopia or with anisocoria, formal visual field testing is usually not necessary, whereas all patients with raised intracranial pressure and papilledema should have formal visual field testing, even when they have no visual symptoms.

Most examination techniques detailed here are best performed with appropriate tools in a neuro-ophthalmologist's or ophthalmologist's office. However, a basic neuro-ophthalmic examination (including evaluation of the vision, pupillary function, ocular motility, and funduscopy) can be performed at the bedside, in the emergency room, or in a neurologist's office with only very few tools (see ▶ Table 1.1 for a list of required tools).

The examination usually follows a specific order, as given in the following discussion (e.g., you have to examine the visual acuity before flashing light into the eyes; the pupils need to be examined before drops are placed in the eyes; funduscopic examination is the last part of the examination).

1.1 Visual Acuity

In examining the patient's visual acuity, each eye is tested separately (▶ Fig. 1.1). Visual acuity is measured with the patient's corrective lenses or a pinhole (▶ Fig. 1.2). There are two types of visual acuity tests: distance and near.

Table 1.1 Tools needed for a neuro-ophthalmic examination at the bedside

- Near card to check visual acuity
- A pair of reading glasses (+ 2.00 or + 3.00)
- A pinhole (made from cardboard or plastic with a few small pinholes)
- A red object, such as a pen or the top from a bottle of dilating drops (used to check for color saturation and for visual fields)
- A striped ribbon or paper to test optokinetic nystagmus
- An Amsler grid
- Short-lasting dilating drops
- A direct ophthalmoscope with spare batteries (used to check the pupils, to perform a penlight examination of the eyes, and to examine the fundus)

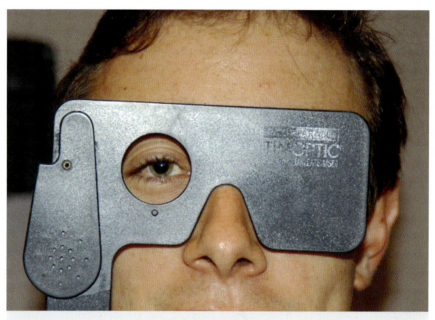

Fig. 1.1 Cover one eye to measure visual acuity. The occluder can be used over the patient's glasses.

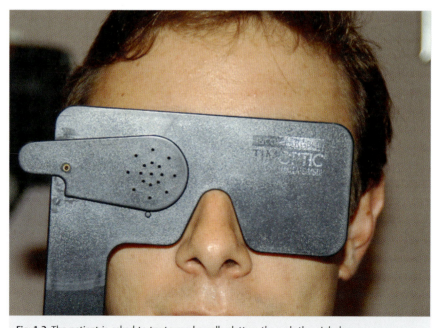

Fig. 1.2 The patient is asked to try to read smaller letters through the pinholes.

Distance visual acuity is tested as follows (▶ Fig. 1.1 and ▶ Fig. 1.2):

1. Place a Snellen chart at 20 feet.
2. Record the smallest letters read by the patient with each eye (e.g., "20/20 right eye with correction; 20/25 left eye with pinhole").
3. If the patient cannot read the largest letter, visual acuity is less than 20/400 and is recorded as "count fingers," "hand motion," "light perception," or "no light perception."

The pinhole is an opaque panel perforated with one or more holes 1.0 to 1.5 mm in diameter. The holes restrict incoming light rays to a narrow path that bypasses refractive irregularities and presents a single, focused image to the fovea of the retina. Refractive errors and visual loss from cataracts improve with a pinhole. If visual acuity cannot be improved with a pinhole, then other media opacities, optic nerve disease, maculopathy, or amblyopia is likely the cause of visual loss. The test may be unreliable with young children, the elderly, and cognitively impaired individuals.

Near visual acuity is tested as follows (▶ Fig. 1.3 and ▶ Fig. 1.4):

1. Hold a near card at 14 inches from the patient. The patient should be tested with reading glasses (or a + 2.00 or + 3.00 lens) if he or she is older than age 50 (because of presbyopia).

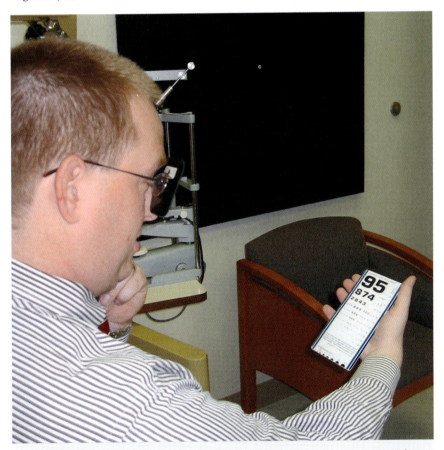

Fig. 1.3 Near vision is tested using a near card held at 14 inches from the patient. It must be tested with the patient's correction for near vision. Most patients older than age 50 will use a + 2.00 or + 3.00 lens to read.

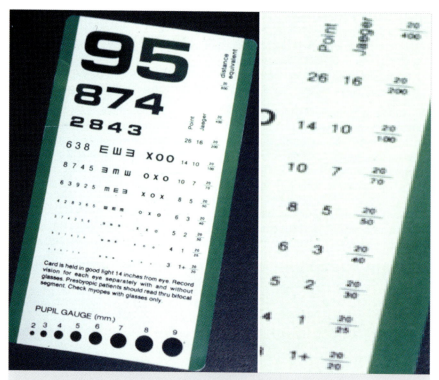

Fig. 1.4 The near card uses numbers or letters. It is usually measured in Jaeger numbers (J1 + corresponds to 20/20, J16 to 20/200).

2. Record the smallest letters or numbers read by the patient with each eye (e.g., "J1 + right eye with correction; J1 left eye with correction").

1.2 Color Vision, Color Saturation

Color vision can be assessed by several methods, and each eye is tested separately. The purpose of color vision testing is to detect acquired unilateral or bilateral color loss, which occurs most commonly with maculopathies, optic neuropathies, chiasmal disorders, and, more rarely, bilateral occipital lesions.

The Ishihara pseudoisochromatic and the Hardy-Rand-Rittler (HRR) color plates are routinely used (▶ Fig. 1.5). The number of plates correctly identified with each eye is recorded (e.g., "14/14 Ishihara color plates right eye; control only left eye"). The control plate can be read by patients with a visual acuity of at least 20/400. Some patients with dementia and simultagnosia may have difficulty using these plates.

When color plates are unavailable, the difference in color perception between the two eyes may be identified using a red object (e.g., the top from a bottle of dilating drops) (▶ Fig. 1.6). Even with normal color plate testing, the patient may recognize a color difference in a red bottle top alternately presented to each eye. The patient should be asked to quantify the red desaturation (percentage of normal).

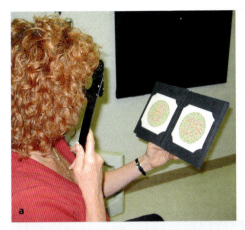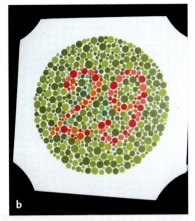

Fig. 1.5 (a,b) Color testing with the Ishihara color plates.

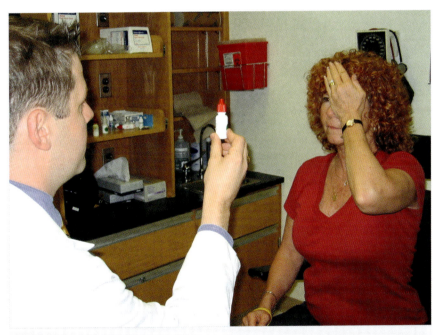

Fig. 1.6 Comparison of color saturation between the two eyes using a red object.

1.3 Contrast Sensitivity

Contrast sensitivity is another measure of visual function and is often abnormal in patients with optic neuropathies. Patients with maculopathies and cataracts also often have decreased contrast sensitivity. It is not tested in all patients but is useful in patients with visual complaints and an otherwise normal examination. It is also used as a measure of visual function in numerous clinical trials, especially multiple sclerosis trials. The test uses a chart with letters or stripes represented in various shades of gray.

1.4 Photostress Recovery Test

Photostress recovery is used to differentiate between macular disease and optic neuropathy. The principle underlying this test is that recovery of retinal sensitivity following exposure to a bright light is based on regeneration of visual pigments that were bleached during exposure to light. A delay in this process occurs in diseases affecting the photoreceptors and is independent of the neural pathways.

Each eye is tested separately:
1. Measure the best corrected visual acuity in each eye.
2. Have the patient look directly into a bright light held a few centimeters from the eye for 10 seconds.
3. Record the time taken for the visual acuity to return to within one line of the best corrected visual acuity.

Most normal patients will have a recovery time of less than 30 seconds, which is symmetric between the two eyes. Macular diseases (but not optic neuropathies) often cause a prolongation in the photostress recovery time. This is particularly useful for unilateral or subtle macular diseases.

1.5 Amsler Grid

The Amsler grid is very useful in detecting macular abnormalities as a cause of visual loss (▶ Fig. 1.7a).

Each eye is tested separately, and the patient is asked to fixate on a central point in a square grid of lines and to draw any area in which the lines disappear or are broken, warped, double, or curved (▶ Fig. 1.7b).

Patients with maculopathy often see the straight lines as curved (metamorphopsia) (▶ Fig. 1.7c).

1.6 Stereo Vision

Stereo vision is tested on a specific book (Titmus test) with both eyes open and polarized glasses placed on the patient's reading corrective lenses. This book shows animals and circles that are seen in stereo with the polarized glasses (▶ Fig. 1.8).

Stereopsis requires binocular vision. Therefore, the presence of stereopsis indicates at least some vision in each eye. This test is very helpful when nonorganic visual loss is suspected.

Stereopsis can be quantified and correlated with visual acuity (▶ Table 1.2).

1.7 Eyelid Examination

An eyelid examination includes evaluation of the following:
- Position of the eyelids
  - Ptosis (droopy eyelid)
  - Retraction
- Lid function
- Swelling
- Mass

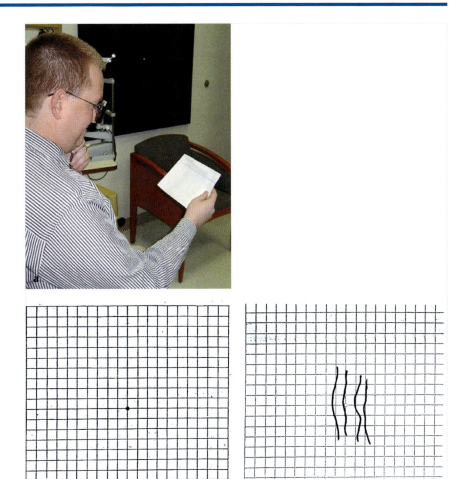

Fig. 1.7 (a) Amsler grid testing. (b) Normal Amsler grid. (c) Amsler grid showing central distortion of the lines.

In normal individuals, the upper lid covers the superior 1 to 2 mm of the iris, while the lower lid just reaches the inferior aspect of the iris (▶ Fig. 1.9). Examination of the eyelids (▶ Fig. 1.10 and ▶ Fig. 1.11) includes measurements of the following:

- Palpebral fissure: distance between the upper and lower eyelid in vertical alignment with the center of the pupil (normal 9–12 mm)
- Margin reflex distance (normal 4–5 mm)
  - Marginal reflex distance-1 (MRD-1): distance between the center of the pupillary light reflex and the upper eyelid margin with the eye in primary gaze
  - Marginal reflex distance-2 (MRD-2): distance between the center of the pupillary light reflex and the lower eyelid margin with the eye in primary gaze

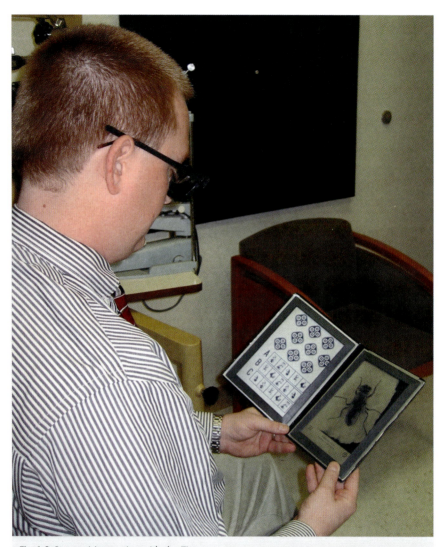

Fig. 1.8 Stereo vision testing with the Titmus test.

Table 1.2 Relationship of visual acuity to stereopsis

Visual acuity in each eye	Stereopsis (arc seconds)[a]
20/20	40
20/25	43
20/30	52
20/40	61
20/50	89
20/70	94
20/100	124
20/200	160

[a]The Titmus test gives results in seconds of arc.

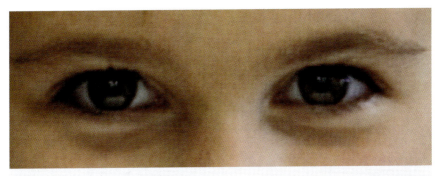

Fig. 1.9 Normal eyelids.

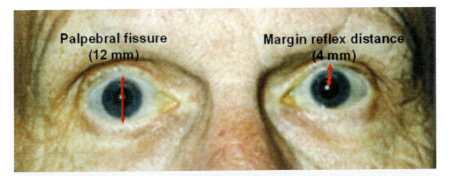

Fig. 1.10 Measurement of palpebral fissure and margin reflex distance.

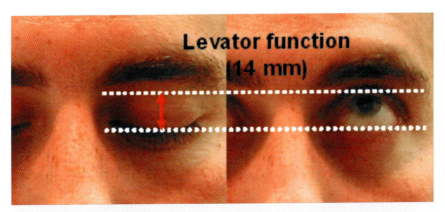

Fig. 1.11 Measurement of levator function.

- Levator function: distance the eyelid travels from downgaze to upgaze while the frontalis muscle is held inactive at the brow. A measurement of greater than 10 mm is considered excellent, whereas 0 to 5 mm is considered poor.

For more information on disorders of the eyelid, see Chapter 17.

1.8 Orbital Examination

An orbital examination includes the following:
- Inspection of the patient's external appearance:
  - Orbital deformations
    - Hypo- or hypertropia of the globes
  - Abnormal position of the eyes within the orbits
    - Proptosis (eye bulging out of the orbit)
    - Enophthalmos (eye sinking into the orbit)
  - Periorbital soft tissues
    - Swelling
    - Redness
    - Hematoma
    - Mass
- Palpation of the orbital rims
- Resistance to retropulsion of the eyes
- Auscultation of the orbital contents (for a bruit)

Proptosis can be measured with the Hertel exophthalmometer (▶ Fig. 1.12) and on neuroimaging (▶ Fig. 1.13). Deformations (▶ Fig. 1.14) and disease (▶ Fig. 1.15) cause various orbital syndromes. For more information on orbital syndromes, see Chapter 14.

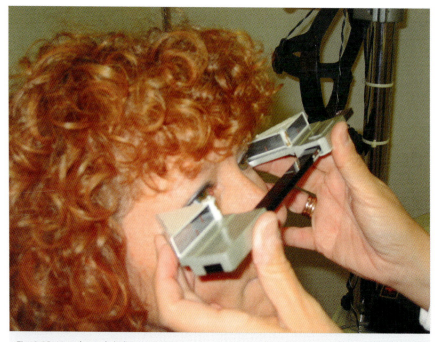

Fig. 1.12 Hertel exophthalmometer.

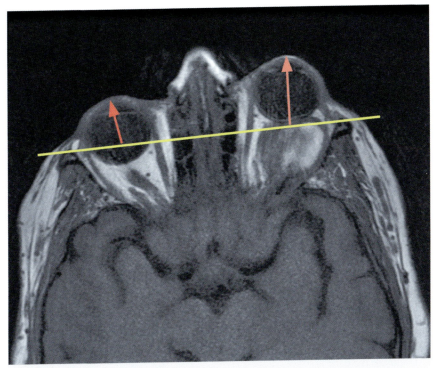

Fig. 1.13 Measurement of proptosis on axial orbital magnetic resonance imaging.

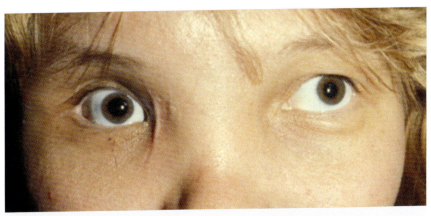

Fig. 1.14 Bilateral orbital deformations from fibrous dysplasia. The right orbit is lower (hypoglobus), and the left eye is deviated out because of bony deformation.

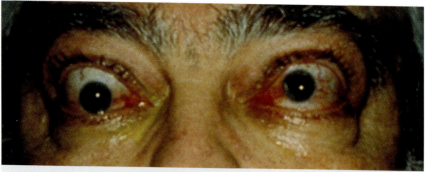

Fig. 1.15 Thyroid eye disease with bilateral proptosis, lid retraction, ocular misalignment, and conjunctival hyperemia over the insertions of the rectus muscles.

1.9 Pupillary Testing

Pupils should be tested in the dark with a bright light and with the patient fixating at a distance (▶ Fig. 1.16). Pupil examination includes the following (▶ Table 1.3):
• Size
• Presence of anisocoria (difference of size between the two pupils)
• Response to light
• Presence of a relative afferent pupillary defect (RAPD)
• Dilation in the dark
• Constriction at near

For a full discussion on the pupil, see Chapter 12.

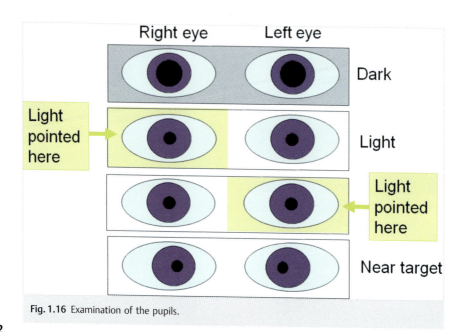

Fig. 1.16 Examination of the pupils.

Table 1.3 Testing the pupils (how to report the results)

	Right eye	Left eye
Dark	6 mm	6 mm
Light	3 mm	3 mm
Reaction to light	Brisk (3+)	Brisk (3+)
RAPD	No	No
Dilation in dark	Normal	Normal
Reaction at near	2 mm	2 mm

Abbreviation: RAPD, relative afferent pupillary defect.

1.9.1 Relative Afferent Pupillary Defect

A RAPD (▶ Fig. 1.17 and ▶ Fig. 1.18) ipsilateral to visual loss indicates an optic neuropathy or severe retinal disease (in which case the retina looks abnormal on funduscopic examination). Ocular diseases, such as corneal abnormalities, cataracts, and most retinal disorders, do not cause RAPDs.

Pathophysiology of the RAPD includes the following:

1. When a light is directed into either eye, both pupils react equally. The brighter the light source, the greater the degree of bilateral pupillary constriction.
2. The amount of pupillary constriction from the same light source directed to either eye should be identical.
3. In unilateral optic nerve (or retinal ganglion cell) dysfunction, the light signal received by the brainstem efferent centers is relatively less than when the same light source is presented to the unaffected eye. Hence, both pupils constrict less when the involved eye is stimulated and more when the normal eye is stimulated.
4. A RAPD will not cause anisocoria.

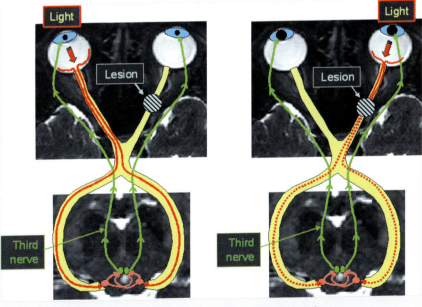

Fig. 1.17 Pathophysiology of a relative afferent pupillary defect in the left eye.

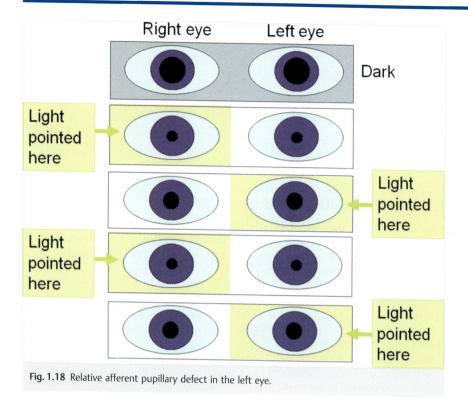

Fig. 1.18 Relative afferent pupillary defect in the left eye.

Testing for a RAPD includes the following:
1. The swinging flashlight test demonstrates a relative afferent pupillary defect in patients with unilateral or asymmetric optic neuropathies (Marcus Gunn pupil):
   - Swinging the light source back and forth emphasizes this difference in transmission of the afferent signal because both pupils will reset at the size appropriate for the amount of light transmitted by the illuminated optic nerve.
   - When the light source swings from the affected eye to the unaffected eye, further constriction of both pupils will be demonstrated; when the light swings back to the involved eye, relative dilation of both pupils will occur. Even though the examiner may look only at the pupil upon which the light is shining, it is important to be aware that both pupils are changing size equally during this maneuver.
2. By placing neutral density filters over the normal eye, the examiner can neutralize the RAPD and quantitate its severity (► Fig. 1.19).

1.9.2 Anisocoria

Anisocoria (unequal pupils; ► Fig. 1.20) means there is an abnormality of the efferent (sympathetic or parasympathetic) portion of the pupil pathways. Lesions of the afferent pathways do not produce anisocoria.

When evaluating a patient with anisocoria, pupil examination in the dark and light allows determination of which pupil is abnormal.

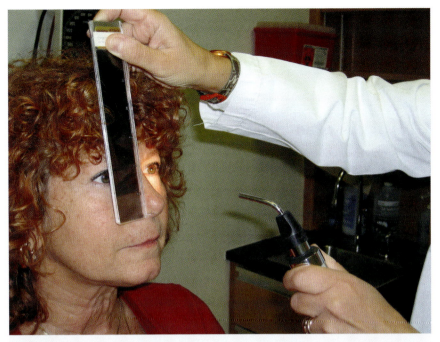

Fig. 1.19 Neutralization of a relative afferent pupillary defect with neutral density filters.

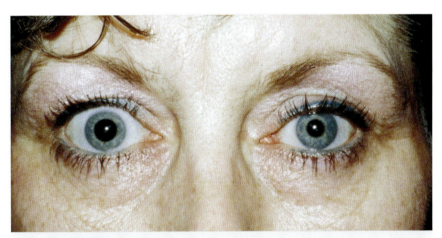

Fig. 1.20 Anisocoria. The left pupil is smaller than the right pupil. The examiner should examine the pupils in the dark and in the light to determine whether the large pupil does not constrict well, or whether the small pupil does not dilate well.

1.10 Ocular Examination

This part of the examination is better performed in an office equipped with a slit lamp, which allows two- and three-dimensional views of the eyes through a microscope. Mirrors and a slit beam allow visualization of the anterior segment of the eye and anterior vitreous when the pupil is dilated (▶ Fig. 1.21 and ▶ Fig. 1.22).

For an examination of the patient at the bedside without the help of a slit lamp, you should look at the eyes with the help of a penlight (or the direct ophthalmoscope):
1. Look at the external appearance of the eye, eyelid, and orbit (▶ Fig. 1.23, ▶ Fig. 1.24, ▶ Fig. 1.25, ▶ Fig. 1.26).
2. Look for abnormalities of the cornea or lens that could be the cause of decreased vision or that could obstruct an adequate view of the fundus.
3. Abnormalities of the ocular media sufficient to cause significant visual loss usually result in a poor view of the ocular fundus. If you can't see in, the patient can't see out.

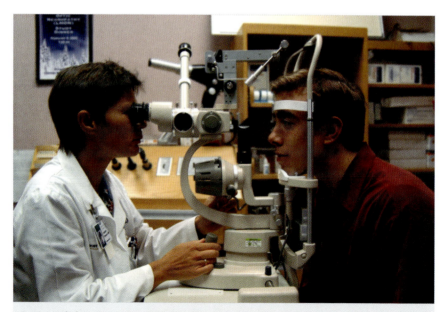

Fig. 1.21 Slit lamp examination. The patient needs to be able to sit up and stay still while looking straight ahead. Portable slit lamps are also available for bedside examination.

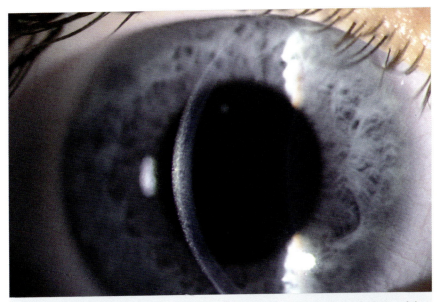

Fig. 1.22 View of the anterior segment with a slit lamp. It allows visualization of the layers of the cornea (most anterior white line), aqueous humor ("empty space" behind the cornea), iris, and lens (centered behind the iris).

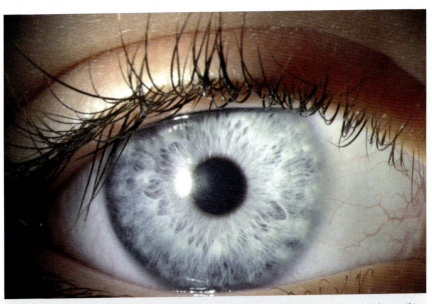

Fig. 1.23 Normal external appearance. The eye is white (quiet), the cornea is clear, and the pupil is round and centered. The eyelid is normal, and the position of the eye is normal. There is no proptosis.

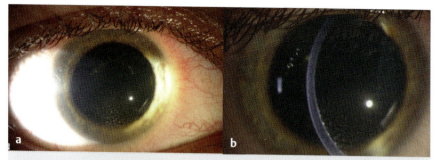

Fig. 1.24 Anterior uveitis with keratoprecipitates on the corneal endothelium. (**a**) View with a penlight placed laterally, allowing good visualization of the precipitates. The conjunctiva is mildly hyperemic. (**b**) View through the slit lamp, demonstrating the precipitates (seen as whitish dots) on the corneal endothelium. When focusing in the anterior chamber (beyond the cornea) with the slit lamp, it would also be possible to see the inflammatory cells in the anterior chamber.

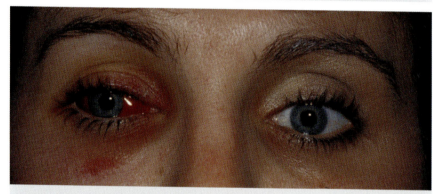

Fig. 1.25 Right orbital inflammatory pseudotumor with painful visual loss. The right eye is red and mildly proptotic, and there is some periorbital edema.

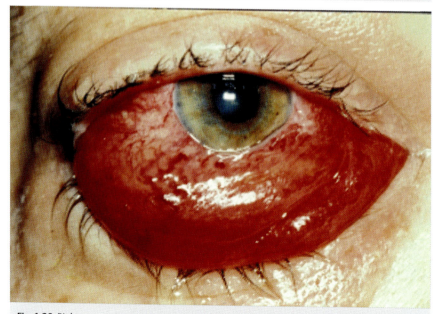

Fig. 1.26 Right traumatic carotid cavernous fistula, with severe chemosis and periorbital edema.

1.11 Ocular Motility

The motility examination evaluates the integrity of the following:
• Extraocular muscles
• Neuromuscular junction
• Ocular motor nerves (third, fourth, and sixth)
• Ocular motor nuclei
• Internuclear pathways
• Supranuclear pathways

The ocular motility examination consists of the following:
• Observation in primary gaze
• Ductions (monocular eye movements)
• Vergence (binocular dysconjugate movements)
• Versions (binocular conjugate eye movements)
  ○ Saccades
  ○ Pursuit
  ○ Oculocephalic responses and vestibulo-ocular reflex (VOR)
  ○ Optokinetic nystagmus
• Detection and measurement (with prisms) of ocular misalignment (strabismus)
• Detection of nystagmus

The various techniques used to examine the extraocular movements, how to interpret abnormal extraocular movements, and their localization value are detailed in Chapter 13.

An optokinetic stimulus produces a jerk nystagmus in patients with good vision and intact ocular motor systems. It coordinates eye movements when the environment moves, such as when looking out from a moving train.

Physiologic optokinetic nystagmus (OKN) can be elicited by rotating a striped drum or moving a striped tape horizontally and vertically and asking the patient to "count the stripes as they go by" (▶ Fig. 1.27).

The slow phases of the OKN are generated as the patient follows a target. The OKN fast phase is a corrective saccade to view the next target.

The OKN response is involuntary and is difficult to suppress. An intact OKN response confirms that visual acuity is at least 20/400. This is very helpful in checking the vision of infants and very young children as well as patients suspected of nonorganic visual loss claiming to have a visual acuity of hand motion, light perception, or no light perception. ▶ Table 1.4 outlines when to test for OKN and why. Testing the OKN is also helpful to elicit subtle adduction weakness in internuclear ophthalmoplegia and convergence retraction nystagmus of the dorsal midbrain syndrome (rotate the drum downward).

1.12 Visual Field Testing

Examination of the visual field is essential in all patients complaining of visual loss. It can be performed at bedside using confrontation techniques and Amsler grid testing. Formal visual field testing requires machines that are available in most ophthalmic clinics and in all neuro-ophthalmology offices. The various techniques used to test

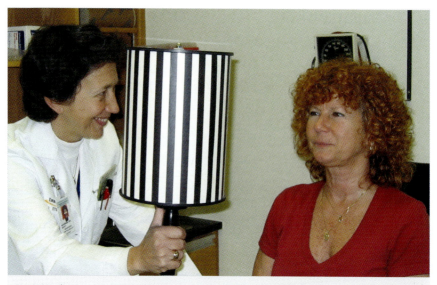

Fig. 1.27 Eliciting optokinetic nystagmus. As the examiner rotates a drum with black and white stripes in the horizontal or vertical direction, the patient is asked to "count the stripes."

Table 1.4 When to test for optokinetic nystagmus (OKN) and why

1. Infants with infantile nystagmus syndrome (congenital nystagmus): preserved vertical OKN = intact vision
2. Infantile nystagmus: characteristic reverse OKN response
3. Patient claiming complete blindness: intact OKN indicates vision of at least 20/400 (can be used on one eye at a time)
4. Deep parietal lesion: reduced response when tape is moved in the direction of a parietal lesion
5. Patient with homonymous hemianopia and symmetric OKN: probably occipital lesion; most likely vascular
6. Patient with homonymous hemianopia and asymmetric OKN: probably parietal lesion; most likely mass

visual fields, how to interpret a visual field test, and the localization value of visual field defects are detailed in Chapter 3.

1.13 Symmetry of Red Reflex

The red reflex is examined with the ophthalmoscope (see Chapter 2). A normal or symmetric red reflex suggests transparency of the ocular media (▸ Fig. 1.28).

Symmetry of a normal red reflex suggests the following:
• Symmetric transparency of the ocular media
• Symmetric refraction and no strabismus
• Grossly attached retina

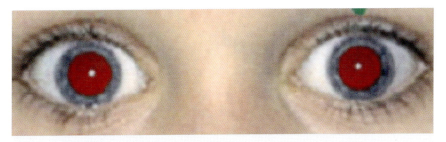

Fig. 1.28 Symmetric red reflex.

1.14 Funduscopic Examination

The ocular fundus can be viewed directly through the pupil with the help of an ophthalmoscope. Pupillary dilation is essential because it allows easier and better visualization of the fundus (see Chapter 2) (▶ Fig. 1.29, ▶ Fig. 1.30, ▶ Fig. 1.31, ▶ Fig. 1.32, ▶ Fig. 1.33). However, new digital fundus cameras allow excellent quality photographs without dilation of the pupils (nonmydriatic digital cameras) (▶ Fig. 1.34). Such cameras are now often routinely used in nonophthalmic settings to visualize the ocular fundus.

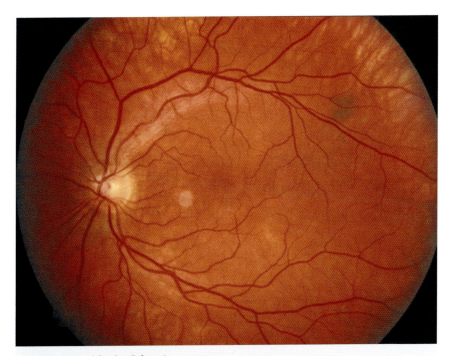

Fig. 1.29 Normal fundus (left eye).

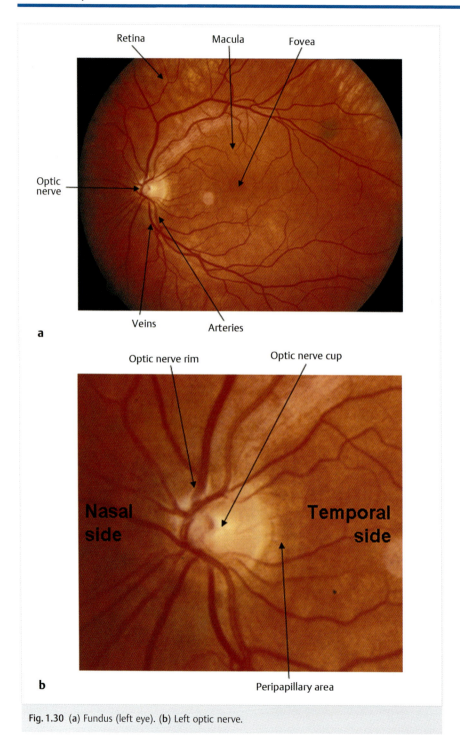

Fig. 1.30 (a) Fundus (left eye). (b) Left optic nerve.

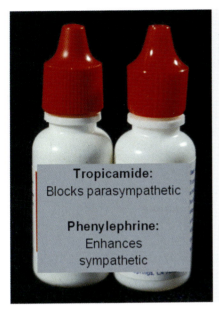

Fig. 1.31 Short-acting dilating drops used to visualize the fundus. Full dilation takes about 30 to 40 minutes and lasts up to 6 hours. Dilating drops all have a red top.

Tropicamide:
Blocks parasympathetic

Phenylephrine:
Enhances
sympathetic

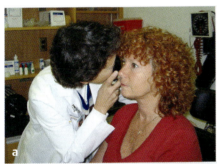
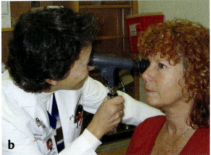

Fig. 1.32 (a) Funduscopic examination with a direct ophthalmoscope. It is essential to be very close to the patient's head to see the fundus. (b) Funduscopic examination with a direct PanOptic (Welsh Allyn, Skaneateles Falls, NY) ophthalmoscope. The field of view is larger, but the magnification is less than with a classic direct ophthalmoscope.

Examination of the fundus includes the following:

- Optic nerve
  - Normal (measure cup-to-disc ratio)
  - Pale
  - Swollen
- Macula and retina
  - Normal
  - Whitening from edema
  - Exudates
  - Hemorrhages
  - Detachment

- ○ Hole
- ○ Mass
- Arteries
- Veins
- Vitreous

The best three-dimensional views of the optic nerve are obtained with lenses and a slit lamp. This technique requires cooperation from the patient and is mostly used in a neuro-ophthalmologist's or ophthalmologist's office.

1.15 General Examination

Depending on the type of complaints, a neurologic examination, including cranial nerves, and general examination, including blood pressure, will complete the neuro-ophthalmic examination.

1.16 Neuro-ophthalmic Examination of the Comatose Patient

By definition, comatose patients have their eyes closed. They are unresponsive to all external stimuli, but there may be nonpurposeful movements or posturing of the limbs.

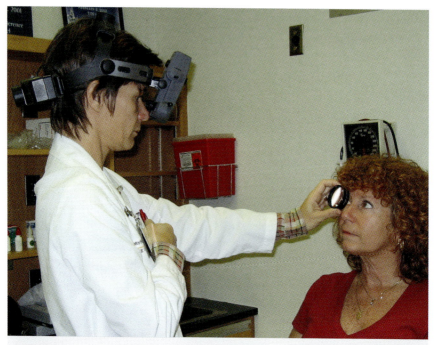

Fig. 1.33 Funduscopic examination with an indirect ophthalmoscope. The field of view is larger, but the magnification is less than with a direct ophthalmoscope. The fundus is seen in stereo.

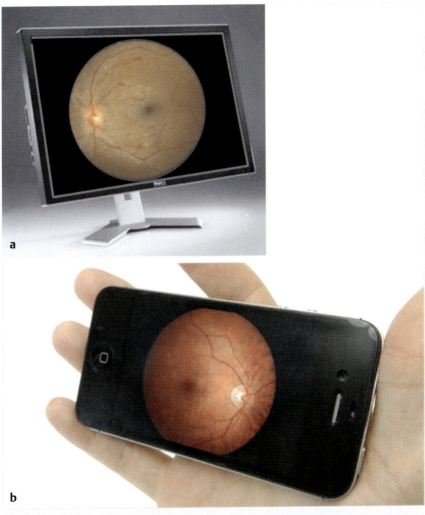

Fig. 1.34 Fundus photograph taken with a nonmydriatic digital camera displayed on a computer monitor (**a**) and on a smartphone (**b**).

Coma results from the following:
- Direct brainstem-diencephalic damage disrupting the reticular formation or nuclei
- Bilateral cerebral dysfunction

Some causes of coma include the following:
- Herniation from brain swelling or mass
- Hydrocephalus
- Intracranial hemorrhage
- Hypoxic-ischemic insult
- Trauma
- Infection
- Toxic/metabolic insult

25

Table 1.5 Glasgow Coma Scale for traumatic brain injuries

Verbal response (score 5 [good]–1 [none])	Mild trauma: total score 14 or 15
Spontaneity of eye opening:	Moderate trauma: score 9–13
4: spontaneous	Severe trauma: 3–8
3: to speech	
2: to pain	
1: none	
Motor function (score 6 [good]–1 [none])	

When evaluating a patient with unexplained coma, differentiating between structural and toxic/metabolic causes is important, given that it influences workup and management.

Neuro-ophthalmic examination is helpful, particularly regarding evaluation of the brainstem. Because the pathways governing ocular motility traverse the entire brainstem, brainstem lesions will most often result in abnormal eye movements, and the lesion can be localized to the midbrain, pons, or medulla; conversely, if the eye movements are normal, the brainstem is likely to be normal, and bilateral hemispheric or thalamic disease should be suspected.

The Glasgow Coma Scale is a neurological score used to record the level of consciousness after a head injury. The patient is assessed against the criteria of the scale (▶ Table 1.5), and the resulting points give a patient score between 3 (deep unconsciousness) and 15 (normal state).

Examination of the comatose patient involves the following:

- Pupils (▶ Fig. 1.35): Metabolic causes of coma usually cause small reactive pupils. Many toxins and drugs administered may also have effects on the size of the pupils, and pharmacologic mydriasis can inadvertently occur in patients treated with aerosols after extubation.
  - Size
  - Shape
  - Reactivity to light
- Eye position
  - Dysconjugate ocular deviation:
    – Horizontal, vertical, or oblique misalignment
    – Often indicates a cranial nerve palsy or skew deviation
  - Conjugate ocular deviation; conjugate lateral eye deviation indicates the following:
    – Large lesion in the ipsilateral frontal lobe (the patient looks at his or her lesion)
    – Lesion in contralateral pons (gaze palsy) (the patient looks away from the lesion)
    – Seizure focus in the contralateral cerebral hemisphere
    – Thalamic lesion, which may cause "wrong-way eyes," with horizontal eye deviation paradoxically looking away from the lesion
- Spontaneous eye movements
  - Roving eye movements: slow ocular conjugate deviations in random directions
    – Indicate intact ocular motility function in the brainstem
  - Periodic alternating ("ping-pong") gaze: slow, repetitive, rhythmic, back-and-forth, horizontal conjugate eye movements
    – Indicates intact ocular motility function in the brainstem

○ Spontaneous nystagmus (unusual in coma)
○ Ocular bobbing: conjugate eye movement beginning with a fast downward movement followed by a slow drift back to the midline (similar to a fish bob in the water)
– Severe pontine lesion
○ Ocular dipping: slow downward movement followed by a quick upward deviation
– Severe pontine lesion

If there are no spontaneous eye movements, perform oculocephalic maneuvering (eliciting eye movements by turning the head horizontally, then vertically). The eyes should deviate in the direction opposite the head turn. *This maneuver should not be performed in trauma patients with possible cervical spine injury.*

If there are no oculocephalic eye movements, test the VOR with the caloric test (apply ice-cold water against the tympanic membranes). The cold water creates convection currents in the endolymph of the horizontal semicircular canals and inhibits the ipsilateral vestibular system.

A normal caloric response in an awake patient is when the eyes move slowly toward the irrigated ear, followed by a fast corrective phase to reset the eyes. With warm water, the eyes move slowly away from the irrigated ear (fast phase is toward the irrigated ear).

A way to remember this is with the mnemonic COWS: cold–opposite; warm–same. Bilateral caloric stimulation with cold water produces a downward slow phase. Bilateral caloric stimulation with warm water produces an upward slow phase.

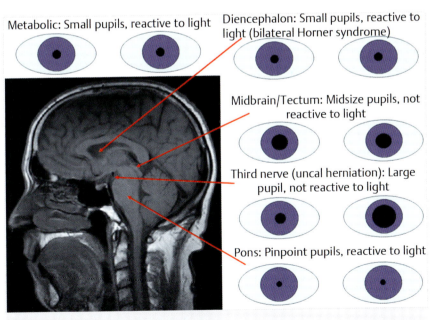

Metabolic: Small pupils, reactive to light

Diencephalon: Small pupils, reactive to light (bilateral Horner syndrome)

Midbrain/Tectum: Midsize pupils, not reactive to light

Third nerve (uncal herniation): Large pupil, not reactive to light

Pons: Pinpoint pupils, reactive to light

Fig. 1.35 Pupillary abnormalities in coma.

Table 1.6 Summary of the neuro-ophthalmic examination

Visual acuity	Distance		Near	
Without correction With correction or pinhole	Right eye	Left eye	Right eye	Left eye
Color vision Color plates Color saturation (%)	Right eye		Left eye	
Amsler grid	Right eye		Left eye	
External examination Orbits Hertel (mm)	Right eye		Left eye	
Lids Palpebral fissure (mm) Margin reflex distance (mm) Levator function (mm)	Right eye		Left eye	
Pupils Size in dark (mm) Size in light (mm) Response to light Dilation in dark RAPD Reaction at near	Right eye		Left eye	
Ocular examination Corneal sensation Conjunctiva Cornea Anterior chamber Lens vitreous	Right eye		Left eye	
Ocular motility Eye movements Pursuit, vergence, saccades Cross cover test Nystagmus	Right eye 		Left eye 	
Fundus Undilated Dilated Time Drops	Right eye 		Left eye 	

Table 1.6 (*continued*)

Visual acuity	Distance	Near

Visual fields
Confrontation
Formal:
  Goldmann
  Automated perimetry
	Left eye	Right eye

Other cranial nerves	Right	Left
Blood pressure Neurologic examination Other		

Abbreviation: IO, inferior oblique; IR, inferior rectus; LR, lateral rectus; MR, medical rectus; RAPD, relative afferent pupillary defect. SO, superior oblique; SR, superior rectus.

Caloric stimulation involves the following steps:

1. Angle the patient's head at 30 degrees to align the horizontal semicircular canal perpendicular to the floor.
2. Inspect the tympanic membrane (otoscopy) to exclude rupture or cerumen impaction.
3. Irrigate 30 to 60 mL of ice water into the external auditory canal using a large syringe and tubing from a butterfly catheter (without the needle); place a basin under the ear to collect the water.
4. The other ear can be tested after a few minutes.

In the comatose patient, cold caloric stimulation indicates a normal brainstem or bilateral hemispheric dysfunction when there is an ipsilateral tonic slow phase. It indicates a complete brainstem injury when there are no slow or fast eye movements.

Corneal reflex may be absent if there is pontine dysfunction.

Funduscopic examination of the comatose patient is usually performed undilated because pupil monitoring may be important in coma. Bilateral disc edema suggests raised intracranial pressure and should raise the possibility of an intracranial mass or hemorrhage, hydrocephalus, cerebral venous thrombosis, or meningitis. Vitreous hemorrhage (uni- or bilateral) suggests Terson syndrome (related to acutely raised intracranial pressure, most commonly with subarachnoid hemorrhage).

1.17 Summary of the Neuro-ophthalmic Examination

▶ Table 1.6 provides a summary of the neuro-ophthalmic examination and can be used as a checklist at bedside.

2 Funduscopic Examination

The ocular fundus can be viewed directly through the pupil with the help of an ophthalmoscope. Examination of the fundus is essential in cases of visual loss, but it is also helpful in detecting numerous systemic and neurologic disorders.

2.1 What Is Seen with an Ophthalmoscope

▶ Fig. 2.1 diagrams what is seen on examination of the fundus with a direct ophthalmoscope. ▶ Fig. 2.2 shows a patient being examined with a direct PanOptic (Welsh Allyn, Skaneates Falls, NY) ophthalmoscope, which features a larger field but less magnification than the classic direct ophthalmoscope.

The following make direct ophthalmoscopy easier:

1. Get close to the patient.
2. Use your right eye to look into the patient's right eye, and use your left eye to look into the patient's left eye.
3. Find the red reflex and get closer until you see the retina.
4. After focusing on the retina, follow the blood vessels toward the patient's nose to find the optic nerve.
5. To easily find the macula, ask the patient to look into the light.
6. Dilate the pupils to allow easier examination (▶ Fig. 2.3).

It is possible to visualize the optic nerve through an undilated pupil. However, it is technically difficult, and it does not allow examination of the entire fundus. Retinal disorders are missed without pupillary dilation.

> **Pearls**
>
> To view the ocular fundus to the best advantage, the pupils should be dilated. To dilate the pupils use a combination of short-acting agents that block parasympathetic transmission (tropicamide) and enhance sympathetic activity (phenylephrine). It also possible to use only one drop. Dilation occurs within 30 minutes and usually resolves within 6 hours. Long-acting dilating drops (used as cycloplegics), such as cyclopentolate, homatropine, and atropine, should not be used to view the fundus (the dilation and cycloplegia may last from 12 hours to up to 14 days).
>
> Be sure to alert the patient that driving may be difficult after dilation, especially in bright sunlight. Young patients will have difficulty reading after pharmacologic dilation because of the blockage of accommodation.
>
> It is always better to dilate both eyes rather than one eye (a unilateral mydriasis is often alarming, whereas most people will not be concerned about bilateral mydriasis if the patient is awake and alert). Always document the time of dilation and the drops used. Do not dilate a neurosurgical or unstable patient, because monitoring of the pupils may be important.
>
> Glaucoma is not a contraindication for pupillary dilation. Patients who know they have a diagnosis of angle closure glaucoma will already have been treated with laser to prevent episodes of angle closure from pupillary dilation and can therefore be dilated without risk. Nearly all patients who say they have glaucoma have open angle glaucoma, which does not contraindicate pupillary dilation.

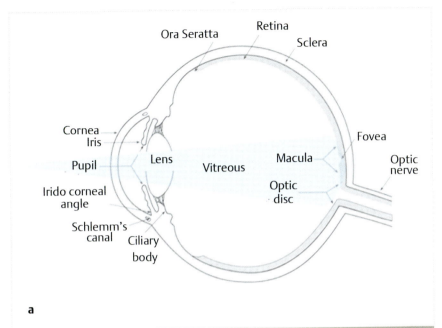

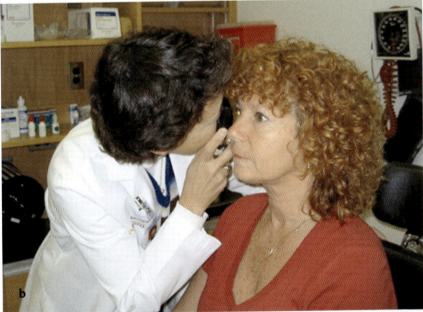

Fig. 2.1 (a) Diagram illustrating what is seen on examination using a direct ophthalmoscope. (b) The direct ophthalmoscope allows visualization of the fundus (posterior pole).

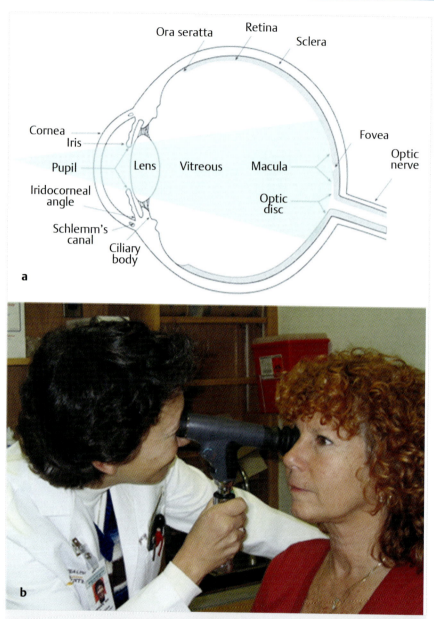

Ora seratta Retina Sclera

Cornea
Iris
Pupil Lens Vitreous Macula
Iridocorneal
angle
Schlemm's
canal
Ciliary
body
Fovea
Optic
nerve
Optic
disc

a

b

Fig. 2.2 (a) Diagram illustrating what is seen on examination using a direct PanOptic (Welsh Allyn, Skaneates Falls, NY) ophthalmoscope. (b) The PanOptic direct ophthalmoscope provides a larger field but less magnification than the classic direct ophthalmoscope.

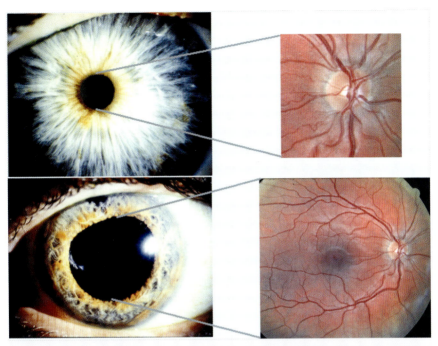

Fig. 2.3 Only the optic nerve can be seen through an undilated pupil (top), whereas the entire posterior pole can be examined through a dilated pupil (bottom)

Funduscopic examination includes the optic nerve (specifically, checking for cup-to-disc ratio, edema, and pallor), the retina around the optic nerve, the macula (specifically, checking for color, edema, hemorrhages, exudates, and masses), and arteries and veins (specifically, checking for size, occlusion, and emboli) (▶ Fig. 2.4).

The cup-to-disc ratio (the size of the cup in relation to the size of the disc) should be measured horizontally and vertically (▶ Fig. 2.5).

2.1.1 If You Cannot See the Fundus

If you are unable to see the fundus on examination, review the following checklist:
1. Is the ophthalmoscope working? (are the batteries charged?)
2. Is the pupil too small? (Did you forget to dilate the patient's pupils?)
3. Are you sure you know how to use the ophthalmoscope?
4. Is there something blocking the view (media opacity)? Many ocular disorders—corneal disorders, anterior uveitis or hyphema, cataracts, and vitreous inflammation or hemorrhage—decrease the normal transparency of the ocular media, thereby obstructing the view of the fundus (▶ Fig. 2.6). Remember that if you can't see in, the patient can't see out.

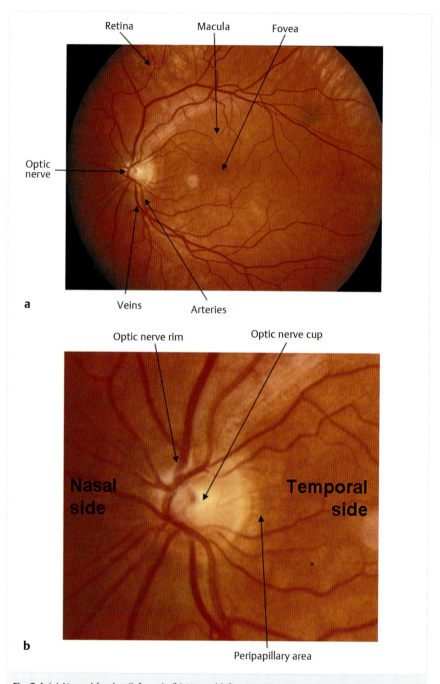

Fig. 2.4 (a) Normal fundus (left eye). (b) Normal left optic nerve. Note that veins are larger and darker than arteries (the normal arteriovenous ratio is 2:3).

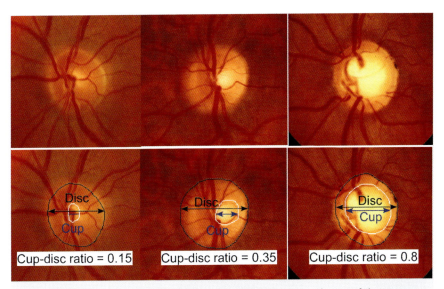

Fig. 2.5 Evaluation of the cup-to-disc ratio in three different patients. The size of the cup is measured in relation to the size of the disc. A small or moderate cup-to-disc ratio (left and middle) is common in normal subjects, whereas a large cup-to-disc ratio (right) is suggestive of glaucoma.

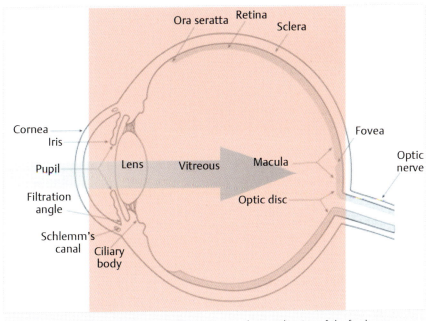

Fig. 2.6 Diagram illustrating how a media opacity can obstruct the view of the fundus.

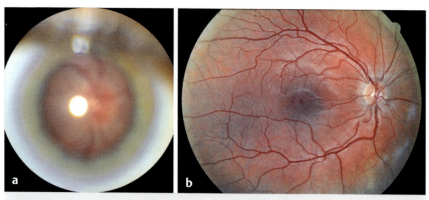

Fig. 2.7 A normal red reflex suggests transparency of the media, allowing good visualization of the fundus. **(a)** The red reflex is first seen at about 2 feet from the patient's eye, then **(b)** the fundus is visualized once you get close to the patient.

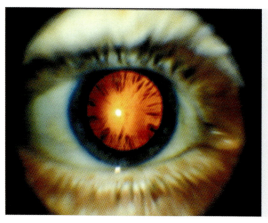

Fig. 2.8 Red reflex with a mild cataract.

An easy way to check for media opacity is to look for the red reflex with the ophthalmoscope (compare both eyes):

1. Look through the ophthalmoscope at about 2 feet from the patient's eye and direct the light straight into the pupil.
2. You should see an orange-red reflex (reflection of the light on the normal orange-red retina) (▶ Fig. 2.7). (This is what you observe when a camera flash gives subjects red eyes.)
3. By retroilluminating the cornea and the lens and using "plus" (green numbers) lenses in the direct ophthalmoscope, you can use the red reflex to look for corneal and lens opacities (cataracts) at the bedside (▶ Fig. 2.8).

When there is a severe retinal disorder involving the posterior pole, or a vitreous hemorrhage (▶ Fig. 2.9), the red reflex can also be abnormal. This is particularly common with a large retinal detachment (▶ Fig. 2.10), an ocular mass (retinoblastoma, melanoma), and large retinal scars.

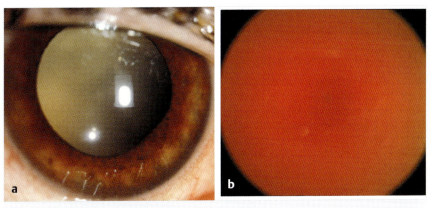

Fig. 2.9 (a) Poor red reflex in a patient with vitreous hemorrhage from subarachnoid hemorrhage as a result of aneurysmal rupture (Terson syndrome). (b) Dense vitreous hemorrhage (same patient) obscuring the view of the fundus.

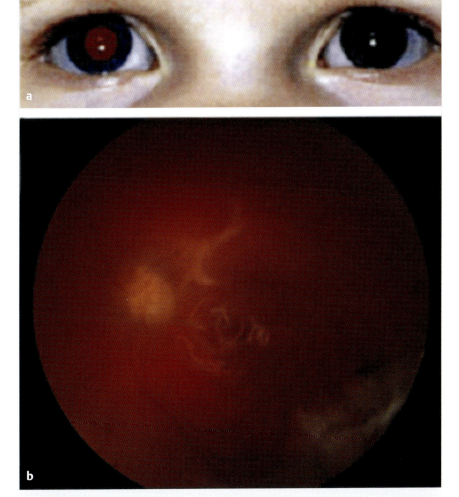

Fig. 2.10 (a) No red reflex in the left eye of a child with a left total retinal detachment. (b) Total retinal detachment with retinal tear.

2.1.2 If You Have a Clear View of the Fundus

Most causes of monocular central visual loss that are not due to media abnormalities result from disorders of either the optic nerve or the macula. Although more peripheral retinal findings may provide important diagnostic clues, it is primarily disease of the optic nerve or the most central retina that results in loss of central visual function, and many of these disorders can be seen with a direct ophthalmoscope.

Pertinent visible abnormalities include the following (▶ Fig. 2.11−2.20):

- Disc edema
- Disc pallor
- Whitening of the inner retinal layers secondary to infarction, as in central and branch retinal artery occlusions
- Hemorrhages and venous dilation in central retinal vein occlusion
- Detachment of the retina or accumulation of subretinal fluid, as in central serous retinopathy
- Degeneration of the retina, as in macular degeneration

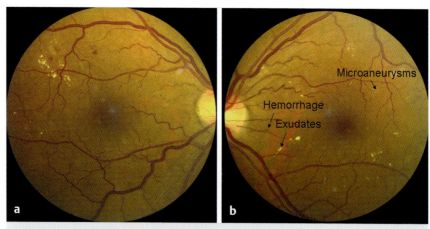

Fig. 2.11 Diabetes mellitus. Nonproliferative diabetic retinopathy is seen in both eyes. Note the small intraretinal hemorrhages, microaneurysms, and yellow exudates **(a)** Right eye **(b)** Left eye.

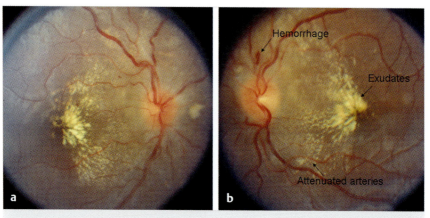

Fig. 2.12 Hypertensive retinopathy. Severe (stage IV) hypertensive retinopathy is seen in both eyes. Note the mild bilateral optic nerve edema, a few intraretinal hemorrhages, extensive yellow exudates, and attenuation of the arteries **(a)** Right eye **(b)** Left eye.

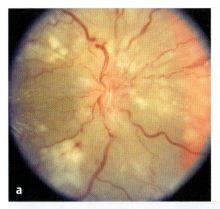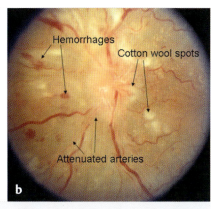

Fig. 2.13 Hypertensive retinopathy with acute bilateral visual loss in the setting of eclampsia. Severe (stage IV) hypertensive retinopathy is seen in both eyes. Note the bilateral optic nerve edema, intraretinal hemorrhages, numerous cotton wool spots, and severe attenuation of the arteries (a) Right eye (b) Left eye.

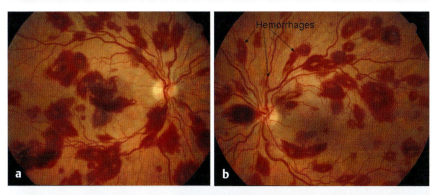

Fig. 2.14 Intraretinal hemorrhages from thrombocytopenia. Note the multiple retinal hemorrhages in both eyes. The optic nerves are normal (a) Right eye (b) Left eye.

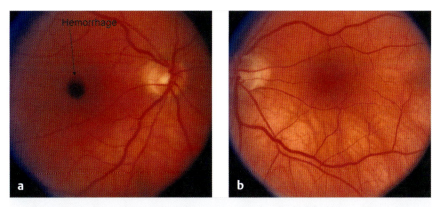

Fig. 2.15 Macular hemorrhage in the right eye. Intraretinal and subhyaloid hemorrhage is seen in the right macula with acute visual loss in the right eye. (a) There is no relative afferent pupillary defect. The optic nerves are normal. The view is hazy in the right eye because of a mild vitreous hemorrhage (b) The left eye is normal.

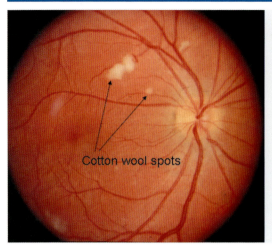

Fig. 2.16 Fat emboli after femur fracture. Note the cotton wool spots.

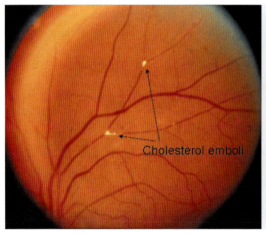

Fig. 2.17 Cholesterol emboli. Refractile, bright emboli are seen at arterial bifurcations.

- Abnormalities of the retinal vasculature, including thrombosis and emboli
- Vasculitis with arterial or venous sheathing or exudate deposition, such as may result from infections like syphilis or systemic inflammatory disorders such as sarcoidosis

2.2 Fundus Photography Is Another Way to Examine the Ocular Fundus

Digital photography of the ocular fundus is widely used to examine the optic nerve and the retina. Nonmydriatic cameras allow excellent-quality photographs without pharmacologic dilation of the pupils and provide very good views of the posterior pole (optic nerve, macula, and vascular arcades). The photographs can be easily analyzed on a computer, a tablet, or even a smartphone (▶ Fig. 2.21); they can also be transmitted electronically for remote consultation (see ▶ Fig. 1.34).

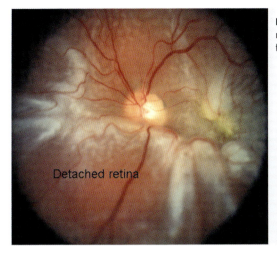

Fig. 2.18 Inferior retinal detachment. The inferior retina is out of focus, elevated, and wrinkled.

Detached retina

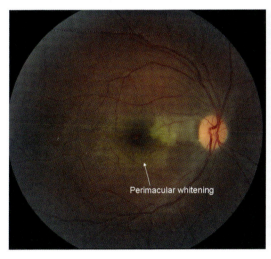

Fig. 2.19 Commotio retina after traumatic brain injury. There is perimacular whitening secondary to retinal edema.

Perimacular whitening

2.3 When to Examine the Fundus

Examples of systemic and neurologic disorders in which examination of the fundus should be systematic, even in the absence of visual symptoms, include the following:
- Systemic hypertension
- Malignant systemic hypertension (hypertensive crisis)
- Diabetes mellitus
- Sickle cell disease
- Human immunodeficiency virus (HIV) infection with low CD4 count
- Severe thrombocytopenia

- Endocarditis, septicemia
- Systemic vasculitis, autoimmune disease
- Headache
- Any cause of raised intracranial pressure
- Intracranial mass
- Any cause of meningeal process
- Subarachnoid hemorrhage
- Stroke

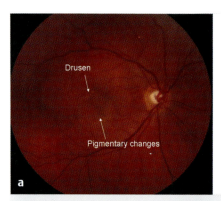
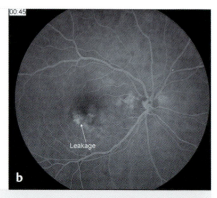

Fig. 2.20 Age-related macular degeneration with choroidal neovascular membrane. (a) On the color fundus photograph, there are pigmentary changes and drusen involving the macula. (b) The central, elevated, whiter area corresponds to early leakage on the fluorescein angiogram, suggesting a classic choroidal neovascular membrane.

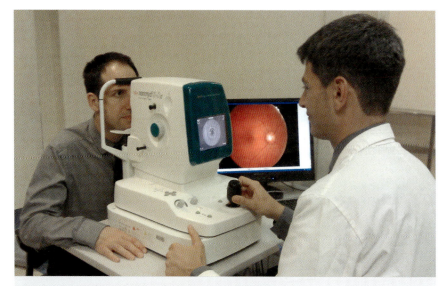

Fig. 2.21 Nonmydriatic digital ocular fundus camera. The camera takes photographs of the ocular fundus that are immediately seen on the computer screen and can be transferred remotely for consultation (see ▶ Fig. 1.34).

3 Visual Fields

Examination of the visual fields helps to localize and identify diseases affecting the visual pathways (▶ Fig. 3.1). Visual field testing is useful when evaluating patients complaining of visual loss (especially when the cause of visual loss is not obvious after ophthalmic examination) or patients with neurologic disorders that may affect the intracranial visual pathways (e.g., pituitary tumors, strokes involving the posterior circulation, and traumatic brain injuries).

Examination allows localization by correlating the shape of defects to the abnormal portion of the visual pathways. It can be repeated to monitor if the defects are growing or shrinking as a measure of whether the disease process is worsening or improving.

3.1 Visual Pathways

The visual field and retina have an inverted and reversed relationship.
Relative to the point of fixation:
- The upper visual field falls on the inferior retina (below the fovea).
- The lower visual field falls on the superior retina (above the fovea).
- The nasal visual field falls on the temporal retina.
- The temporal visual field falls on the nasal retina.

The nasal fibers of the ipsilateral eye (53% of all fibers) cross in the chiasm to join the uncrossed temporal fibers (47% of all fibers) of the contralateral eye. They form the optic tract, which synapses in the lateral geniculate nucleus to form the optic radiations, which terminate in the visual cortex (area 17) of the occipital lobe. Because more fibers in the optic tract come from the opposite eye (crossed fibers), a relative afferent pupillary defect (RAPD) is often observed in the eye contralateral to an optic tract lesion (see discussion later in this chapter).

At the level of the chiasm, the crossing inferonasal fibers travel anteriorly toward the contralateral optic nerve before passing into the optic tract. This is called Wilbrand's knee and is responsible for the "junctional scotoma" in lesions of the posterior optic nerve. Although the anatomical presence of Wilbrand's knee is debated, junctional scotomas are observed clinically.

The visual field of each eye overlaps centrally. The normal visual field in each eye is approximately (▶ Fig. 3.2)
- 60 degrees superiorly
- 70 to 75 degrees inferiorly
- 60 degrees nasally
- 100 to 110 degrees temporally

The physiologic blind spot corresponds to the optic disc (which has no overlying photoreceptors) and is located approximately 15 degrees temporally in each eye.

3.2 Techniques to Evaluate the Visual Field

Current methods of visual field testing all require the subject to indicate whether the stimulus is seen or not. You cannot reliably test the visual field of an uncooperative or very sick patient. There have been attempts to develop an "objective perimetry" by

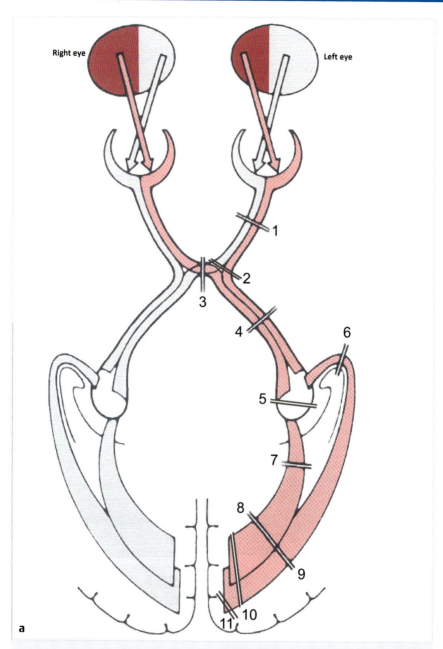

Fig. 3.1 a–b (a) Lesions of the visual pathways (Adapted Rokhamm R. Color Atlas of Neurology. New York, NY: Thieme; 2004:81). (b) Types of visual field defects secondary to lesions along the visual pathways. Note that the visual pathways (a) are shown with the right eye on the left and the left eye on the right (similar to a computed tomographic or magnetic resonance imaging scan). (*continued*)

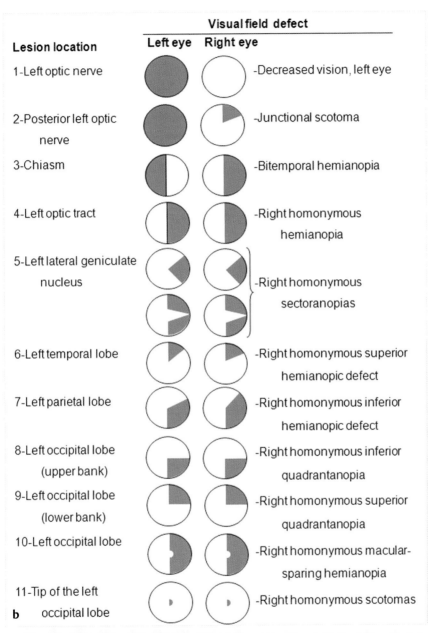

Lesion location	Visual field defect		
	Left eye	Right eye	
1-Left optic nerve			-Decreased vision, left eye
2-Posterior left optic nerve			-Junctional scotoma
3-Chiasm			-Bitemporal hemianopia
4-Left optic tract			-Right homonymous hemianopia
5-Left lateral geniculate nucleus			-Right homonymous sectoranopias
6-Left temporal lobe			-Right homonymous superior hemianopic defect
7-Left parietal lobe			-Right homonymous inferior hemianopic defect
8-Left occipital lobe (upper bank)			-Right homonymous inferior quadrantanopia
9-Left occipital lobe (lower bank)			-Right homonymous superior quadrantanopia
10-Left occipital lobe			-Right homonymous macular-sparing hemianopia
11-Tip of the left occipital lobe			-Right homonymous scotomas

b

Fig. 3.1 (*continued*) The visual field defects (**b**) are by convention shown with the right eye on the right and the left eye on the left.

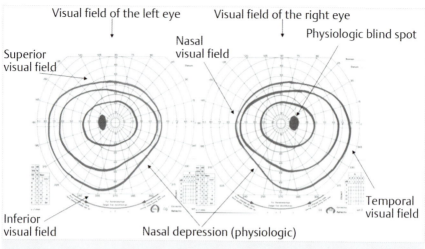

Fig. 3.2 Normal visual fields (Goldmann visual fields). By convention, the visual field of the right eye is placed on the right, and the visual field of the left eye is placed on the left (as if the patient were looking at his or her own visual field). Although the visual field of each eye overlaps, each eye is examined separately and is represented separately.

projecting stimuli onto discrete areas of the retina and using electroretinographic or pupillometric responses as end points, but these methods remain experimental.

Visual fields should be tested monocularly given that the overlap in binocular fields may mask visual field defects.

3.2.1 Visual Field Testing at Bedside

Bedside visual field testing is quick and easy but has relatively poor reliability, depending on the patient's ability to identify and describe the visual field defect.

Face: Ask the patient to look at your nose and tell you if any parts of your face are missing.

Grid: Present a square grid of lines and ask the patient to fixate on a central point and to draw any area in which the lines disappear (▶ Fig. 3.3)

Finger confrontation: This is useful in identifying dense hemianopic or altitudinal defects (▶ Fig. 3.4).

The test involves the following steps:

1. Line up the patient across from you.
2. Have the patient cover one eye and stare into the opposite eye on your face with his or her open eye to maintain central fixation.
3. Instruct the patient to count fingers presented within the central 30 degrees (in each of four quadrants around fixation). Special attention should be directed to the horizontal and vertical axes of the visual field to see if there is a change in vision across an axis. The patient should perform the task equally well in all four quadrants.
4. Ask the patient to count fingers in two quadrants simultaneously. If a quadrant of the visual field is consistently ignored, a subtle field defect (or neglect) has been revealed.
5. The far periphery can be assessed by finger wiggle.
6. A consistent difference in color perception (use a red object) across the horizontal or vertical meridian may be the only sign of an altitudinal or hemianopic defect, respectively.

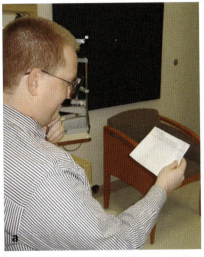

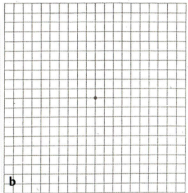

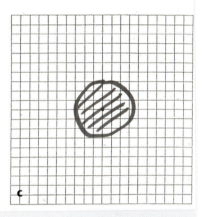

Fig. 3.3 (a) Amsler grid testing. (b) Normal Amsler grid (evaluates the central 10 degrees). (c) Amsler grid showing a small central scotoma in one eye.

3.2.2 Visual Field Testing in the Office

Tangent Screen

The tangent screen is rarely used and is primarily helpful for evaluating patients suspected of nonorganic constriction of the visual field (▶ Fig. 3.5).

The test involves the following steps:
1. The patient sits 1 m from a black screen (mounted on a wall) on which there are concentric circles.
2. While the patient is asked to fixate on a central target, a white or colored circular stimulus is slowly moved from the periphery toward the center of the screen until the patient reports seeing the stimulus.
3. By repeating this in various parts of the visual field, an isopter can be plotted and then drawn on the screen with chalk or pins.

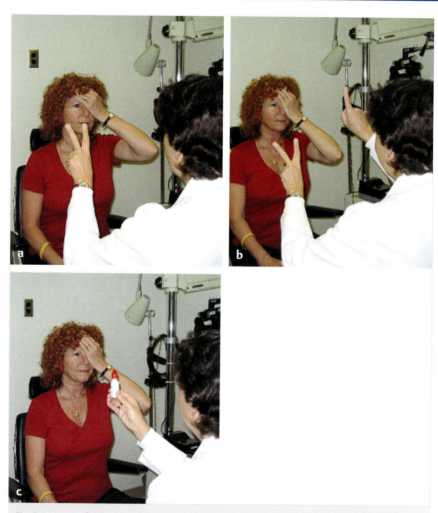

Fig. 3.4 a–c Confrontation visual field testing. See text for a description of the technique.

By varying the distance of the patient from the screen, it is possible to differentiate organic from nonorganic constriction of the visual field: in organic patients, the visual field enlarges when the patient is placed farther away from the screen (see Chapter 18).

Goldmann (Kinetic) Perimetry

Goldmann perimetry has the advantage of charting the entire visual field and includes the far temporal periphery (▶ Fig. 3.2, ▶ Fig. 3.3, ▶ Fig. 3.4, ▶ Fig. 3.5, ▶ Fig. 3.6, ▶ Fig. 3.7). It can quickly establish the pattern of visual field loss in the ill, poorly attentive, or elderly patient who requires continued encouragement to maintain fixation and respond appropriately.

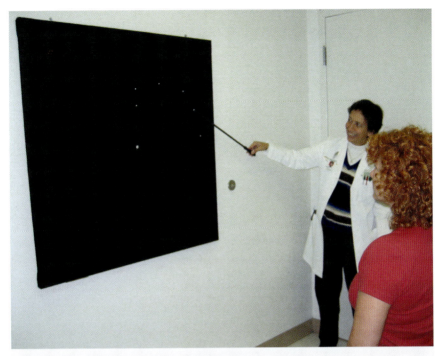

Fig. 3.5 Tangent screen. See text for a description of the technique.

The test involves the following steps:
1. Place the patient's head on a chin rest on the open side of a white hemispheric bowl.
2. Cover one of the patient's eyes.
3. Tell the patient to fixate on a central spot.
4. Present stimuli consisting of dots of white light projected one at a time onto the inner surface of the bowl, usually moving from the unseen periphery into the patient's field of view.
5. Ask the patient to signal detection of the white dot by pressing a buzzer. Note the responses on a chart representing the visual field.
6. Lights of different sizes and brightness allow the drawing of isopters.

The quality of the field is examiner-dependent, and it does not detect subtle changes. Defects are more difficult to quantify than with automated perimetry.

Automated Static Perimetry

Automated perimetry is more sensitive, quantitative, and reproducible, but it is more time consuming and requires good patient cooperation and attention (▶ Fig. 3.8). It is the technique of choice for patients with optic nerve lesions, papilledema, chiasmal compressive lesions, and other progressive visual disorders. Although numerous automated perimetries are available, the Humphrey strategies, in particular, the Swedish Interactive Thresholding Algorithm (SITA) standard and SITA fast programs, are the

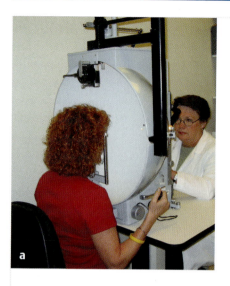
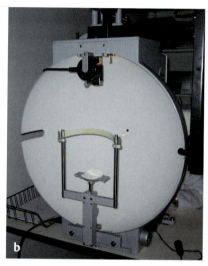
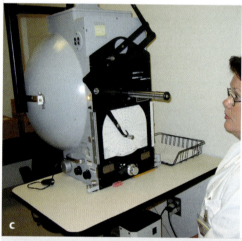

Fig. 3.6 a–c Goldmann perimetry. See text for a description of the technique.

most commonly used. These tests average about 3 minutes (fast) and 6 minutes (standard) per eye.

The test involves the following steps:
1. Place the patient's head on a chin rest in front of a computer screen.
2. Cover one of the patient's eyes.
3. Tell the patient to fixate on a central spot.
4. Present stimuli consisting of dots of white light projected one at a time onto the screen, randomly presented (not moving).
5. Ask the patient to signal detection of the white dot by pressing a buzzer.
6. The stimulus size is kept the same, but the brightness varies.
7. Only the central 10, 24, or 30 degrees is usually tested.

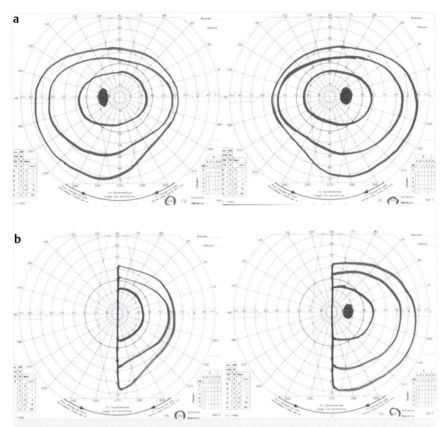

Fig. 3.7 (a) Normal Goldmann visual field test. The right eye is on the right, and the left eye is on the left. Note the normal physiologic blind spot in the temporal field of each eye. (b) Goldmann visual field test showing a left homonymous hemianopia.

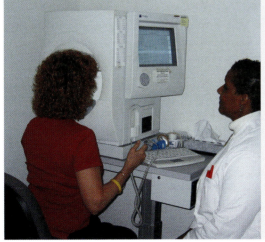

Fig. 3.8 Automated perimetry. See text for a description of the technique.

3.3 Interpretation of a Visual Field Defect

3.3.1 Understanding a Humphrey Visual Field Printout

Humphrey perimetry uses computerized programs to randomly test points in the patient's central visual field with a standard stimulus size but varying stimulus intensities (▶ Fig. 3.9). It uses a threshold strategy, in which the stimulus intensity varies and is presented multiple times at each location so that the level of detection of the dimmest stimulus is determined. This is then reported on a computerized printout in various ways, some numerical, others pictorial.

3.3.2 Assessing the Quality of the Visual Field

The ability of the patient to perform the test can be evaluated by measurements of reliability reported on the printout. In the example provided in ▶ Fig. 3.10, the left eye was tested (as indicated by the word *left* in the upper right corner). Reliability measurements are reported in the upper left corner and include the number of fixation losses (2/13), false-positive errors (0%), and false-negative errors (3%) during the test. A large number of fixation losses (> 33% of false-positive or false-negative responses) indicates an unreliable test.

3.3.3 Interpreting the Visual Field Test

The numeric grid just to the right of the measurements of reliability is a presentation of the threshold level in decibels for all points checked in the patient's visual field. A recorded number of 0 indicates that the patient could not detect even the brightest stimulus at that point. The higher the number, the better the vision at that point in the field.

These numbers are then converted to a gray scale representation of the field (upper right, ▶ Fig. 3.10), which provides a gross picture of the size and severity of the field defects present.

A comparative scale on the bottom relates the degree of grayness on the gray scale to the change in decibel levels from the numeric grid. The number scale labeled "Total Deviation" in ▶ Fig. 3.10 indicates the amount each point deviates from the age-adjusted normal values. In this case, the more negative a number, the more abnormal that point. The number scale to the right in ▶ Fig. 3.10 labeled "Pattern Deviation" highlights focal abnormalities in the visual field, helping to emphasize the pattern of visual field loss.

Pearls

In interpreting a visual field test, you need to ask the following questions (▶ Fig. 3.11):
1. Is the test reliable (as indicated by the technician for Goldmann visual fields and by the reliability parameters for automated perimetry)?
2. Is the test normal or not?
3. Does the visual field defect involve one eye or two eyes?
4. If binocular, does the defect respect the vertical meridian?
5. If it respects the vertical meridian, is the defect bitemporal (temporal side of the vertical meridian in each eye) or homonymous (on the same side of the vertical meridian in each eye)?
6. If it is homonymous, is the defect complete or incomplete?
7. If it is homonymous and incomplete, is the defect congruent (same defect shape and size in each eye)?

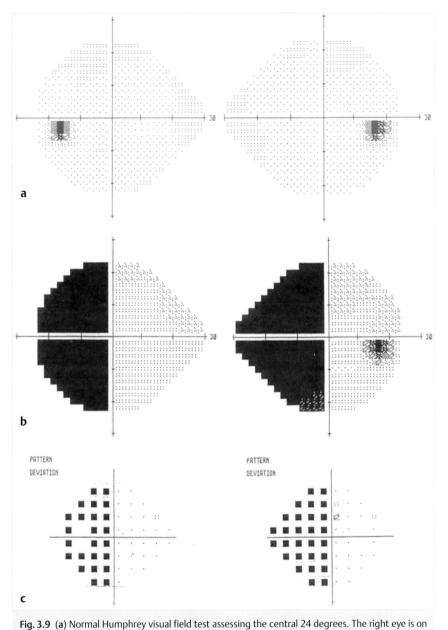

Fig. 3.9 (a) Normal Humphrey visual field test assessing the central 24 degrees. The right eye is on the right, and the left eye is on the left. Note the normal physiologic blind spot in the temporal field of each eye. (b, c) Humphrey visual field test showing a complete left homonymous hemianopia. (There is a temporal defect in the left eye and a nasal defect in the right eye; both defects respect the vertical meridian. The gray scale (b) and the pattern deviation (c) are shown.)

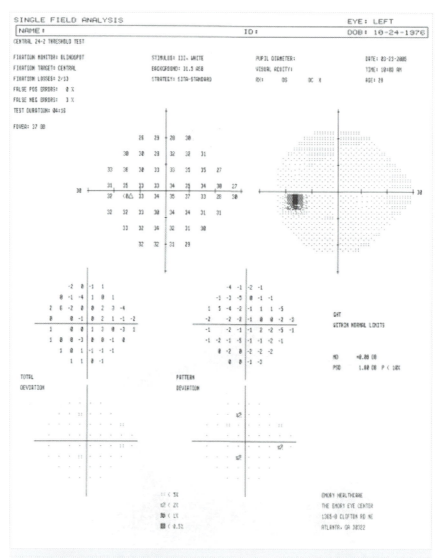

Fig. 3.10 Normal Humphrey visual field in the left eye (24–2 Swedish Interactive Thresholding Algorithm, SITA, standard program).

3.4 Topographic Diagnosis of Visual Field Defects

Characterization of the visual field defect often allows precise localization of the lesion along the visual pathways. Once the lesion is localized anatomically, a directed workup looks for an etiology.

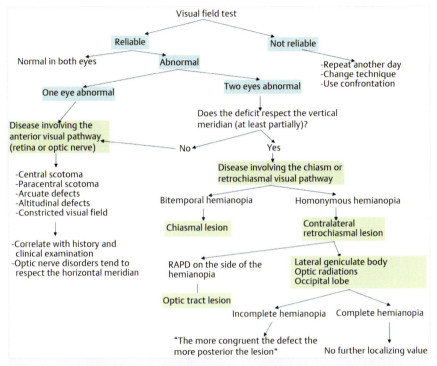

Fig. 3.11 Interpretation of a visual field test. RAPD, relative afferent pupillary defect.

3.4.1 Anterior Visual Pathways

Retina

Macular lesions produce central or paracentral defects, whereas most degenerative retinopathies, such as retinitis pigmentosa, produce progressive constriction of the peripheral and midperipheral visual field (▶ Fig. 3.12 and ▶ Fig. 3.13).

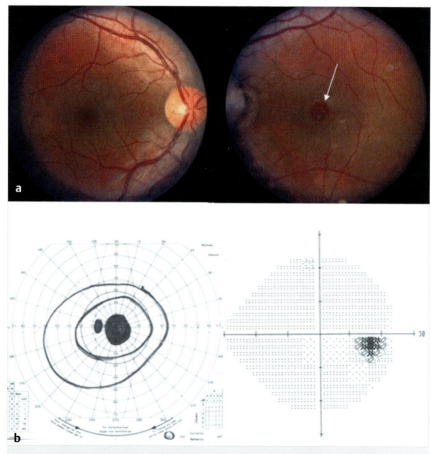

Fig. 3.12 **(a)** Macular hole in the left eye (arrow). Visual acuity is 20/20 in the right eye and count fingers in the left eye. There is no relative afferent pupillary defect. (By convention, the fundus photograph of the right eye is shown on the left, and the fundus photograph of the left eye is shown on the right.) **(b)** Central scotoma in the left eye (Goldmann visual field). The right eye is normal (Humphrey visual field). (By convention, the visual field test of the right eye is shown on the right, and the visual field test of the left eye is shown on the left.)

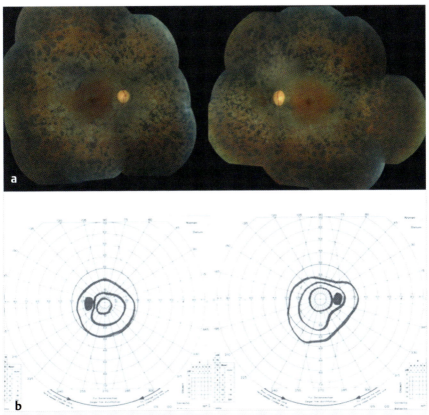

Fig. 3.13 (a) Retinitis pigmentosa with peripheral loss of vision. (b) Goldmann visual field test showing peripheral constriction of all isopters.

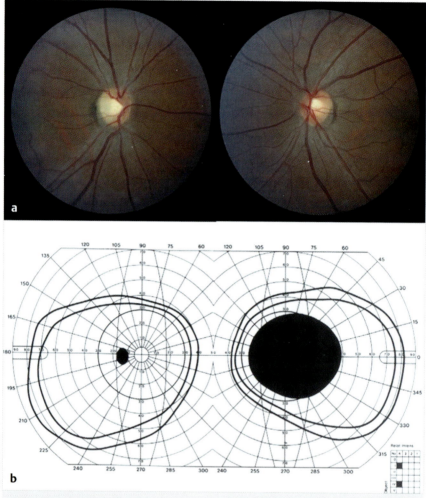

Fig. 3.14 (a) Right optic neuropathy (optic neuritis) with optic nerve pallor. (b) Right central scotoma (Goldmann visual field test). The left eye is normal.

Optic Nerve

Optic neuropathies typically produce nerve fiber bundle defects within the central 30 degrees of the visual field. Depending on the etiology of the optic neuropathy, arcuate defects, altitudinal defects, and central, paracentral, or centrocecal scotomas are observed (▶ Fig. 3.14, ▶ Fig. 3.15, ▶ Fig. 3.16).

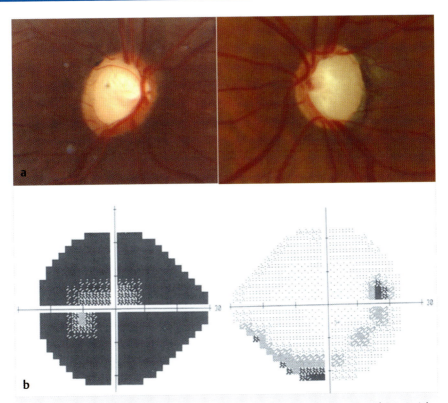

Fig. 3.15 (a) Bilateral glaucomatous optic neuropathy. Very large cup-to-disc ratio with intact pink rims, worse in the left eye. (b) Humphrey visual field test showing an inferior arcuate defect in the right eye and severe constriction in the left eye from advanced glaucoma.

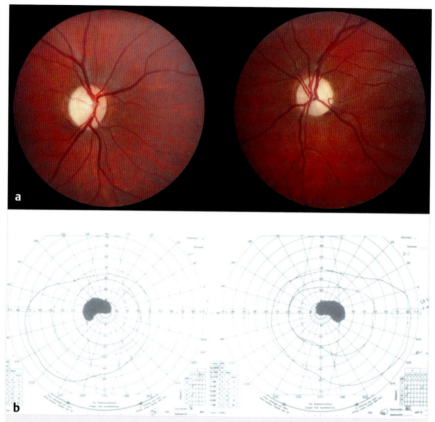

Fig. 3.16 (a) Bilateral optic atrophy secondary to hereditary optic neuropathies. (b) Goldmann visual field test showing bilateral centrocecal scotomas.

Chiasm

The nasal retinal fibers of each eye cross in the chiasm to the contralateral optic tracts, and the temporal fibers remain uncrossed. Thus a chiasmal lesion will cause a bitemporal hemianopia due to interruption of decussating nasal fibers (▶ Fig. 3.17 and ▶ Fig. 3.18).

3.4.2 Retrochiasmal Visual Pathways

Retrochiasmal lesions involving the visual pathways produce a contralateral homonymous hemianopia.

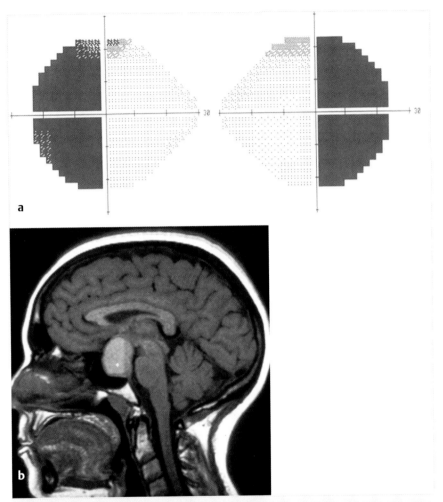

Fig. 3.17 (a) Humphrey visual field test showing a dense bitemporal hemianopia in a patient with pituitary apoplexy. (b) T1-sagittal magnetic resonance imaging (MRI) showing a hemorrhage (*) within a pituitary adenoma (pituitary apoplexy) compressing the chiasm.

Complete homonymous hemianopias may occur with any lesion of the retrochiasmal visual pathways and do not allow precise localization of the lesion along the retrochiasmal visual pathways. Incomplete homonymous hemianopias may help localize the lesion based on their congruity:

- Hemianopia is incongruent when visual field defects are different in each eye.
- Hemianopia is congruent when visual field defects are identical in each eye. The rule of congruency states that the more congruent the homonymous hemianopia, the more posterior the lesion. (This rule does not apply to optic tract lesions that are suspected when the homonymous hemianopia is associated with a RAPD on the side of the hemianopia and bilateral optic nerve pallor). ▶ Fig. 3.19, ▶ Fig. 3.20, and ▶ Fig. 3.21 show different homonymous hemianopias.

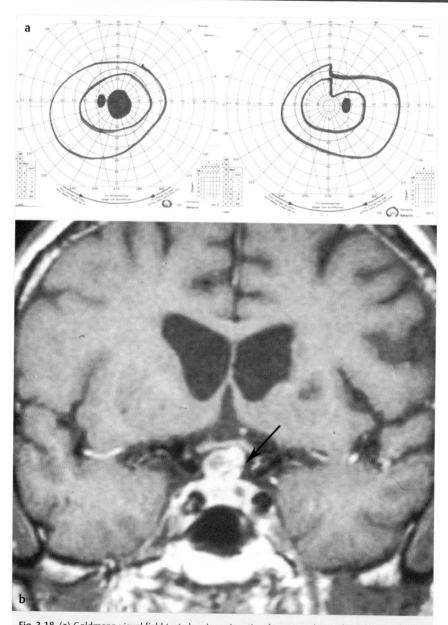

Fig. 3.18 (a) Goldmann visual field test showing a junctional scotoma (central scotoma in the left eye and superior temporal defect respecting the vertical meridian in the right eye, suggesting compression of the left optic nerve at its junction with the chiasm). (b) Coronal T1-weighted magnetic resonance imaging with contrast showing a pituitary tumor pressing on the chiasm (*arrow*) and left optic nerve.

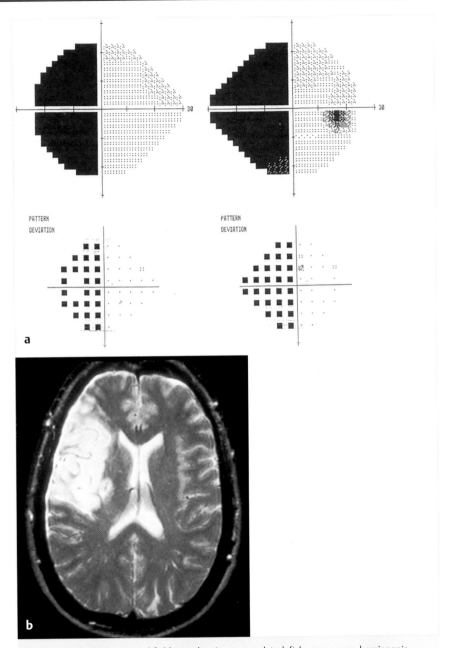

Fig. 3.19 (a) Humphrey visual field test showing a complete left homonymous hemianopia. (b) T2-weighted magnetic resonance imaging shows a large infarction in the territory of the right middle cerebral artery disrupting the right optic radiations.

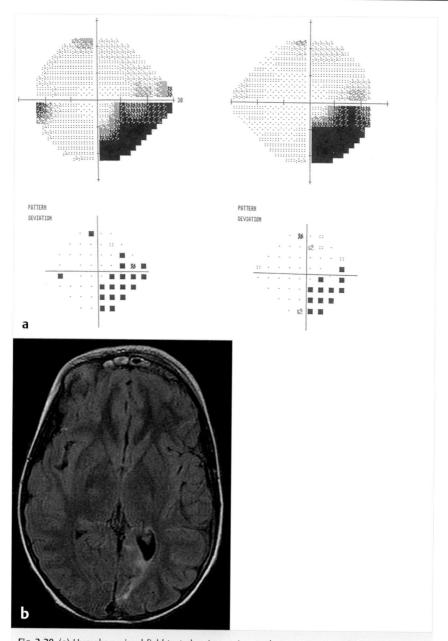

Fig. 3.20 (a) Humphrey visual field test showing an incomplete, congruent right homonymous hemianopia. (b) Fluid-attenuated inversion recovery magnetic resonance imaging showing a left occipital infarction.

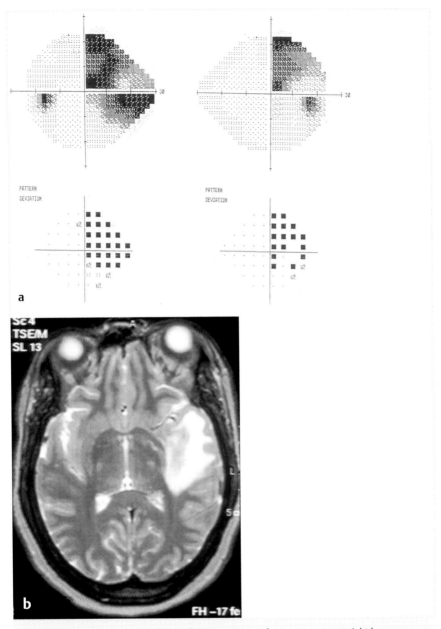

Fig. 3.21 (a) Humphrey visual field test showing an incomplete, noncongruent right homonymous hemianopia. (b) T2-weighted magnetic resonance imaging showing a left temporal lobe tumor.

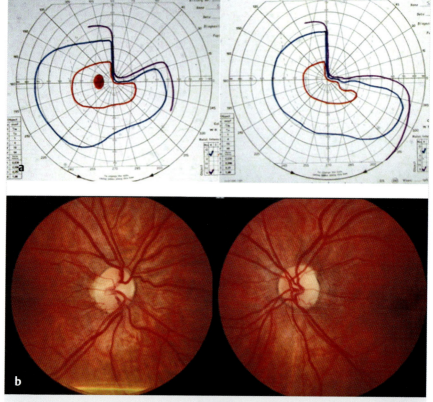

Fig. 3.22 a–d (a) Goldmann visual field test showing a partial right homonymous hemianopia from a left optic tract lesion. There is a right relative afferent pupillary defect (RAPD). (b) Fundus showing "bow-tie" pallor of the right optic nerve (on the left) and temporal pallor of the left optic nerve (on the right). (*continued*)

Optic Tract

Lesions of the optic tract cause a contralateral homonymous hemianopia, which may or may not be congruent.

Optic tract fibers are the axons of the ganglion cells originating in the inner layers of the retina. These axons are destined for the lateral geniculate nucleus, where they synapse with neurons whose axons then form the optic radiations. Therefore, chronic optic tract lesions will cause optic atrophy, often in a characteristic pattern.

Lesions of the optic tract (left optic tract lesion in the example in ▶ Fig. 3.22) produce atrophy of three groups of retinal ganglion cell fibers:
1. Nasal half of the macula of the right eye ([1–red] in ▶ Fig. 3.22d)
2. Nasal retina of the right eye ([2–red]) in ▶ Fig. 3.22d)
3. Temporal retina in the left eye ([3–green] in ▶ Fig. 3.22d)

Lesion groups 1 and 2 result in a bowtie pattern of optic atrophy (▶ Fig. 3.22b) of the right optic nerve. Lesion group 3 results in mostly temporal atrophy of the left optic

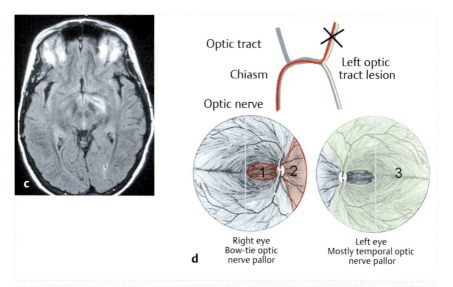

Fig. 3.22 (*continued*) (**c**) Axial fluid-attenuated inversion recovery magnetic resonance imaging showing a lesion of the left optic tract in a patient with multiple sclerosis. (**d**) Diagram showing the effect of a chronic left optic tract lesion on the retinal ganglion cell fibers.

nerve (▶ Fig. 3.22b). A RAPD is often observed in the eye contralateral to the optic tract lesion. This is because more fibers in the optic tract come from the opposite eye, having crossed in the chiasm. This greater contribution from the opposite eye is because the nasal retina is bigger than the temporal retina (the temporal visual field is bigger than the nasal visual field in each eye). The resultant RAPD will be in the eye that has contributed the most fibers to the damaged optic tract (i.e., the eye opposite the lesion, on the same side as the homonymous hemianopia).

> **Pearls**
>
> A left optic tract syndrome includes the following:
> - Right homonymous hemianopia
> - Right RAPD
> - Bowtie atrophy of the right optic nerve
> - Mostly temporal pallor of the left optic nerve

Lateral Geniculate Nucleus

Lesions of the lateral geniculate nucleus typically cause a contralateral homonymous hemianopia. Two patterns of visual field loss occur when the lesion is secondary to an ischemic lesion in the territory of the choroidal arteries (anterior or posterior) (▶ Fig. 3.23).

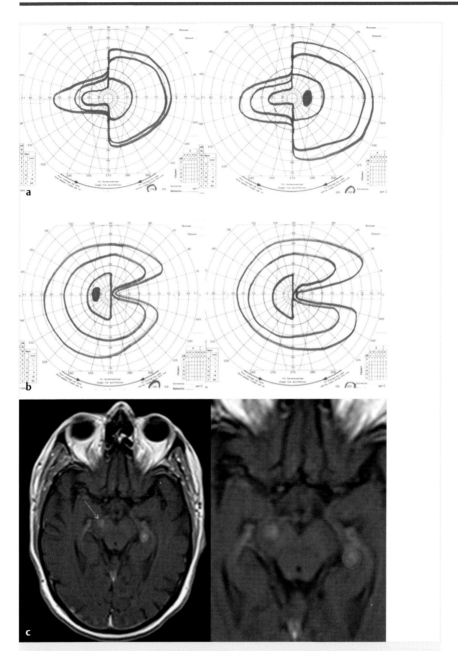

Fig. 3.23 (a) Goldmann visual field test showing an incomplete left homonymous hemianopia (sectoranopia) resulting from a right *anterior* choroidal artery infarction. (b) Goldmann visual field test showing an incomplete right homonymous hemianopia (sectoranopia) resulting from a left *posterior* choroidal artery infarction. (c) Axial magnetic resonance imaging with contrast showing a metastasis on the left lateral geniculate nucleus. The patient had a visual field defect similar to the one shown in (b).

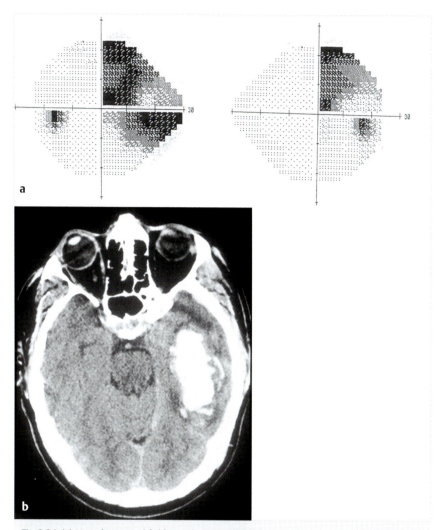

Fig. 3.24 (a) Humphrey visual field test showing a right superior incongruent homonymous hemianopia. (b) Axial computed tomography without contrast showing a left temporal lobe hemorrhage.

Optic Radiations

Lesions of the optic radiations typically produce a contralateral homonymous hemianopia, worse superiorly when the lesion is in the temporal lobe and worse inferiorly when the lesion is in the parietal lobe.

Postsynaptic fibers from the lateral geniculate nucleus form the optic radiations, which separate into the inferior fibers (temporal lobe) and the superior fibers (parietal lobe) as they progress posteriorly toward the occipital cortex (▶ Fig. 3.24). Lesions of

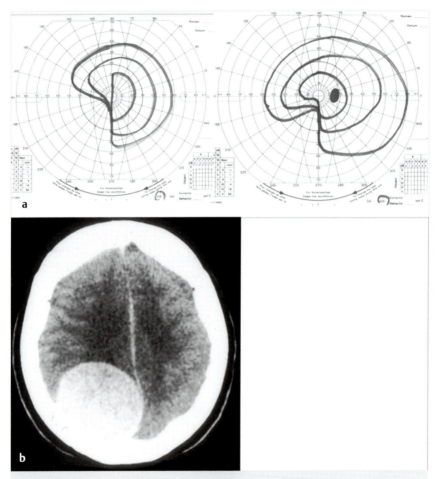

Fig. 3.25 (a) Goldmann visual field test showing a left inferior incongruent homonymous hemianopia secondary to a lesion of the right superior optic radiations. (b) Axial computed tomography with contrast showing a right parietal tumor (meningioma).

the parietal lobe often impair optokinetic nystagmus (see ▶ Fig. 1.27) when stimuli are moved in the direction of the damaged parietal lobe (▶ Fig. 3.25).

Occipital Lobe: Unilateral

Lesions of the occipital lobe produce a contralateral homonymous hemianopia, which is most often congruent. Most isolated congruent homonymous hemianopias are due to an occipital infarction in the territory of the posterior cerebral artery (PCA).

The tip of the occipital lobe, where the macular or central homonymous hemifields are represented, often has a dual blood supply from terminal branches of the PCA and of the middle cerebral artery (MCA). Depending on anatomical variations of the blood supply and of the circle of Willis, the tip of the occipital lobe is often a watershed area

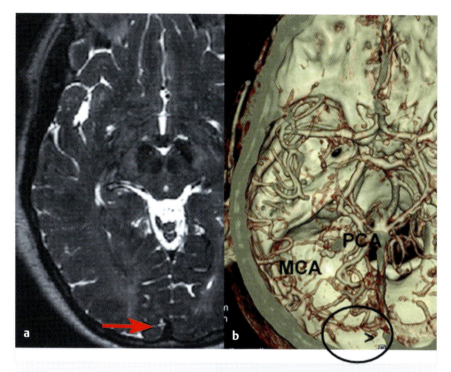

Fig. 3.26 (a) T2-axial magnetic resonance imaging showing the occipital lobe (*red arrow*). (b) Three-dimensional reconstruction of a computed tomographic angiogram showing the blood supply of the occipital lobe. The circle shows the potential watershed area of blood supply from the middle cerebral artery (MCA) and posterior cerebral artery (PCA) to the most posterior tip of the occipital lobe.

(▶ Fig. 3.26). Occlusion of the PCA often results in sparing of the tip of the occipital lobe, thereby sparing the macular representation, which is vascularized by terminal branches of the MCA (▶ Fig. 3.27).

An embolic infarction of either a distal MCA or PCA branch can result in exclusive ischemia of the tip of the occipital lobe, thereby producing a small homonymous scotomatous defect if there is inadequate collateral circulation (▶ Fig. 3.28).

Occipital Lobe: Sparing the Temporal Crescent

When we fixate with both eyes, there is superimposition of the central 60 degrees of visual fields in both eyes. There remains in each eye a temporal crescent of visual field for which there are no corresponding points in the other eye. The representation of this most peripheral 20 to 30 degrees is located in the anteriormost portion of the contralateral occipital cortex. Lesions of the occipital lobe sparing this anteriormost portion of the occipital cortex will spare the temporal crescent (▶ Fig. 3.29).

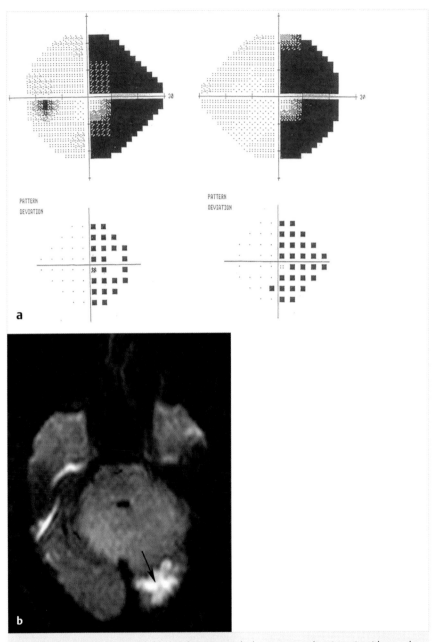

Fig. 3.27 (a) Humphrey visual field test showing a right homonymous hemianopia with macular sparing. (b) Axial magnetic resonance imaging (diffusion-weighted imaging) showing a left occipital infarction (*arrow*) (cardiac emboli), sparing the most posterior tip of the occipital lobe.

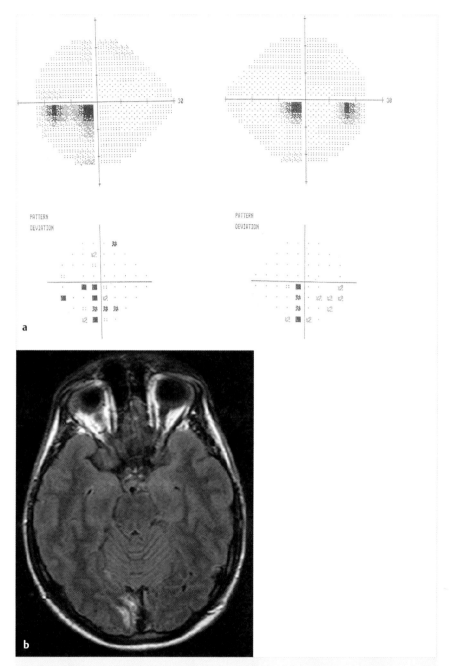

Fig. 3.28 (a) Humphrey visual field test showing a congruent left homonymous scotomatous defect. (b) Fluid-attenuated inversion recovery axial magnetic resonance imaging showing an infarction in the right tip of the occipital lobe (in the setting of complicated cardiac surgery).

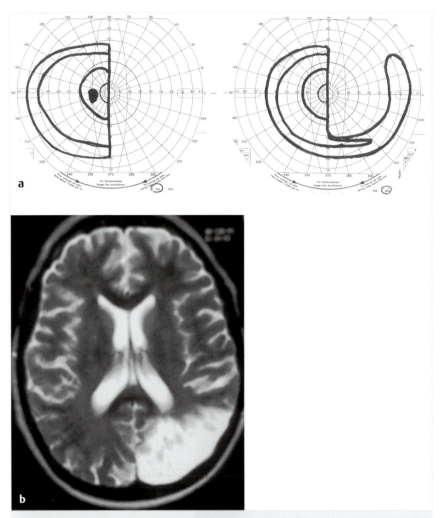

Fig. 3.29 (a) Goldmann visual field test showing a partial right homonymous hemianopia sparing the temporal crescent. (b) T2-axial magnetic resonance imaging showing a left occipital infarction, sparing the anteriormost part of the occipital lobe.

Occipital Lobe: Bilateral

Bilateral occipital lobe lesions will produce bilateral homonymous hemianopias, which may be asymmetric (▶ Fig. 3.30). In addition to the visual field defects, there may be decreased visual acuity, which is always the same in both eyes (▶ Fig. 3.31).

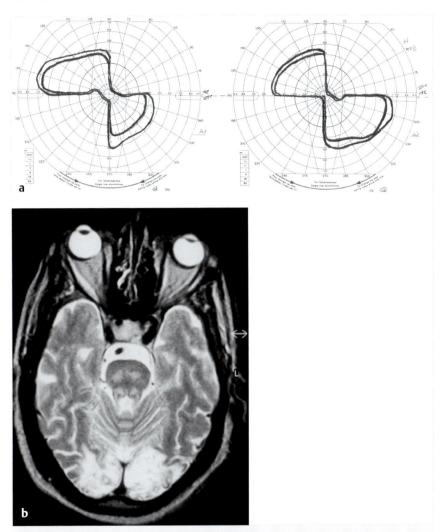

Fig. 3.30 (a) Goldmann visual field test showing bilateral homonymous hemianopias (left inferior homonymous quadrantanopia and right superior homonymous quadrantanopia). (b) T2-weighted axial magnetic resonance imaging showing bilateral occipital infarctions.

Pearls

When bilateral lesions of the retrochiasmal visual pathways produce a decrease in visual acuity, the degree of visual acuity loss is always symmetric in both eyes, unless there are other, more anterior, reasons for a decrease in visual acuity (e.g., asymmetric refractive errors, cataracts, or a superimposed asymmetric or unilateral retinopathy or optic neuropathy).

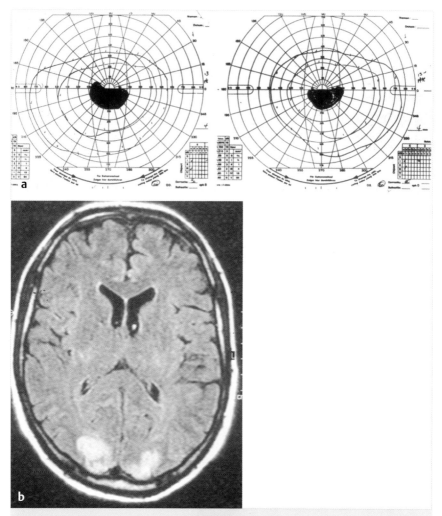

Fig. 3.31 (a) Goldmann visual field test showing bilateral homonymous inferior scotomatous defects. (b) Fluid-attenuated inversion recovery axial magnetic resonance imaging showing bilateral superior occipital lesions from hypertensive encephalopathy.

4 Ancillary Testing Commonly Used in Neuro-ophthalmology

In most cases, decisions regarding lesion localization and presumed etiology are determined based on the clinical history and examination. Ancillary testing should be obtained only to confirm or to document a clinical impression, not to "go fishing" for an answer.

Knowing what to look for before ordering ancillary testing will allow you to recommend the appropriate test and interpret that test correctly. For example, brain imaging obtained for the evaluation of a third nerve palsy may demonstrate a Chiari malformation. In this case, the Chiari malformation should be considered an incidental finding that is asymptomatic and that does not need to be treated or investigated further.

4.1 Electrophysiologic Testing

Electrophysiologic testing can help differentiate retinal from optic nerve disease in selected cases. It is also helpful in documenting occult abnormalities of the optic nerve or retinal function.

4.1.1 Visual Evoked Responses (or Visual Evoked Potentials)

Visual evoked responses (or visual evoked potentials) are measurements of the electrical signal recorded at the scalp over the occipital cortex in response to visual stimuli. In the test, the patient is asked to look at a TV screen on which various stimuli are provided; electrodes placed on the scalp over the occipital cortex record the responses. Each eye is tested separately.

This test is not accurate if the patient does not cooperate. Abnormal responses may occur if the patient does not look at the screen, does not focus on the screen, moves the tested eye, or is tired. Appropriate refraction is necessary.

The visual evoked response reflects the integrity of the afferent visual pathway (damage anywhere from the retina to the occipital cortex may alter the signal). It is primarily a function of central visual function because such a large region of the occipital cortex near the recording electrodes is devoted to macular projections.

Two techniques are used to record visual evoked responses: pattern stimulus, which provides a quantifiable and reliable waveform but may be absent in patients with poor vision, and flash stimulus, which is useful for patients with very poor vision in whom the pattern stimulus response is absent. The recorded responses for each eye are then compared (▶ Fig. 4.1), with the focus on the amplitude and peak latency of the waveform (P100). Classically, the P100 waveform is delayed in patients with demyelinating optic neuritis.

In most clinical situations, the visual evoked responses are of limited usefulness and are not necessary to make the diagnosis of optic neuropathy.

Visual evoked responses are most useful in evaluating the integrity of the visual pathway in infants and inarticulate adults. A preserved flash or pattern response confirms intact pathways, whereas an abnormal flash response indicates gross impairment

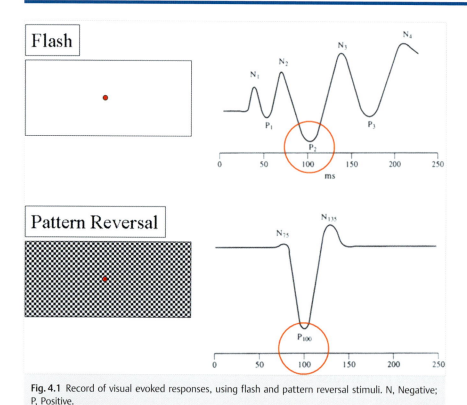

Fig. 4.1 Record of visual evoked responses, using flash and pattern reversal stimuli. N, Negative; P, Positive.

(▶ Fig. 4.2). An abnormal pattern response is less useful: it may indicate damage, or it may be falsely abnormal.

Visual evoked responses are also useful in confirming intact visual pathways in patients with markedly abnormal subjective visual responses of suspected nonorganic origin. A response with an intact pattern not only confirms intact visual pathways but also provides an estimate of visual acuity when stimuli of various sizes are used. A response with an abnormal or absent pattern does not confirm organic disease because voluntary inattention or defocusing can markedly alter the pattern waveform.

4.1.2 Electroretinogram

The electroretinogram (ERG) is a measurement of electrical activity of the retina in response to light stimulus. It is measured at the corneal surface by electrodes embedded in a corneal contact lens worn for testing. The ERG is normal in optic neuropathies.

Full-Field Electroretinogram

A full-field ERG is generated by stimulating the entire retina with a flash light source under varying conditions of retinal adaptation to dark and light (▶ Fig. 4.3).

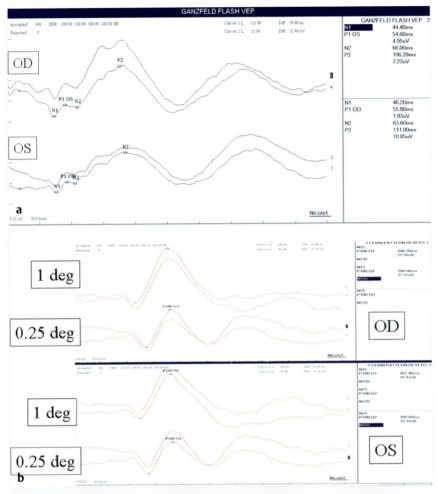

Fig. 4.2 **(a)** Normal and symmetric flash visual evoked responses in an infant with shaken baby syndrome, indicating intact visual pathways bilaterally. **(b)** Normal pattern visual evoked responses in a patient claiming poor vision in both eyes after a traumatic brain injury. This test confirms that the visual pathways are intact and proves normal central vision. N, Negative; P, Positive.

Major components of the electrical waveform generated and measured include the following:

- *A wave (negative):* primarily derived from the photoreceptor layer (outer retina)
- *B wave (positive):* derived from the inner retina (Müller and bipolar cells)
- Two other waveforms that are sometimes recorded are the *c-wave* originating in the pigment epithelium and the *d-wave* indicating activity of the OFF bipolar cells.

Rod and cone photoreceptors can be separated by varying stimuli and the state of retinal adaptation during testing.

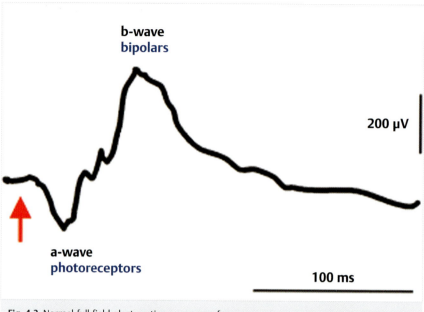

Fig. 4.3 Normal full-field electroretinogram wave form.

Full-field ERG is useful in detecting diffuse retinal disease in the setting of generalized or peripheral vision loss. Disorders such as retinitis pigmentosa, cone–rod dystrophy, toxic retinopathies, and retinal paraneoplastic syndromes may present with variably severe visual loss and minimally visible retinal abnormalities. The ERG is invariably severely depressed by the time patients complain of visual loss, making full-field ERG testing very useful. Although poorly cooperative patients can make interpretation of the full-field ERG more difficult (there can be background noise due to frequent blinking and squeezing), the responses cannot be substantially altered voluntarily (unlike visual evoked responses).

Because the full-field ERG measures only a mass response of the entire retina, it may be normal in minor or localized retinal disease, particularly maculopathies, even with severe visual acuity loss.

Multifocal Electroretinogram

Multifocal ERG simultaneously records ERG signals from up to 250 focal retinal locations within the central 30 degrees. The individual responses are mapped topographically (▶ Fig. 4.4).

This technique is extremely helpful in detecting occult focal retinal abnormalities within the macula. Unlike full-field ERG, however, uncooperative patients can alter the responses on a multifocal ERG by not fixating accurately.

4.2 Fundus Autofluorescence Imaging

Fundus autofluorescence (FAF) imaging is helpful in diagnosing retinal conditions at an early stage by showing abnormalities that are often invisible to standard fundus

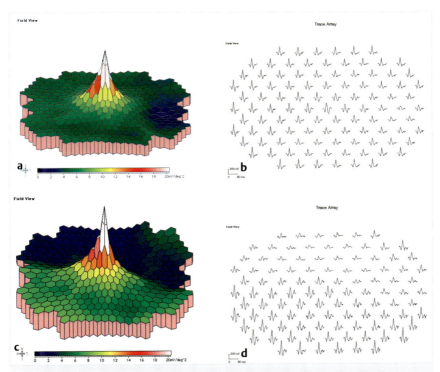

Fig. 4.4 (a,b) Normal multifocal electroretinogram (ERG) showing the normal foveal peak. (c,d) Abnormal multifocal ERG showing a decreased superior foveal peak in a patient with a superior branch retinal artery occlusion. (Courtesy of Dr. M. S. Lee.)

photography and ophthalmoscopy (▶ Fig. 4.5). Autofluorescence is caused by the presence of lipofuscin, an aging pigment fluorophore produced by the outer segments of the photoreceptors and stored at the level of the retinal pigment epithelium. Two abnormal states of lipofuscin exist, hyperautofluorescence and hypoautofluorescence (▶ Fig. 4.5b); both are associated with various retinal disorders. Optic nerve head drusen are also usually hyperautofluorescent (▶ Fig. 4.6).

4.3 Retinal Fluorescein Angiography

Intravenous (IV) fluorescein angiography is a photographic method of angiography that does not rely on radiation. After IV injection of fluorescein solution (in an arm vein), rapid-sequence retinal photography is performed by using a camera with spectrally appropriate excitation and filters (the fluorescein absorbs blue light and becomes fluorescent, which can be captured on photographs).

Fluorescein angiography is helpful in studying the vascular filling patterns of the choroidal, retinal, and optic nerve head arteries and veins. It can also help differentiate macular from optic nerve–related visual loss by showing macular changes that are not always easily visible on funduscopic examination. However, imaging of the macula with optical coherence tomography has now replaced fluorescein angiography for most of these cases.

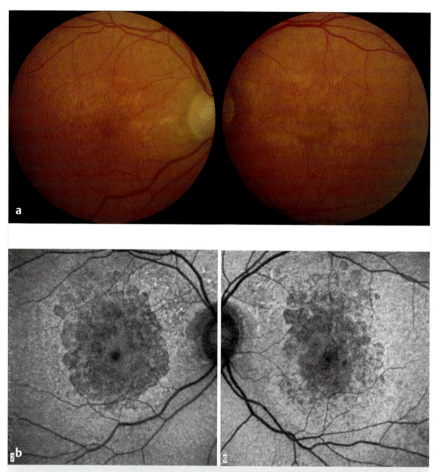

Fig. 4.5 Autofluorescence imaging of the macula showing extensive bilateral maculopathies. (a) On the color fundus photo, the macula has an abnormal mottled appearance with pigmentary changes. (b) The autofluorescence imaging demonstrates large areas of hypofluorescence (dark) involving both maculae.

The test requires the cooperation of the patient, who needs to be able to sit up and fixate. It also requires relatively clear ocular media.

Fluorescein angiography is usually well tolerated, although side effects include nausea, vomiting, and vasovagal responses. True allergic reactions are rare. The fluorescein is excreted in the urine (which becomes yellow and fluorescent) within 24 to 36 hours.

The technique for fluorescein angiography is as follows. Color photos and red-free photos are taken prior to the injection of fluorescein. Once the fluorescein is injected, multiple retinal photos are taken on the same eye (chosen by the clinician) to study the choroidal and retinal vascular filling dynamic. A time (since the injection) is noted on each photo (▶ Fig. 4.7). Delay in the choroidal filling, as well as delay or asymmetry in the retinal vascular filling, is indicative of vascular disease. Photos are then taken of both eyes depending on the reason for the test. Abnormal fluorescence of the retina

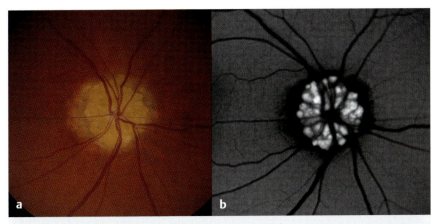

Fig. 4.6 Autofluorescence imaging of the optic nerve in optic nerve head drusen. (**a**) Superficial optic nerve drusen appearing as multiple small round calcifications in the optic nerve head on a color fundus photo. (**b**) The same optic nerve head in autofluorescence imaging showing the drusen as hyperfluorescent.

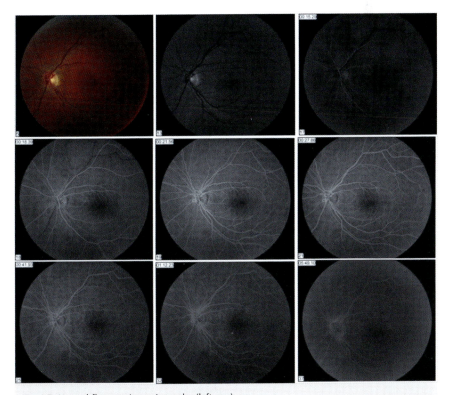

Fig. 4.7 Normal fluorescein angiography (left eye).

(indicating staining, pooling, or leakage of the fluorescein or blockage of the fluorescence) is indicative of retinal or choroidal disorders. Late photos may show leakage of the vessels (as in vasculitis) or of the optic nerve (as in optic nerve edema) (▶ Fig. 4.8 and ▶ Fig. 4.9).

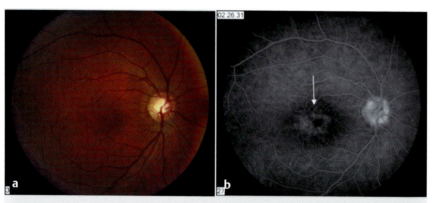

Fig. 4.8 Cystoid macular edema in the right eye responsible for central visual loss. (**a**) The macula looks relatively normal on the color photo. (**b**) The fluorescein angiogram demonstrates a characteristic leakage (*arrow*) at the level of the macula.

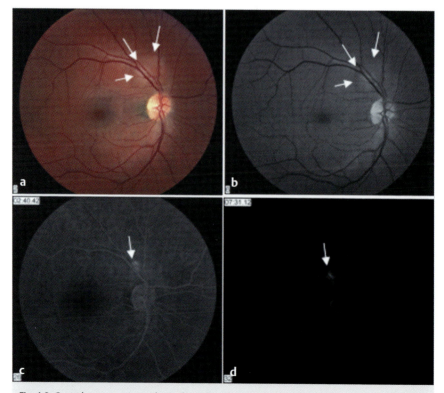

Fig. 4.9 Central serous retinopathy in the right eye presenting with a small paracentral scotoma. There is a bullous serous detachment on the color (**a**) and red-free photos (**b**) (*arrows*). (**c,d**) The fluorescein angiography shows dye leakage at the same level (*arrows*).

Demonstration of retinal small vessel vasculopathy such as vasculitis is best done with retinal fluorescein angiography. The abnormal vessels leak, and vascular abnormalities may be missed on fundus examination (▶ Fig. 4.10).

Fluorescein angiography is also very helpful for the diagnosis of giant cell arteritis. Photographs should be taken of both eyes with transit (early images after injection of IV fluorescein) on the most affected eye (▶ Fig. 4.11).

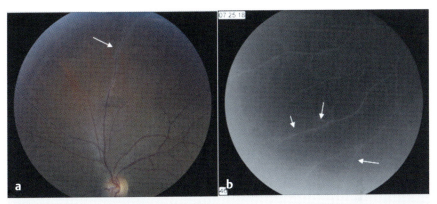

Fig. 4.10 Retinal vasculitis with sheathing (*arrow*) of the vessels on the color photo (**a**) and leakage of the dye on the fluorescein angiogram (**b**) (*arrows*).

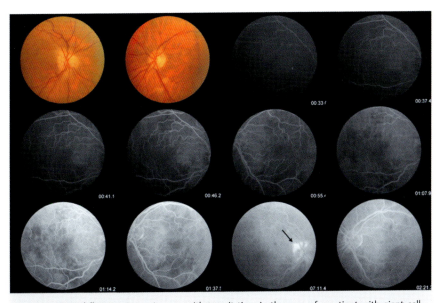

Fig. 4.11 Retinal fluorescein angiogram with transit time in the eyes of a patient with giant cell arteritis. There is an anterior ischemic optic neuropathy in the right eye with disc edema, and there are two cotton wool spots inferiorly in the left eye that are asymptomatic (color photos). The angiography shows early photos of the right eye with delayed and patchy choroidal filling. There is progressive and heterogeneous filling of the choroid, then of the retinal vessels on successive images. The late phase shows leakage of the fluorescein at the level of the right optic nerve, which is swollen (*arrow*).

4.4 Optical Coherence Tomography

Optical coherence tomography (OCT) is routinely performed in ophthalmology. It is a noninvasive transpupillary ophthalmic imaging technology that can image retinal and optic nerve structures in vivo with a resolution of 4 μm.

Cross-sectional images of the retina, the optic nerve, and peripapillary areas are produced using the optical backscattering of light similar to what is obtained with a B-scan ultrasound (OCT uses low-coherence near-infrared light). The anatomical layers within the retina can be differentiated, and retinal thickness can be measured (▶ Fig. 4.12). OCT is particularly useful for macular diseases (▶ Fig. 4.13); however, it requires a patient's ability to fixate and relatively clear ocular media. The quality is often better when the pupils are pharmacologically dilated.

OCT is very useful in demonstrating anatomical changes in the macular, such as edema (▶ Fig. 4.13), holes, cysts, macular traction, and an epiretinal membrane. Additionally, individual retinal layers can be analyzed and the retinal nerve fiber layer thickness and macular volume can be measured with OCT (▶ Fig. 4.14). This is important because peripapillary nerve fiber thickness and macular volume are decreased in glaucoma and other diseases of the optic nerve, such as optic neuritis. They are used to monitor disease activity in numerous optic neuropathies.

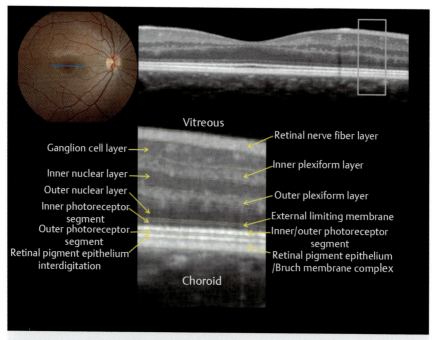

Fig. 4.12 Normal optical coherence tomography (OCT) of the macula. This high-resolution horizontal scan centered on the fovea allows visualization of each retinal layer.

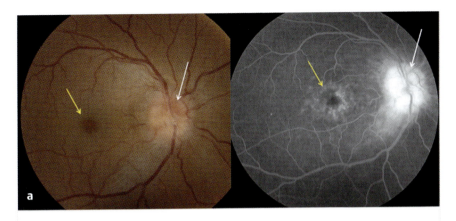

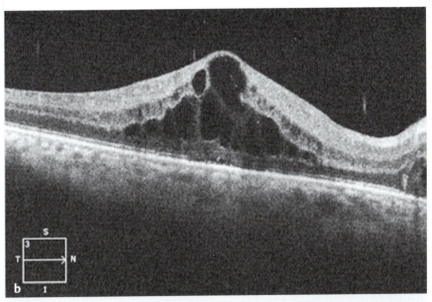

Fig. 4.13 **a–c** Posterior scleritis with thickening of the posterior pole and macular and disc edema. (**a**) Color fundus photo showing disc edema (*white arrow*) and abnormal edematous macula (*yellow arrow*), and fluorescein angiography (image taken at 3 min, 18 s after intravenous injection of fluorescein) demonstrating leakage of dye at the optic nerve and macula. (**b**) Optical coherence tomographic (OCT) imaging of the macula demonstrates cystoid macular edema consistent with the leakage of dye that was noted in the fluorescein angiogram. (*continued*)

4.5 Ocular/Orbital Echography

Echography, or ultrasound, is a technique that uses high-frequency sound waves to image tissue. Tissue characteristics such as increased cell density and reflective surfaces determine the specific echographic pattern.

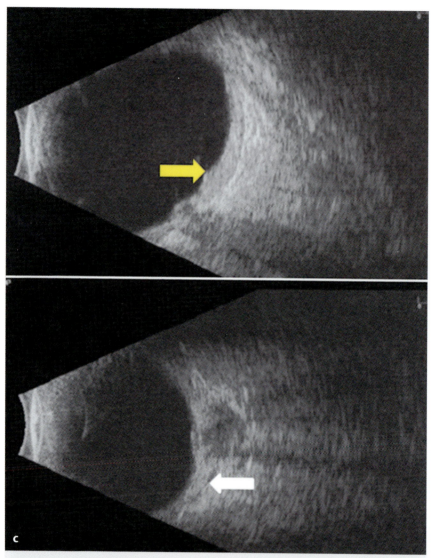

Fig. 4.13 (*continued*) (**c**) Thickening of the choroid and posterior scleral wall (*yellow arrow*) and fluid in the Tenon capsule (*white arrow*).

Ocular and orbital echography is performed by applying a probe directly to the eye (on the eyelid or directly on the corneal surface). The amount of energy returned to and detected by the probe determines the height (A scan) or intensity (B scan) of the resultant image.

A-scan echography is usually not used in neuro-ophthalmology (it allows measurement of ocular axial length such as for calculation of intraocular lens power before cataract surgery, as well as analysis of choroidal tumors).

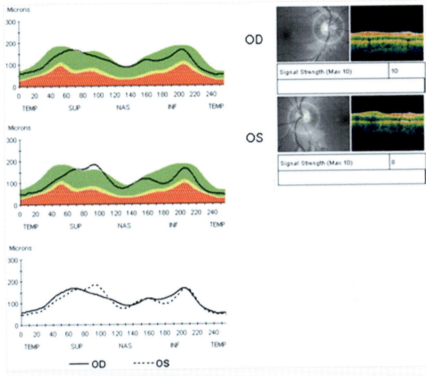

Fig. 4.14 Measurement of the retinal nerve fiber layer thickness in each eye with optical coherence tomography (OCT). It allows reproducible quantification of the peripapillary nerve fiber layer thickness. The average thickness is within normal limits in each eye (within the normal green layer). INF, inferior; NAS, nasal; OD, right eye; OS, left eye; SUP, superior; TEMP, temporal.

B-scan echography shows a two-dimensional image representing a "slice" through the globe. It is therefore particularly useful in examining the posterior pole in patients with vitreous opacities in whom the retina cannot be visualized, or to visualize calcified optic nerve drusen, and to evaluate a choroidal mass. It can also evaluate the anterior orbit and is used to measure the extraocular muscles in suspected thyroid eye disease and the superior ophthalmic vein when a carotid cavernous fistula is suspected.

Indications for B-scan echography in neuro-ophthalmology include the following:

- Optic nerve head drusen (may not be seen on fundus examination when buried) (▶ Fig. 4.15)
- Trauma with poor view of the fundus to demonstrate vitreous hemorrhage (▶ Fig. 4.16) or retinal detachment (▶ Fig. 4.17)
- Identification of an intraocular foreign body
- Analysis of posterior pole tumors
- Examination of the extraocular muscles when thyroid eye disease is suspected
- Examination of the superior ophthalmic vein when a carotid-cavernous fistula is suspected (▶ Fig. 4.18)
- Posterior scleritis (T sign) (see ▶ Fig. 4.13c)

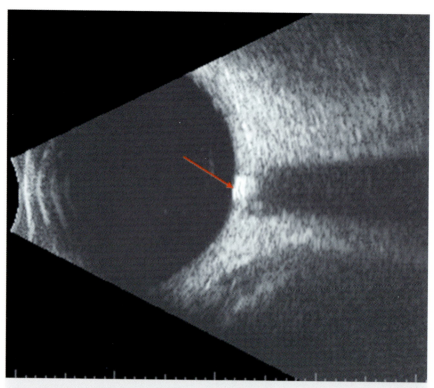

Fig. 4.15 Optic nerve head drusen on B-scan echography. The calcified drusen appear as an ovoid echogenic lesion (*arrow*) with a posterior acoustic shadowing.

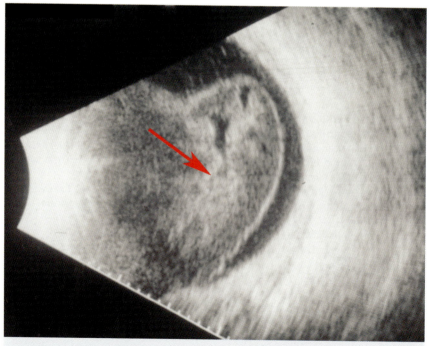

Fig. 4.16 Vitreous hemorrhage on B-scan echography. Note the white opacities in the vitreous (*arrow*).

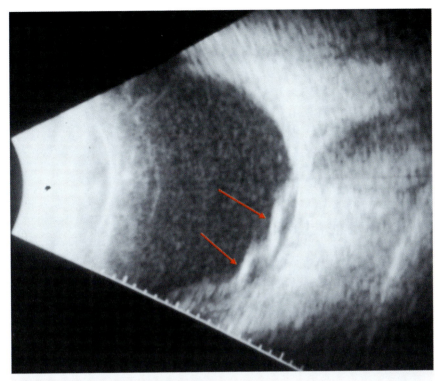

Fig. 4.17 Retinal detachment on B-scan echography (*arrows*).

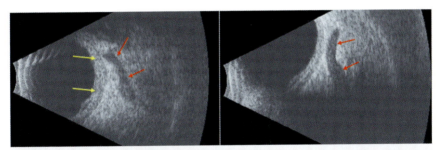

Fig. 4.18 Carotid cavernous fistula on B-scan echography. The congested choroid is thickened (*yellow arrows*), and the superior ophthalmic vein is dilated (*red arrows*).

4.6 Imaging of the Orbits and Visual Pathways

▶ Table 4.1 presents the advantages and disadvantages of computed tomography (CT) and magnetic resonance (MR) for imaging the orbits and visual pathways.

Table 4.1 Advantages (+) and disadvantages (−) of computed tomography and magnetic resonance imaging

Computed tomography	Magnetic resonance imaging
− Uses X-rays (radiation exposure) − Should not be used during pregnancy	+ No X-ray + Can be used during pregnancy
Contrast is iodine (administered intravenously during the test) − Should not be used during pregnancy − Common allergies − Renal toxicity (should not be used for patients with renal insufficiency and for diabetics)	Contrast is gadolinium (administered intravenously during the test) − Should not be used during pregnancy + Very rare allergies + Rare renal toxicity
+ Readily available + Test is very quick (a few minutes) + Can be done in confused or claustrophobic patients + Not expensive	− Less readily available − Test is long (30–45 minutes) − Cannot be done in a confused, uncooperative, or claustrophobic patient (very sensitive to movement artifacts) − Expensive − Incompatible with magnetic materials or pacemakers
− Limited multiplanar reformatting capability − Low resolution for soft tissue of the brain	+ Multiplanar reformatting capability (allows cuts in any directions) + High resolution for soft tissue of the brain
Ideal to image + Fresh blood + Calcium + Bone + Orbit + Facial sinuses, ears, skull base + All foreign bodies (except wood) + CT angiography good for imaging extracranial and intracranial circulations + Very accurate for aneurysms + CT venography good for imaging extracranial and intracranial veins + Very accurate for venous sinuses	Ideal to image + Soft tissues (brain parenchyma) + Meninges + Optic nerves and orbital apex + Cavernous sinus + Cranial nerves + Wood foreign bodies + MR angiography good for imaging extracranial and intracranial circulations − Less accurate for small aneurysms + MR venography good for imaging extracranial and intracranial veins − Common artifacts on venous sinuses

4.6.1 Computed Tomography

Because bone, calcification, fat, and blood all have unique X-ray absorption patterns, CT is a very effective technique for orbital imaging (▶ Table 4.2). Specific absorption patterns can be highlighted on CT to emphasize bone, soft tissues, or blood.

CT images are classically obtained in the axial planes. It is possible to also request images in the coronal plane by repositioning the patient. Sagittal images may be obtained by computer reformatting.

Routine studies are done at 3 or 5 mm slice intervals, but it is possible to obtain 1 mm slice intervals (better resolution).

A head CT without contrast takes only a few minutes and is readily available. It is commonly performed in the emergency room and is extremely valuable in trauma patients (who may have a bone fracture or an orbital foreign body), in stroke patients (▶ Fig. 4.19 and ▶ Fig. 4.20), and when an acute intracranial or intraorbital hemorrhage

Table 4.2 Appearance of tissues on computed tomography

Normal brain	Isodense (gray)
Edema Necrosis Infarction	Hypodense (dark gray or black)
Fresh blood Acute clot in a large vessel Bone Calcium Fat	Hyperdense (white)
Contrast	Enhancement of (appear white): Blood vessels Inflammatory lesions Neoplasms Breakdown of the normal blood–brain barrier (e.g., from cerebral ischemia)

is suspected (e.g., to detect a subarachnoid hemorrhage in a patient with an explosive headache). However, a normal head CT without contrast is insufficient in almost all other situations. It is falsely reassuring and often misses serious disorders.

The following are good indications for orbital CT:

- Orbital trauma (suspected fractures or foreign body)
- Ocular trauma to rule out a foreign body (ruptured globe)
- Infectious or noninfectious orbital inflammation (▶ Fig. 4.21 and ▶ Fig. 4.22)

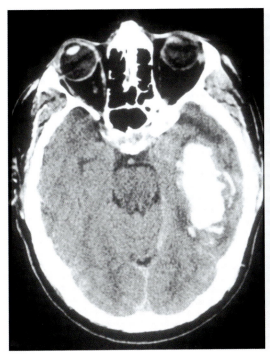

Fig. 4.19 Head computed tomography (CT) without contrast showing a large hyperdensity in the left temporal lobe consistent with a cerebral hemorrhage.

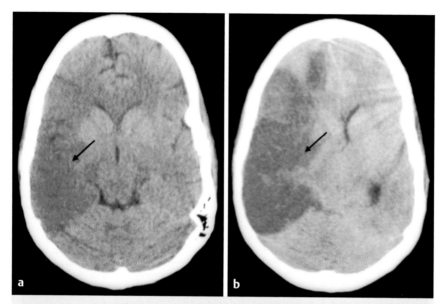

Fig. 4.20 (a) Head computed tomography (CT) without contrast performed 6 hours after a right hemispheric cerebral infarction (seen as mild hypodensity) (*arrow*). (b) Head CT without contrast performed 24 hours after a right hemispheric cerebral infarction (same patient) (seen as pronounced hypodensity, *arrow*). Note the interval development of mass effect on the ventricles.

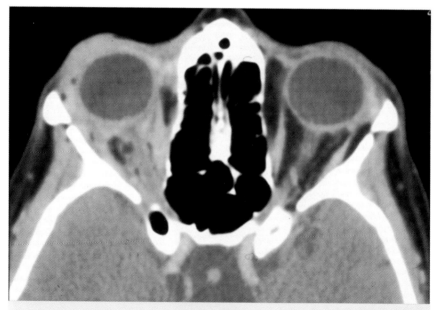

Fig. 4.21 Axial computed tomography of the orbits with contrast showing enhancement of the orbital contents on the right. This patient had a metastasis from breast cancer.

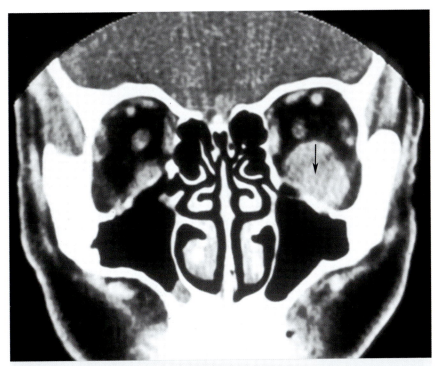

Fig. 4.22 Coronal computed tomography of the orbits with contrast showing a large metastasis from melanoma in the inferior left orbit (*arrow*).

- Bone lesions (osteoma, fibrous dysplasia, suspected metastatic disease, etc.)
- Preoperative imaging for orbital disease (when imaging of the facial sinuses is very important)
- Lesions that may contain calcium (retinoblastoma, optic nerve drusen, orbital varix, meningioma, etc.)
- Lacrimal gland lesions

4.6.2 Magnetic Resonance Imaging

MRI offers many advantages over CT and is the most commonly obtained ancillary test in neuro-ophthalmology. It provides excellent contrast resolution between soft tissues, and multiplanar imaging can be done without repositioning the patient.

Various sequences are obtained that allow visualization of different tissues. The appearance of the tissues varies based on the sequence used.

T1-weighted images provide good anatomical details. Fat looks bright (hyperintense), vitreous looks black (hypointense), cerebrospinal fluid (CSF) looks black (hypointense), and subacute blood appears white (hyperintense). On T1-weighted images, brain gray matter is gray, and brain white matter is lighter. Most cerebral parenchymal lesions appear dark (hypointense), unless gadolinium contrast is given; in that case, and if there is a breakdown in the blood–brain barrier, they may appear white (hyperintense).

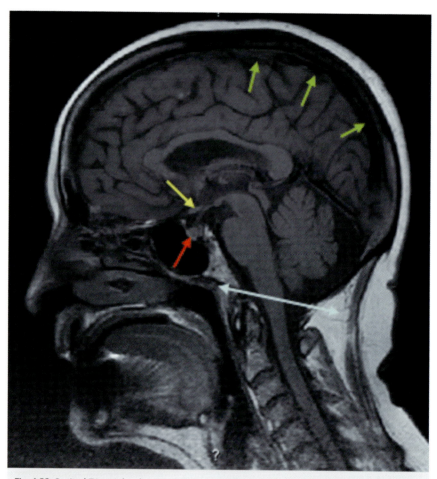

Fig. 4.23 Sagittal T1-weighted magnetic resonance imaging. See text for identification of arrows.

The T1-weighted midline sagittal view is the first sequence systematically obtained on MRI, and it is very helpful in neuro-ophthalmology (▶ Fig. 4.23). It provides information on the absence of cerebellar tonsillar herniation (Chiari malformation) (blue line in ▶ Fig. 4.23), the pituitary gland (red arrow), the chiasm (yellow arrow), and the superior sagittal venous sinus (green arrows).

Because the orbits are filled with fat, a regular T1 sequence does not allow good evaluation of the orbits. In addition, administration of contrast results in enhancement of normal extraocular muscles and abnormal intraorbital structures; these appear brighter and therefore cannot be distinguished from the white orbital fat on a regular T1 sequence. A *T1 sequence with fat suppression* transforms the bright signal of the fat into a black signal and allows for very good orbital studies, before and after contrast administration (▶ Fig. 4.24).

The orbits are best studied with a combination of axial and coronal views. Thin cuts are necessary.

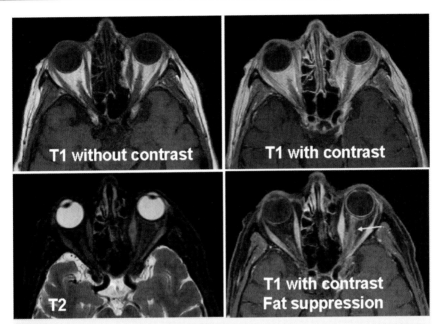

Fig. 4.24 Appearance of the orbits on various magnetic resonance imaging sequences. The fat appears bright on T1, and the T1 sequence with contrast is helpful only if it is performed with fat suppression. Thin cuts are necessary to allow good studies of the orbit. In this example, there is a left optic neuritis with enhancement of the left optic nerve and optic nerve sheath, seen on the T1 fat-suppressed enhanced image (*arrow*). On the T2 sequence, the orbital fat is dark.

Orbital MRI should include the following:
- Axial T1 sequence
- Axial T1 sequence with fat suppression
- Axial T1 sequence with fat suppression after injection of contrast
- Coronal T1 sequence with fat suppression
- Coronal T1 sequence with fat suppression after injection of contrast (▶ Fig. 4.25)

T2-weighted images are ideal for screening for brain parenchymal abnormalities. On T2-weighted images, fat looks darker (hypointense), vitreous looks bright (hyperintense), ventricles (CSF) look bright (hyperintense), and brain gray matter is lighter than brain white matter. Additionally, most cerebral parenchymal lesions appear bright (hyperintense), especially inflammatory or ischemic lesions.

Because the ventricles are filled with CSF, a regular T2 sequence shows the ventricles, and the subarachnoid space as very bright and does not allow for good evaluation of periventricular lesions, such as the white matter lesions from multiple sclerosis. A specific sequence called *fluid-attenuated inversion recovery (FLAIR)* allows transformation of the bright CSF signal into black signal, while maintaining the other characteristics of a T2-weighted image. FLAIR images are therefore "black CSF" T2-weighted images (▶ Fig. 4.26).

Specific T2 sequences (*gradient echo*) also allow better visualization of blood products, such as hemosiderin. These sequences are particularly helpful when evaluating patients with cerebral vascular malformations, tumors, trauma, or infarctions.

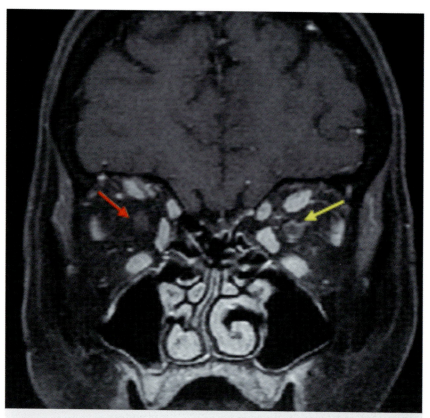

Fig. 4.25 Coronal T1-weighted magnetic resonance imaging of the orbits with contrast and fat suppression. The right optic nerve (*red arrow*) is normal, and the left optic nerve and optic nerve sheath (*yellow arrow*) enhance.

Diffusion-weighted images are ideal in detecting acute cerebral ischemia. They demonstrate restricted diffusion within hours of acute cerebral ischemia (while CT and other MRI sequences are often still normal) and should be obtained in all patients with acute neurologic deficits or when cerebral ischemia is suspected (▶ Fig. 4.27). The appearance of lesions varies on diffusion-weighted images based on the time elapsed since the infarction. Old ischemic lesions do not show restricted diffusion, whereas acute ischemic lesions appear hyperintense on diffusion-weighted images and hypointense on the apparent diffusion coefficient (ADC) map (▶ Fig. 4.28).

It is important to know which type of MRI to order. For example, with suspicion of cerebral infarction, a stroke protocol MRI of the brain should be ordered. This typically includes MRI without contrast (including sagittal T1-weighted sequence, axial T1-weighted sequence, axial FLAIR sequence, T2-weighted sequence, and often gradient echo to detect blood), MRI with diffusion weighted images (shows very acute infarctions), and MRI with magnetic resonance angiography (MRA) of the head (circle of Willis) and neck (extracranial cervical arteries).

In the case of optic neuropathy, MRI of the brain and orbits with contrast should be ordered. This includes regular MRI of the brain with contrast (including

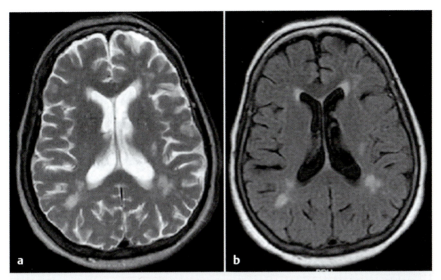

Fig. 4.26 (a) Axial T2-weighted sequence and (b) fluid- attenuated inversion recovery (FLAIR) sequence. Both sequences are T2-weighted, but the cerebrospinal fluid (ventricles and subarachnoid spaces) appears dark on the FLAIR sequence, thereby facilitating observation of periventricular hyperintensities.

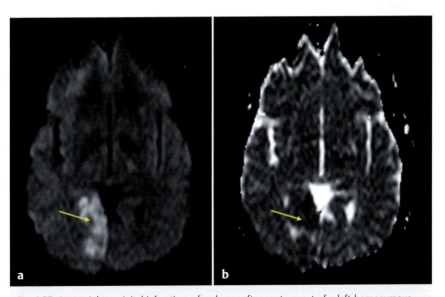

Fig. 4.27 Acute right occipital infarction a few hours after acute onset of a left homonymous hemianopia. Head computed tomography and T1- and T2-weighted brain magnetic resonance imaging were normal. (a) The diffusion-weighted image shows a hyperintensity in the territory of the right posterior cerebral artery (*arrow*), suggesting restricted diffusion. (b) The apparent diffusion coefficient map shows a hypointensity (*arrow*) in the same area, confirming the acute infarction.

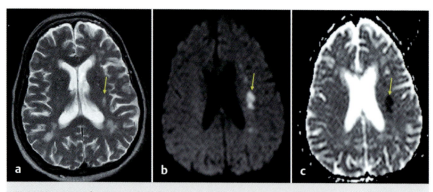

Fig. 4.28 Acute infarction in the left corona radiata. (a) The T2-weighted image shows numerous hypersignals in the white matter. (b) The diffusion-weighted image and (c) the apparent diffusion coefficient map show, respectively, a hyperintensity and a hypointensity (*arrow*) demonstrating that this lesion is acute.

sagittal T1-weighted sequence, axial T1-weighted sequence, axial FLAIR sequence, and T1- weighted sequence with contrast) and dedicated orbital views (including axial and coronal T1-weighted sequence with and without fat suppression, as well as axial and coronal T1-weighted sequence with fat suppression and with contrast).

In the case of chiasmal syndrome, the examiner should order an MRI scan of the brain and orbits with contrast, with special attention to the pituitary gland. T1, T2, and T1 axial, coronal, and sagittal views of the sella turcica and pituitary gland with contrast should also be ordered.

In the case of cranial nerve deficit, the examiner should order an MRI scan of the brain with contrast, with special attention to the specific cranial nerve. Imaging should also include very thin axial and coronal cuts in T1, T2, and T1 with contrast, covering the anatomical course of the cranial nerve in question.

The following are good indications for MRI:
- Optic neuropathy
- Suspected optic nerve tumor
- Wooden foreign body
- Orbital apex or cavernous sinus syndrome
- Chiasmal syndrome
- Brain lesion
- Fungal sinusitis

4.7 Vascular Imaging

Imaging of the intracranial and extracranial arteries and veins can be performed noninvasively with ultrasound, CT, and MRI. However, the gold standard for vascular imaging remains the catheter angiogram.

4.7.1 Vascular Ultrasound

Ultrasound allows reliable imaging of the extracranial carotid and vertebral arteries (▶ Fig. 4.29 and ▶ Fig. 4.30). It combines Doppler imaging (which provides information

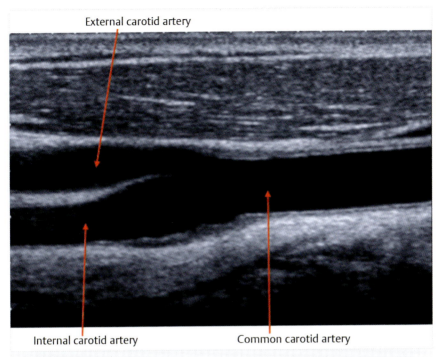

Fig. 4.29 Carotid ultrasound showing normal common, internal, and external carotid arteries.

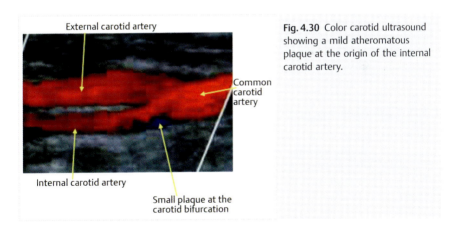

Fig. 4.30 Color carotid ultrasound showing a mild atheromatous plaque at the origin of the internal carotid artery.

on the flow within a blood vessel) and imaging of the vessels (often with color), thereby allowing quantification of the stenosis and evaluation of the hemodynamic significance of the stenosis.

Transcranial Doppler (TCD) is used for evaluation of the intracranial cerebral circulation and of the ophthalmic artery. The transorbital, transtemporal, and transforaminal windows are used to detect flow within large intracranial arteries.

101

TCD is routinely used for detection of intracranial vessel stenosis, early identification of vasospasm in subarachnoid hemorrhage, and evaluation of intracranial hemodynamic impairment in patients with cervical artery stenosis and occlusion.

Doppler of the ophthalmic artery is helpful when there is ocular ischemia or to evaluate the collateral circulation in patients with severe carotid artery stenosis or carotid occlusion. It may show the following:

- Normal or attenuated flow in the ophthalmic artery
- No flow in the ophthalmic artery (indicating occlusion of the ophthalmic artery)
- Reversed flow in the ophthalmic artery (indicating that the ipsilateral cerebral anterior circulation is coming from branches of the external carotid artery in a patient with ipsilateral occlusion of the internal carotid artery). These patients have a high risk of hemodynamic cerebral infarction and chronic ocular ischemia.

4.7.2 Computed Tomographic Angiography and Venography

CT angiography (CTA) and CT venography (CTV) allow very good evaluation of the intracranial and extracranial arteries and veins. These tests require high volumes of contrast and may be problematic in patients with renal insufficiency or diabetes mellitus.

Examination of the source images, as well as three-dimensional (3D) reconstructions, provides a very reliable screening for arterial stenosis, aneurysms, and venous stenosis or occlusion (▶ Fig. 4.31, ▶ Fig. 4.32, ▶ Fig. 4.33).

4.7.3 Magnetic Resonance Angiography and Venography

MR angiography (MRA) and MR venography (MRV) of the brain are often performed without contrast, although contrast can also be used with specific MRA and MRV techniques. The source images should be examined in addition to 3D reconstruction images (▶ Fig. 4.34, ▶ Fig. 4.35, ▶ Fig. 4.36).

Interpretation of vascular imaging with MRA or CTA is difficult (▶ Fig. 4.37). The radiologist often has to look at hundreds of images (the slice spacing is very small), and only a good clinical correlation allows accurate interpretation. Communication with the radiologist is essential.

4.7.4 Catheter Angiography

Catheter angiography is an invasive test that requires an experienced interventional radiologist. It is performed under local anesthesia and requires puncture of the femoral artery, along with selective catheterization of the cervical and intracranial arteries, with a catheter brought into the aorta. It also requires injection of a large volume of contrast.

Complications are rare when the test is performed by an experienced radiologist (< 1% of procedures). However, the complications can be devastating and include the following:

- Groin hematoma
- Femoral artery pseudoaneurysm
- Aortic dissection
- Cervical artery dissection
- Disruption of atheromatous plaques present in the aorta with resultant distal emboli
- Cerebral infarction

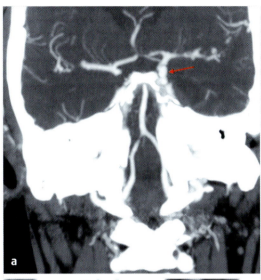

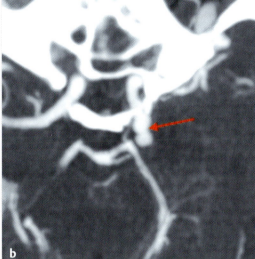

Fig. 4.31 **(a)** Computed tomographic angiogram (CTA; coronal view, source images) showing a large left posterior communicating artery aneurysm (*arrow*) in a patient with a painful left third nerve palsy. **(b)** CTA (axial view, source image) showing the left posterior communicating aneurysm (*arrow*).

Despite advancement in noninvasive imaging, a catheter angiogram is still obtained in specific situations, such as carotid cavernous fistulas, aneurysms, and intracranial stenoses (▶ Fig. 4.38 and ▶ Fig. 4.39).

As for CTA, 3D reconstructions can be obtained with catheter angiography (▶ Fig. 4.40). They allow better views of the circle of Willis as well as rotation of images. However, artifacts are possible, and these images should be correlated with conventional images.

Endovascular treatment of the aneurysm is often possible during the diagnostic catheter angiography performed emergently in a patient with a subarachnoid hemorrhage (▶ Fig. 4.41a). Whenever possible (depending on the location, the size and shape of the aneurysm, and the size and shape of its neck), the aneurysm is occluded with coils

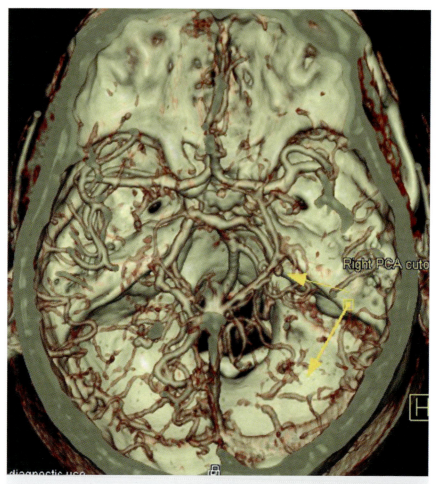

Fig. 4.32 Computed tomographic angiography of the circle of Willis with three-dimensional reconstruction. The right posterior cerebral artery is occluded (*arrows*).

brought via the catheter used to perform the angiography. The coils promote thrombosis of the aneurysm sac (and therefore prevent rebleeding) and reduce the mass effect of the aneurysm.

The coils are made of platinum and are seen on plain X-ray (▶ Fig. 4.41b). They produce artifact on CT or MRI scans, making subsequent noninvasive imaging of the brain and of the aneurysm difficult. It is thus usually necessary to obtain repeat catheter angiograms to image the intracranial vasculature in patients with a coiled aneurysm.

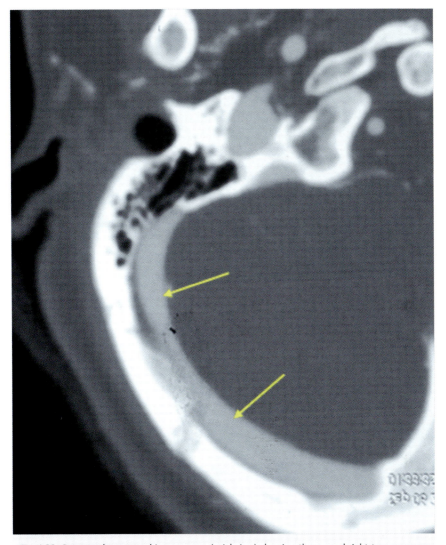

Fig. 4.33 Computed tomographic venogram (axial view) showing the normal right transverse sinus (*arrows*).

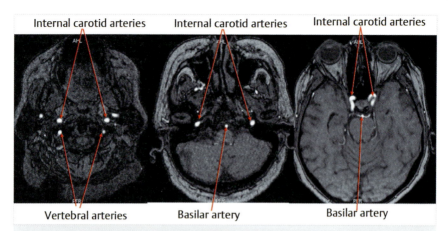

Fig. 4.34 Source images of the magnetic resonance angiogram at three different levels, showing the normal intracranial vessels.

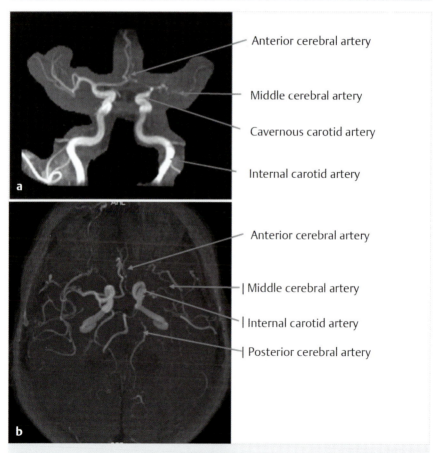

Fig. 4.35 Reconstruction magnetic resonance angiogram of the circle of Willis. (a) View from the front. (b) View from above.

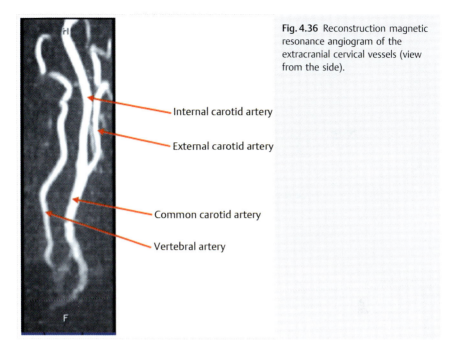

Internal carotid artery

External carotid artery

Common carotid artery

Vertebral artery

Fig. 4.36 Reconstruction magnetic resonance angiogram of the extracranial cervical vessels (view from the side).

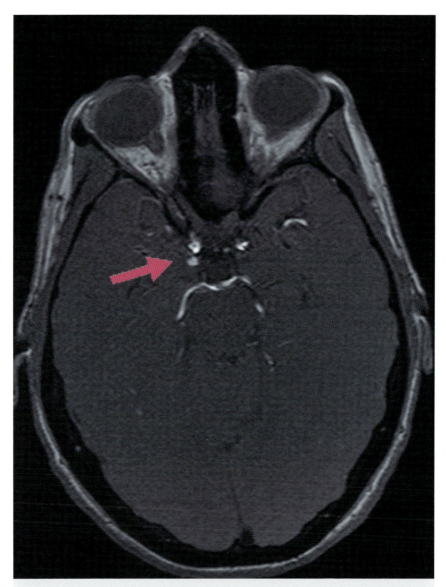

Fig. 4.37 Source image of a head magnetic resonance angiogram (MRA) showing a right posterior communicating aneurysm in a patient with a painful right third nerve palsy (*arrow*). The reconstruction MRA of the circle of Willis failed to show this small aneurysm.

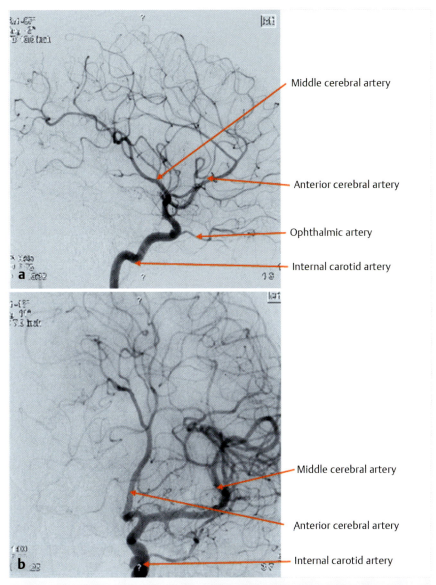

Fig. 4.38 Anterior circulation as seen with selective catheterization of the carotid artery during catheter angiogram. (a) Lateral view. (b) Anterior view.

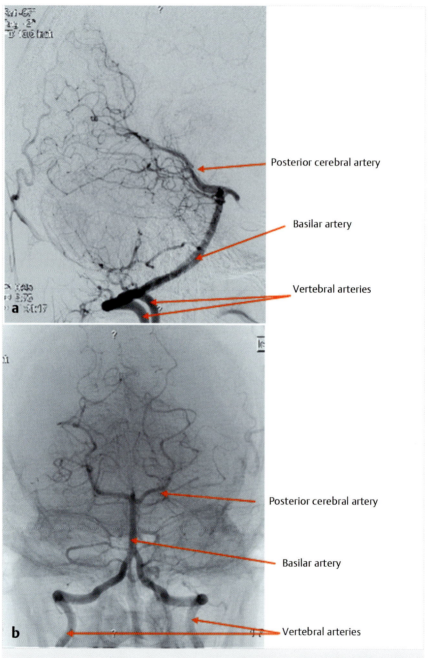

Fig. 4.39 Posterior circulation as seen with selective catheterization of a vertebral artery during catheter angiogram. (a) Lateral view. (b) Anterior view.

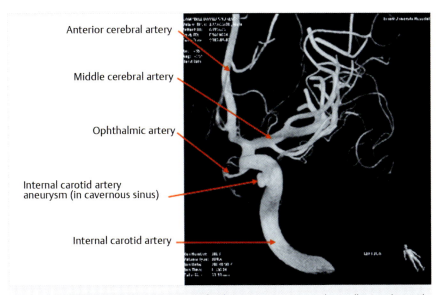

Anterior cerebral artery

Middle cerebral artery

Ophthalmic artery

Internal carotid artery
aneurysm (in cavernous sinus)

Internal carotid artery

Fig. 4.40 Three-dimensional reconstruction of catheter angiogram. Note the small internal carotid aneurysm at the level of the cavernous sinus.

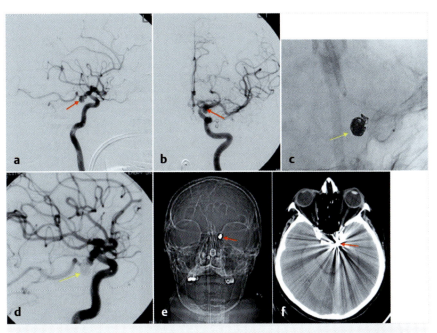

Fig. 4.41 (a–d) Catheter angiogram in a patient presenting with a left third nerve palsy, who developed a subarachnoid hemorrhage a few hours later. There is a large aneurysm at the level of the left posterior communicating artery (*red arrows*). The aneurysm was occluded with coils (*yellow arrows*). Coil seen on a plain X-ray (e) and on a head computed tomographic (CT) scan (f). Note the artifacts seen on the CT scan.

111

5 Visual Loss: An Overview

Transient or permanent visual loss is a common complaint and may result from an ocular disorder, an optic neuropathy, or a lesion involving the intracranial visual pathways. The visual pathways (▶ Fig. 5.1) represent one third of the supratentorial brain mass and are frequently affected by structural lesions and a wide range of neurologic disorders.

This chapter gives a brief review of the approach to the patient with visual loss, then provides an overview of the many causes of monocular and binocular visual loss.

5.1 Approach to the Patient with Visual Loss

The most important part of the history, when evaluating a patient with visual loss, is to establish whether the visual loss is monocular or binocular. Monocular visual loss results from lesions anterior to the chiasm (i.e., the eye itself or the optic nerve), whereas binocular visual loss results from either bilateral anterior lesions or chiasmal or retrochiasmal lesions.

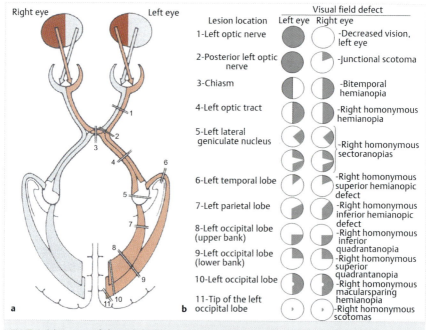

Fig. 5.1 (a) Lesions of the visual pathways. (Adapted from Rohkamm R. Color Atlas of Neurology. New York, NY: Thieme; 2004:81.) (b) Types of visual field defects secondary to lesions along the visual pathways. Note that the visual pathways (a) are shown with the right eye on the left and the left eye on the right (similar to a computed tomographic or magnetic resonance imaging scan); the visual field defects (b) are by convention shown with the right eye on the right and the left eye on the left.

Clinical examination allows for anatomical localization of the lesion and determination of the mechanism of visual loss. Further workup looks for a specific cause.

Evaluation of the patient with visual loss also involves determining whether the loss is transient or permanent, acute or progressive. Identification of any associated symptoms, such as ocular pain, red eye, proptosis, chemosis, diplopia, and headache, as well as neurologic symptoms and elevated blood pressure, is essential.

Pearls

- If visual acuity can be improved by the patient looking through a pinhole, the problem is refractive or ocular, not neurologic in origin.
- Reduction in the saturation or brightness of colors may be an early sign of optic nerve disease.
- A relative afferent pupillary defect (RAPD) ipsilateral to visual loss indicates an optic neuropathy or severe retinal disease (in which case the retina looks abnormal on funduscopic examination). Ocular disease, such as corneal abnormalities, cataracts, and most retinal disorders, do not cause RAPDs.
- If nonorganic visual loss is suspected, stereovision should be tested first: normal stereovision implies 20/20 visual acuity in both eyes.
- A positive response to the optokinetic nystagmus stimulus indicates a visual acuity of at least 20/400 in the eye tested.

5.2 Monocular Visual Loss

Monocular visual loss always results from lesions anterior to the chiasm (the eye or the optic nerve). Transient or permanent monocular visual loss may result from various mechanisms. Those resulting from disorders of the eye itself are usually easily diagnosed by the ophthalmologist. Optic neuropathies and some retinal and ocular vascular disorders that cause monocular visual loss may present to the neurologist.

Any lesion involving the eye (▶ Fig. 5.2) or optic nerve may produce monocular visual loss, including the following:
- Refractive errors
- Corneal diseases
- Anterior chamber inflammation (anterior uveitis)
- Anterior chamber hemorrhage (hyphema)
- Lens opacities (cataract), dislocation
- Vitreous hemorrhage
- Vitreous inflammation (posterior uveitis)
- Retinal diseases
- Choroidal diseases
- Optic neuropathies

5.2.1 Causes of Transient Monocular Visual Loss

Numerous ocular disorders as well as transient ocular ischemia may produce episodes of transient monocular visual loss (TMVL) (see Chapter 6).

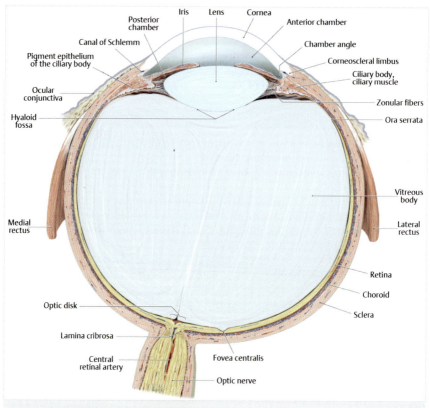

Fig. 5.2 Anatomy of the eye. (From Schuenke M, Schulte E, Schumacher U, Ross LM, Lamperti ED, Voll M. THIEME Atlas of Anatomy, Head and Neuroanatomy. Stuttgart, Germany: Thieme; 2007. Illustration by Karl Wesker.)

There are three main causes of TMVL: vascular disorders, ocular diseases, and optic nerve disorders:

- The most common vascular disorder of the eye is sometimes referred to as amaurosis fugax, the temporary loss of vision of one eye caused by decreased blood flow (ischemia) to the retina.
- Orbital (ophthalmic artery), retinal (central retinal artery and its branches), optic nerve (short posterior ciliary arteries), and choroidal (posterior ciliary arteries) ischemia can all produce TMVL.
- Ocular diseases involving the anterior segment of the eye that can cause TMVL include dry eyes, keratoconus, hyphema, and angle closure glaucoma. Retinal detachment can also rarely produce transient visual loss.
- Optic nerve disorders that can cause TMVL include papilledema, optic disc drusen, and congenitally anomalous optic discs, all of which can produce transient visual obscurations. Gaze-evoked transient monocular visual loss can be the result of optic nerve compression. The Uhthoff phenomenon occurs in patients with optic neuropathies, (especially of demyelinating etiology), whose vision may worsen with heat or exercise.

5.2.2 Ocular Causes of Permanent Monocular Visual Loss

In cases of permanent visual loss, the ocular examination usually allows direct visualization of the cause of visual loss. It is when the eye itself appears normal, or when the optic nerve is not normal, that a neuro-ophthalmic disorder is suspected.

Permanent visual loss may result from disorders involving the anterior segment of the eye (seen with a penlight or direct ophthalmoscope at bedside, or with a slit lamp) or from disorders involving the posterior segment of the eye (seen with a direct ophthalmoscope, with a slit lamp, or with an indirect ophthalmoscope).

▶ Fig. 5.3, ▶ Fig. 5.4, ▶ Fig. 5.5, ▶ Fig. 5.6, ▶ Fig. 5.7, and ▶ Fig. 5.8 show examples of anterior segment disorders presenting with acute or chronic visual loss.

Funduscopic examination is essential in patients with visual loss (see Chapter 2). Optic neuropathies and retinal disorders involving the macula are common causes of central visual loss in patients with clear ocular media. Neurologists need to be able to reliably examine the optic nerve and the macula, which can be done with a direct ophthalmoscope at the bedside (▶ Fig. 5.9). Ophthalmologists use the slit lamp and lenses of various powers to visualize the optic nerve and macula (posterior pole) and an indirect ophthalmoscope to examine the entire retina and its vasculature. The slit lamp and the indirect ophthalmoscope require more practice than the direct ophthalmoscope and are only rarely used by neurologists. These techniques allow stereo views of the fundus and therefore better appreciation of optic nerve elevation, cupping, and contour, as well as macular thickness and edema.

The red reflex is the first step of the funduscopic examination (▶ Fig. 5.10; see Chapter 2) and is used to screen for opacities or irregularities in the cornea, lens, or vitreous. An abnormal red reflex suggests a problem with the ocular media or severe retinal disease involving the posterior pole (▶ Fig. 5.11). Patients with optic neuropathies have

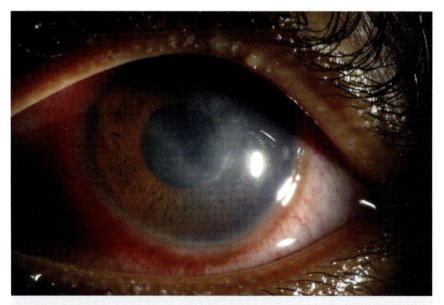

Fig. 5.3 Infectious keratitis. Visual loss with pain and ocular redness from infectious keratitis and conjunctivitis. Illumination of the eye shows conjunctival hyperemia with discharge and hazy cornea.

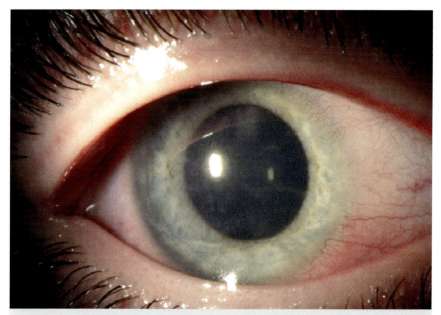

Fig. 5.4 Acanthamoeba keratitis. Visual loss with severe pain and ocular redness from infectious keratitis related to acanthamoeba infection. The infection is a classic complication of contact lens wear. Illumination of the eye shows mild conjunctival hyperemia and hazy cornea.

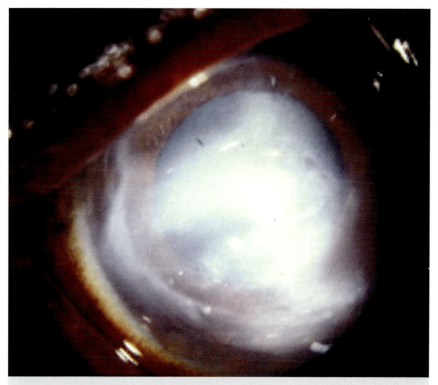

Fig. 5.5 Corneal ulcer. Severe visual loss with pain and ocular redness secondary to infectious corneal ulcer. The cornea is opaque.

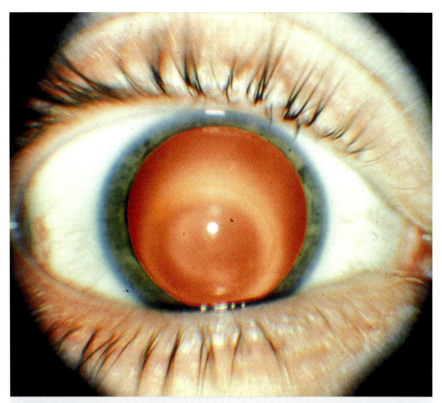

Fig. 5.6 Keratoconus. Chronic, painless visual loss. Examination of the red reflex (focus on the cornea) shows an abnormal reflection with a conical deformation of the cornea.

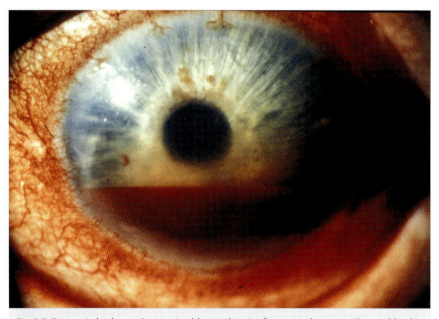

Fig. 5.7 Traumatic hyphema. Severe visual loss with pain after an ocular injury. There is blood in the anterior chamber (hyphema).

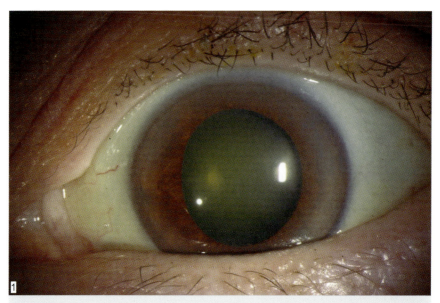

Fig. 5.8 Cataract (nuclear sclerosis). Progressive, painless visual loss secondary to a cataract. The lens is yellow and opaque. The eye is quiet (no redness).

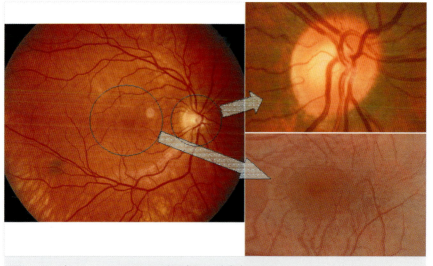

Fig. 5.9 Funduscopic examination with a direct ophthalmoscope in neuro-ophthalmology focuses on the optic nerve (*short arrow*) and the macula (*long arrow*).

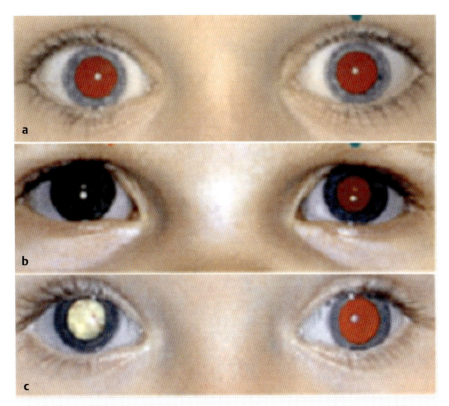

Fig. 5.10 Examples of red reflexes. (a) Normal and symmetric red reflex; (b) absence of right red reflex from a right retinal detachment; (c) and right leukocoria from a retinoblastoma.

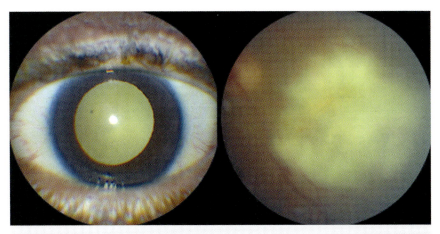

Fig. 5.11 Abnormal red reflex from vitritis related to infectious retinitis (toxoplasmosis).

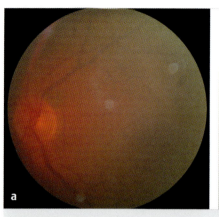
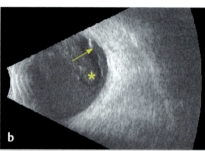

Fig. 5.12 (a) Hazy view of the fundus related to a vitreous hemorrhage. (b) B-scan ultrasound confirms the vitreous hemorrhage (*) and demonstrates a retinal tear (*arrow*).

a normal red reflex. When the red reflex is abnormal and the fundus cannot be visualized (hazy or no view), then a media opacity is obstructing the view (▶ Fig. 5.12a), and B-scan ultrasonography of the eye is helpful in this setting as it may provide an explanation for the media opacity and allow examination of the retina to see if it is attached or not and if there is a retinal tear (▶ Fig. 5.12b) (see Chapter 4).

Pearls

- Use the red reflex (with the ophthalmoscope) to look for media opacities or to screen for visual abnormalities in young children.
- A normal red reflex indicates transparent ocular media (see ▶ Fig. 5.10).
- An asymmetric red reflex indicates a problem with the ocular media, a retinal disorder, high refractive error, or ocular misalignment (strabismus). Checking for asymmetry of the red reflex is therefore a good way to screen young children for ocular disorders and amblyopia.
- A white reflex (also called leukocoria) suggests that something "white" is in the way. Retinoblastoma, congenital cataract, and retrolental fibroplasia are the most important causes of leukocoria in children.

▶ Fig. 5.13 provides an anatomical approach to the patient with monocular visual loss.

5.2.3 Retinal Masqueraders of Optic Neuropathies

Retinal disorders involving the inner retinal layers (i.e., near the vitreous), such as central retinal artery occlusion, are usually easily identified on funduscopic examination (see Chapter 7).

When the outer retina (deeper layers of the retina, including the photoreceptors and the underlying retinal pigment epithelium; ▶ Fig. 5.14) is affected, the fundus is often normal initially.

Some retinal disorders, especially those involving the macula and the outer layers of the retina, can mimic a unilateral or bilateral optic neuropathy. The absence of a RAPD

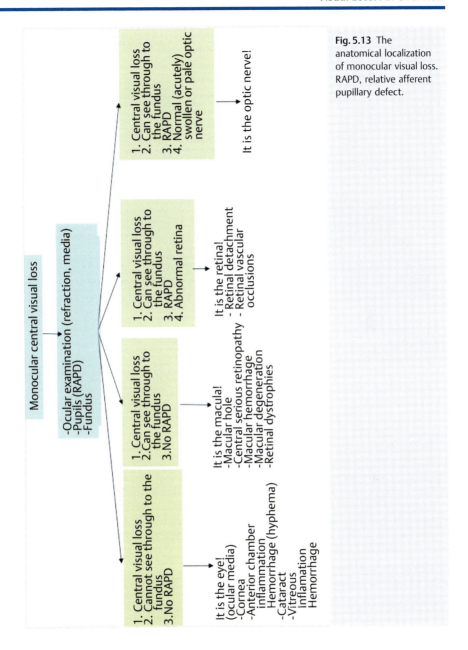

Fig. 5.13 The anatomical localization of monocular visual loss. RAPD, relative afferent pupillary defect.

should lead the examiner to suspect a problem removed from the optic nerve in cases of unilateral or asymmetric visual loss (▶ Table 5.1).

In general, maculopathies produce visible fundus abnormalities that allow a correct diagnosis. However, they may be missed, subtle, or absent. Fluorescein angiography, optical coherence tomography (OCT), and electroretinogram (especially multifocal electroretinogram) can be very helpful in this setting (see Chapter 4).

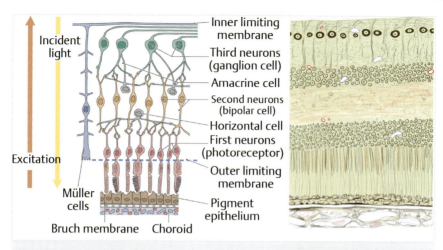

Fig. 5.14 Representations of the inner and outer retina. (From Schuenke M, Schulte E, Schumacher U, Ross LM, Lamperti ED, Voll M. THIEME Atlas of Anatomy, Head and Neuroanatomy. Stuttgart, Germany: Thieme; 2007. Illustration by Karl Wesker.)

Examples of retinal disorders that may mimic optic neuropathies are central serous retinopathy, macular degeneration, macular hole, cystoid macular edema, and acquired enlargement of the physiologic blind spot.

Central serous retinopathy is common, particularly in young men (▶ Fig. 5.15). In this condition, fluid accumulates in the macular subretinal space and produces central visual loss. Visual loss is acute, painless, and associated with metamorphopsia and a central scotoma. OCT (▶ Fig. 5.15c) and fluorescein angiography have a characteristic appearance and will confirm the diagnosis.

Macular degeneration is common in elderly patients. It is bilateral, progressive, and associated with macular drusen (yellow-white deposits with irregular borders—different from the drusen found in optic nerves) and retinal pigment epithelium (RPE) changes (hypo- or hyperpigmentation) (dry age-related macular degeneration) (▶ Fig. 5.16). Progressive deterioration of the deeper retinal layers and RPE may result in serous retinal detachment, RPE detachment, or subretinal neovascularization with hemorrhage and fibrosis (wet age-related macular degeneration), which are best identified with OCT and fluorescein angiography.

Table 5.1 Clinical characteristics of macular and optic nerve lesions

Characteristics	Macular lesions	Optic nerve lesions
Reduced central acuity	Yes	Yes
Metamorphopsias	Yes	No
Photostress test	Long recovery	Normal recovery
Central scotoma	Yes	Yes
Reduced color vision	Moderate	Often severe
Pain	No	Yes if inflammatory
RAPD	No	Yes

Abbreviation: RAPD, relative afferent pupillary defect.

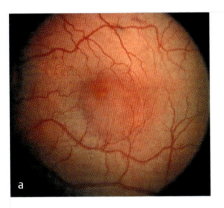
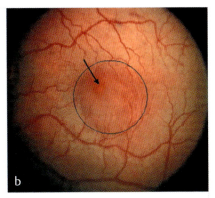
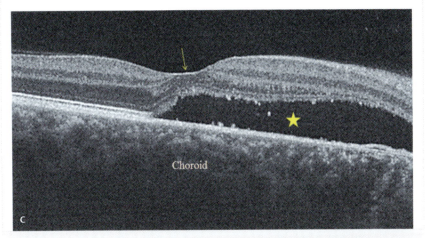

Fig. 5.15 (a) Central serous retinopathy in the left eye. (b) The macula is elevated like a blister. (c) Optical coherence tomography (OCT) of the macula shows the blister (*star*), which elevates and distorts the fovea (*arrow*).

A macular hole is a hole in the center of the macula overlying the foveola and responsible for central visual loss (▶ Fig. 5.17). It is secondary to vitreoretinal traction and occurs most often in elderly patients or after ocular trauma.

Cystoid macular edema (CME) occurs mostly in ocular inflammation and after cataract surgery (▶ Fig. 5.18a). It results from perifoveal capillary leakage. There is thickening of the macular region by edema. OCT and fluorescein angiography are often obtained to confirm CME (▶ Fig. 5.18b).

Acquired enlargement of the physiologic blind spot, both symptomatic and asymptomatic, is usually the result of swelling of the optic nerve head. Occasionally, however, blind spot enlargement may occur with a normal-appearing optic nerve in the setting of outer retinal dysfunction, the so-called acute idiopathic blind spot enlargement (AIBSE) syndrome (part of the group of disorders included in acute zonal occult outer retinopathy [AZOOR]).

AIBSE (▶ Fig. 5.19) is characterized by sudden onset of enlargement of the physiologic blind spot (the patient is aware of a monocular scotoma temporally) and photopsias in the scotomatous field. It affects mostly women between the ages of 20

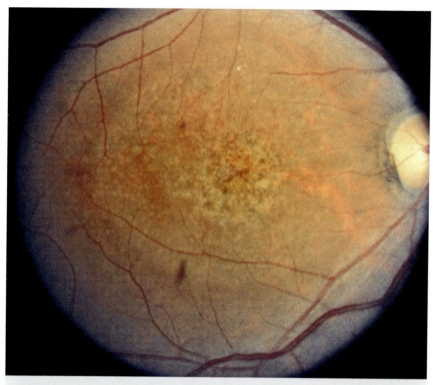

Fig. 5.16 Age-related macular degeneration (dry) with macular drusen and retinal pigment epithelium changes involving the entire macula.

and 40 years. Visual acuity and color vision are typically spared, and there may or may not be a RAPD (present < 50% of the time). Ophthalmoscopy and fluorescein angiography are often normal. However, subtle grayish discoloration of the peripapillary retina (around the disc) may be seen over time. The electroretinogram is often abnormal. AIBSE generally resolves over several weeks or months but occasionally will recur in the same or opposite eye.

5.2.4 Amblyopia

In cases of unexplained monocular visual loss, previously unrecognized amblyopia must be considered.

Amblyopia is defined as reduction of best corrected central visual acuity in the absence of a visible organic lesion corresponding to the degree of visual loss. It will have been present since early childhood and represents the normal brain "not listening" as well to one of the two different afferent inputs.

Causes of amblyopia include the following:
- Uncorrected anisometropia (a difference in refractive error between the two eyes)
- Uncorrected astigmatism
- Strabismus (misalignment of the two eyes, resulting in suppression of one eye's vision)
- Ocular occlusion (e.g., from congenital ptosis)

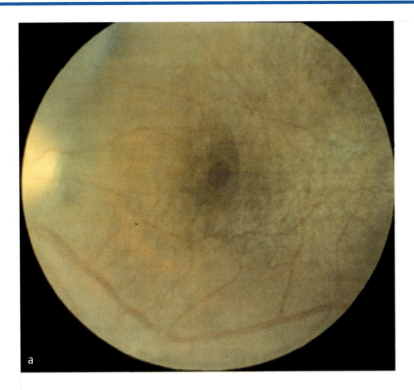

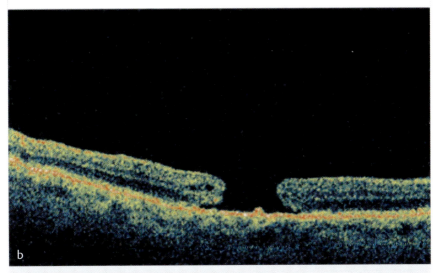

Fig. 5.17 (a) Macular hole in the left eye. (b) Optical coherence tomography (OCT) showing a full-thickness macular hole.

125

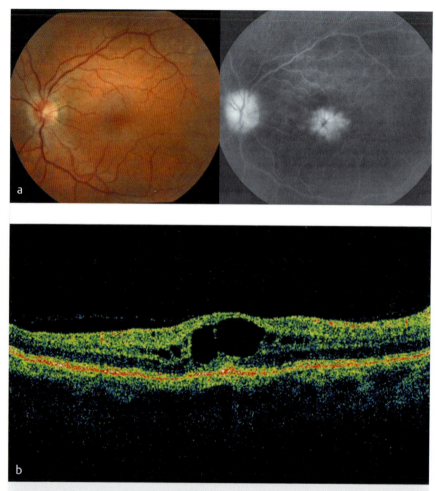

Fig. 5.18 (a) Cystoid macular edema (CME) in the left eye. Note the thickening of the macular region with dull foveal reflex (shown on left). The fluorescein angiogram (shown on right) shows the characteristic petalloid appearance of CME. **(b)** Optical coherence tomography (OCT) showing cysts within the macula.

Consider amblyopia in a patient with unexplained monocular visual loss with normal ocular appearance and a history of uncorrected refractive error, "lazy eye," strabismus surgery, or patching during childhood; improvement of visual acuity with testing of isolated letters (crowding phenomenon); no or small RAPD (0.3–0.6 log unit at most); and a normal visual field (or mild generalized depression).

5.3 Binocular Visual Loss

Binocular visual loss results from lesions of both eyes, of both optic nerves, or of the chiasm or retrochiasmal visual pathways (▶ Fig. 5.20; see also Chapter 3).

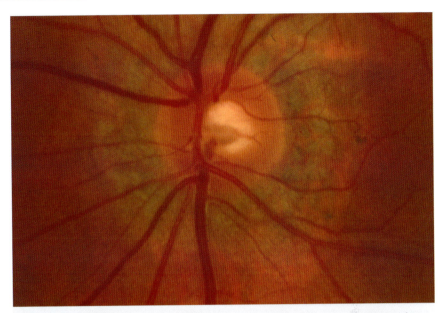

Fig. 5.19 Peripapillary changes in a patient with acute idiopathic blind spot enlargement. The patient complained of photopsias in the left eye and noticed enlargement of the blind spot.

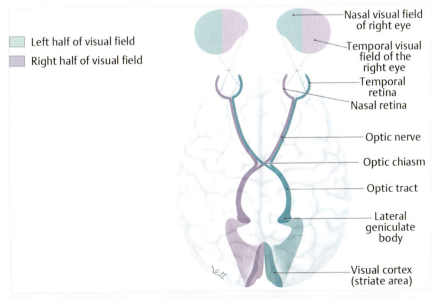

Left half of visual field

Right half of visual field

Nasal visual field of right eye

Temporal visual field of the right eye

Temporal retina

Nasal retina

Optic nerve

Optic chiasm

Optic tract

Lateral geniculate body

Visual cortex (striate area)

Fig. 5.20 Anatomy of the intracranial visual pathways. (From Schuenke M, Schulte E, Schumacher U, Ross LM, Lamperti ED, Voll M. THIEME Atlas of Anatomy, Head and Neuroanatomy. Stuttgart, Germany: Thieme; 2007. Illustration by Markus Voll.)

Acute lesions involving both eyes, or both optic nerves, simultaneously are very rare. Any lesion involving the chiasm or the intracranial visual pathways will produce binocular visual loss or visual field defects, including lesions of the optic tract, lateral geniculate body, optic radiations, and occipital lobe.

Pearl

Lesions involving one side of the intracranial visual pathways produce a contralateral homonymous hemianopia, but the visual acuity is not affected. Lesions involving both occipital lobes may be responsible for severely decreased visual acuity in both eyes; the amount of visual acuity loss is symmetric in both eyes unless there is a superimposed ocular reason for decreased visual acuity.

5.3.1 Bilateral Retinopathies Relevant to Neuro-ophthalmologists

Bilateral retinal disorders may be difficult to distinguish from bilateral symmetric primary optic neuropathies because a RAPD will also be absent. There is a group of retinal disorders, commonly designated retinal degenerations or dystrophies, in which secondary optic disc pallor occurs bilaterally. Arterial attenuation is common in these retinal disorders. Macular changes may be delayed, and the diagnosis may be difficult without electroretinography. Fundus autofluorescence photography of the macula is often helpful to demonstrate early macular changes (see ▶ Fig. 4.5; ▶ Fig. 5.21).

These retinopathies include the following:
- Vitamin A deficiency retinopathy
- Toxic retinopathies (e.g., hydroxychloroquine) (see ▶ Fig. 5.21)
- Carcinoma- and melanoma-associated paraneoplastic retinopathies
- Retinal dystrophies (especially cone dystrophies)

Cone dystrophies are characterized by bilateral loss of central vision (visual acuities typically slowly deteriorate to the 20/200 to 20/400 level) (▶ Fig. 5.22 and ▶ Fig. 5.23), profound color vision deficits, photophobia, and an inability to see as well in bright as in dim light (hemeralopia), a relatively normal-appearing fundus examination except for bilateral temporal disc pallor, and retinal arterial attenuation. Changes in the appearance of the macula, often resembling a bull's-eye, can be delayed. Cone dystrophies are usually sporadic, although inherited forms have been reported.

Electroretinogram is diagnostic in these disorders. When anomalies are limited to the macula, a full-field electroretinogram may be normal, whereas a multifocal electroretinogram is diagnostic.

Paraneoplastic retinopathies (cancer-associated retinopathy [CAR] and melanoma- associated retinopathy [MAR]) follow a more rapid course than the other degenerative retinopathies (▶ Fig. 5.24). CAR may cause early central or paracentral loss of vision. However, initial presentation is often that of bilateral visual loss with minimal or no funduscopic findings. The electroretinogram confirms the retinopathy. Serum antibodies (CAR antibodies) and discovery of a primary neoplasm confirm the diagnosis.

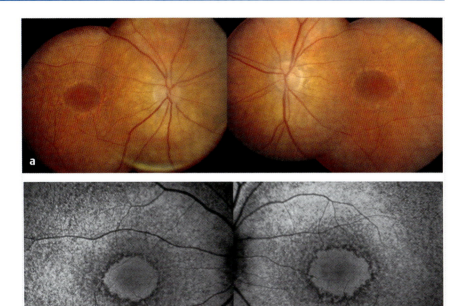

Fig. 5.21 **a–d** Bilateral bull's eye maculopathy from hydroxychloroquine toxicity. (**a**) Bilateral macular changes with a ring of increased pigment surrounding the central fovea. (**b**) Fundus autofluorescence imaging showing an increase in signal in the parafoveal region of both eyes. (*continued*)

5.3.2 Causes of Transient or Permanent Binocular Visual Loss

Causes of transient or permanent binocular visual loss from retrochiasmal lesions are as follows:

- Vascular
  - Vertebrobasilar ischemia (posterior cerebral artery territory)
  - Cerebral anoxia
  - Cerebral venous thrombosis (superior sagittal sinus)
  - Hypertensive encephalopathy
  - Malignant systemic hypertension (▶ Fig. 5.25)
  - Eclampsia
- Head trauma
- Occipital mass (e.g., tumor, abscess, or hemorrhage)
- Demyelinating disease
- Infection
  - Occipital abscess
  - Meningitis

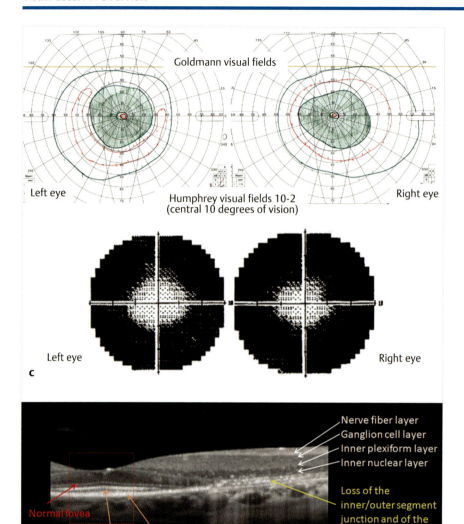

Fig. 5.21 (*continued*) (**c**) Visual field tests (Goldmann visual field test above and central 10–2 Swedish Interactive Thresholding Algorithm (SITA) standard test below) showing a ring scotoma in both eyes. (**d**) Spectral optical coherence tomography (OCT) of the macula demonstrates loss of the inner/outer segment junction and thinning of the outer retina in the parafoveal region, with preservation of these structures in the fovea, highly suggestive of hydroxychloroquine toxicity.

- ○ Progressive multifocal leukoencephalopathy
- ○ Creutzfeldt–Jakob disease
- • Central nervous system toxicity
  - ○ Cyclosporine
  - ○ Tacrolimus (FK-506)
  - ○ Mercury

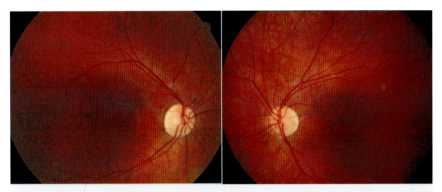

Fig. 5.22 Bilateral optic nerve pallor and retinal arterial attenuation in a patient with cone dystrophy. Macular changes are subtle at this stage. Visual acuity and color vision are reduced bilaterally. There is no relative afferent pupillary defect.

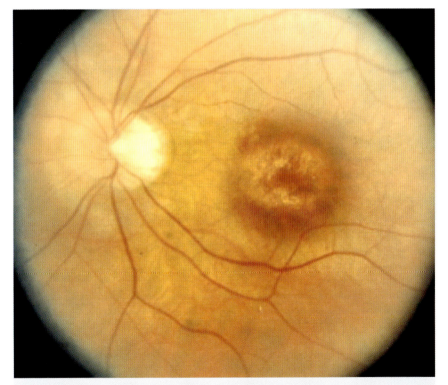

Fig. 5.23 Macular changes typical of bull's-eye maculopathy in a patient with cone dystrophy. The nerve is pale temporally.

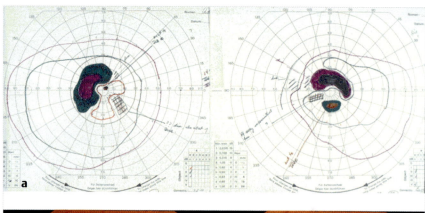

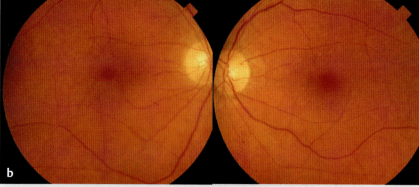

Fig. 5.24 Paraneoplastic retinopathy with cancer-associated retinopathy antibodies in a patient with malignant thymoma. (**a**) Goldmann visual field showing bilateral ring scotomas. (**b**) The fundus shows attenuated arteries. The electroretinogram was abnormal.

- Metabolic
  - Hypoglycemia
  - Porphyria
  - Hepatic encephalopathy
- Migraine (visual aura)
- Occipital lobe seizures
- Degenerative
  - Alzheimer disease
  - Posterior cortical atrophy

Reversible posterior leukoencephalopathy most often results from malignant systemic hypertension, eclampsia, or central nervous system toxicity from cyclosporine or tacrolimus.

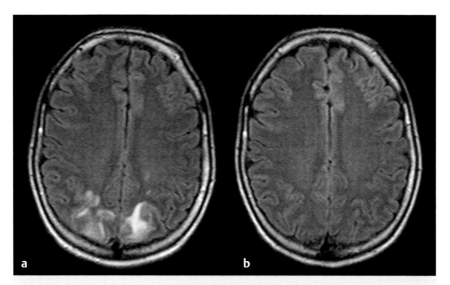

Fig. 5.25 (a) Axial fluid-attenuated inversion recovery (FLAIR) magnetic resonance imaging (MRI) showing bi-occipital lesions from malignant hypertension. The patient experienced acute bilateral visual loss with headaches and confusion. (b) Two weeks after normalization of the blood pressure, the visual function is normal, and the MRI changes have resolved.

6 Transient Visual Loss

It is sometimes difficult to decide whether an episode of transient visual loss occurred in one eye (monocular) or both (binocular). Very few patients realize that binocular hemifield (homonymous) visual field loss affects the fields of both eyes. They will usually localize it to the eye that lost its temporal field. The best clues to the fact that transient visual loss was actually binocular are reading impairment (monocular visual loss does not impair reading unless the unaffected eye had prior vision impairment) and visual loss confined to a lateral hemifield, that is, to the right or left of midline with respect to the vertical meridian (monocular visual loss does not usually cause that pattern of visual loss).

This chapter complements the overview of visual loss given in Chapter 5 and provides differential diagnoses and suggested management for transient monocular and binocular visual loss.

> **Pearls**
>
> The most important step in evaluating a patient with transient visual loss is to establish whether or not the visual loss is *monocular* (lesions of the eye or anterior visual pathways) or *binocular* (lesions of the chiasm or retrochiasmal visual pathways).

6.1 Transient Binocular Visual Loss

6.1.1 Differential Diagnosis

Migrainous Visual Aura

Visual aura associated with migraine is the most common cause of transient binocular visual loss (▶ Fig. 6.1). The patient typically notes a small scotoma in homonymous portions of the visual field, surrounded by jagged, luminous, shimmering edges. The scotoma enlarges over several minutes, then gradually disappears. The visual loss may enlarge to a complete homonymous hemianopia. A hemicranial throbbing headache characteristically follows (see Chapter 19).

Some patients experience the visual aura of migraine without associated headache. The vision and visual fields return to normal after the aura, usually within 20 to 30 minutes (always less than 1 hour).

> **Pearls**
>
> Although migrainous visual aura is binocular by definition (since it originates from the occipital lobe), many patients do not recognize the visual phenomena as being in both eyes, especially when they involve only one hemifield. The relatively long duration of visual phenomena, the progressive buildup of symptoms ("migrainous march"), and the richness of visual phenomena strongly suggest migrainous visual auras, even when the patient thinks the visual symptoms were only in one eye.

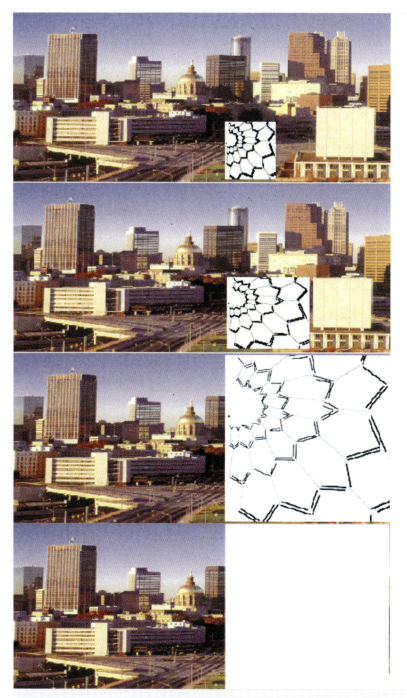

Fig. 6.1 Progression of visual changes during migrainous visual aura (from top to bottom).

Occipital Transient Ischemic Attack

In older patients, episodes of transient, complete binocular visual loss may represent a transient ischemic attack (TIA) in the distribution of the basilar artery or of the posterior cerebral arteries. A unilateral occipital TIA manifests as a transient homonymous hemianopia.

As opposed to migraine, hemianopic events of ischemic origin are typically sudden in onset and last only a few minutes. There may be associated headache, especially over the brow contralateral to the visual field loss, but the pain is usually coincident with the visual loss, rather than following the visual loss as in migraine. TIAs in the anterior circulation produce ipsilateral monocular visual loss, whereas TIAs in the posterior circulation produce binocular visual loss (often contralateral homonymous hemianopia). This is explained by the anatomy of the blood supply to the brain (▶ Fig. 6.2 and ▶ Fig. 6.3).

The internal carotid arteries provide the blood supply to the anterior part of both cerebral hemispheres and to the eyes. The vertebrobasilar system provides the blood

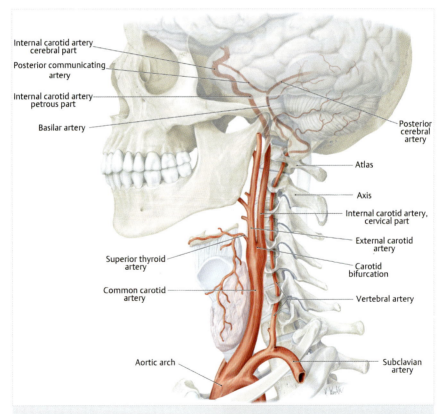

Fig. 6.2 Blood supply of the brain. (From Schuenke M, Schulte E, Schumacher U, Ross LM, Lamperti ED, Voll M. THIEME Atlas of Anatomy, Head and Neuroanatomy. Stuttgart, Germany: Thieme; 2007. Illustration by Karl Wesker.)

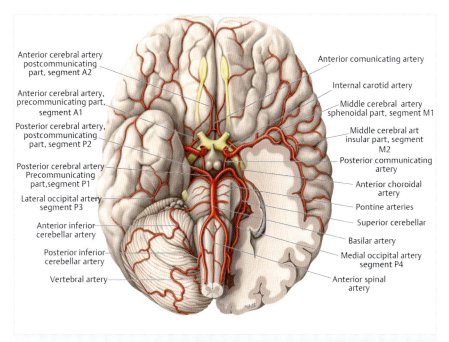

Anterior cerebral artery postcommunicating part, segment A2

Anterior cerebral artery, precommunicating part, segment A1

Posterior cerebral artery, postcommunicating part, segment P2

Posterior cerebral artery Precommunicating part, segment P1

Lateral occipital artery segment P3

Anterior inferior cerebellar artery

Posterior inferior cerebellar artery

Vertebral artery

Anterior comunicating artery

Internal carotid artery

Middle cerebral artery sphenoidal part, segment M1

Middle cerebral art insular part, segment M2

Posterior communicating artery

Anterior choroidal artery

Pontine arteries

Superior cerebellar

Basilar artery

Medial occipital artery segment P4

Anterior spinal artery

Fig. 6.3 Circle of Willis at the skull base. (From Schuenke M, Schulte E, Schumacher U, Ross LM, Lamperti ED, Voll M. THIEME Atlas of Anatomy, Head and Neuroanatomy. Stuttgart, Germany: Thieme; 2007. Illustration by Markus Voll.)

supply to the posterior part of both cerebral hemispheres (including the occipital lobes) and to the posterior fossa (brainstem and cerebellum) (▶ Fig. 6.2).

The occipital lobes are vascularized by the posterior cerebral arteries, which originate from the basilar artery (▶ Fig. 6.3). Basilar artery stenosis or occlusion may result in bilateral occipital ischemia and bilateral complete visual loss (cerebral blindness). Posterior cerebral artery occlusion usually produces unilateral occipital ischemia with contralateral homonymous hemianopia.

Occipital Seizure

Occipital seizures can occur at any age but are more common in children. They may be primary or secondary to an occipital lesion. The patient typically complains of recurrent and brief, simple, positive visual phenomena, such as flashes of light or bubbles. They are binocular and they may be localized to a hemifield or diffuse within the entire field of vision.

▶ Table 6.1 compares the characteristics of migrainous visual aura, occipital TIA, and occipital seizure.

Other less common causes of transient binocular visual loss are head trauma, especially in children; hypertensive encephalopathy; toxemia of pregnancy; and toxicity of drugs, such as cyclosporine, which may result in cerebral blindness lasting hours or days (see ▶ Fig. 5.25).

Table 6.1 Characteristics of the three most common causes of binocular transient visual loss

	Migrainous visual aura	Occipital transient ischemic attack	Occipital seizures
Visual symptoms	Positive; very rich, moving; often black and white, scintillating, shimmering, jagged edges	Negative (hemianopia or blindness)	Positive; simple visual phenomena (phosphenes, bubbles) Colored Ictal blindness
Progression of symptoms	Typical migrainous march, with progression of symptoms over time	Sudden onset and disappearance	Usually not progressive
Duration of visual symptoms	Typically 20 to 30 minutes	A few minutes	Usually brief (seconds) Often repeated
Headache	Migrainous headache typically follows the aura; may be absent	Brow headache possible at the time of visual symptoms	None
Associated symptoms	Headache follows; visual aura may be followed by other migrainous aura (mostly sensory)	Vertebrobasilar ischemia: • Vertigo, dizziness • Imbalance • Diplopia • Bilateral extremity weakness	Often none May be associated with other seizures

6.2 Transient Monocular Visual Loss

Transient monocular visual loss (TMVL) is the preferred term for abrupt and temporary visual loss in one eye. TMVL most often results from transient ocular ischemia (so-called amaurosis fugax;), but it may also result from other mechanisms such as disc edema and numerous ocular diseases. See the discussion in Chapter 5.

6.2.1 Differential Diagnosis

TMVL can be vascular (transient ischemia in the territories of the ophthalmic artery, central retinal artery and its branches, posterior ciliary arteries, or central retinal vein), can be ocular in origin (such as from dry eyes or attacks of angle closure glaucoma), or can result from optic nerve head anomalies.

> **Pearls**
>
> Transient visual obscurations (TVOs) are characterized by brief blackouts or "gray-outs" of vision and are precipitated by changes in posture, such as bending over. They usually indicate underlying optic nerve head edema or optic nerve anomalies causing high tissue pressure at the optic nerve head. Although disc edema results from a variety of disorders, the most likely cause of TVOs is papilledema from raised intracranial pressure.

An orbital mass may produce gaze-evoked episodes of TMVL. The examination may be normal between episodes when the mass is relatively small. Movements of the eye

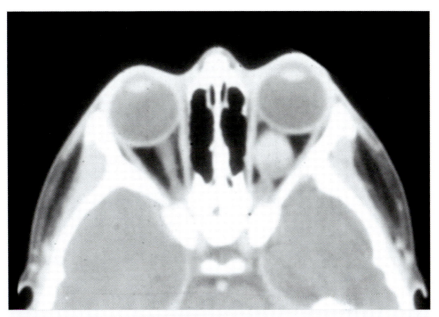

Fig. 6.4 Axial computed tomographic scan of the orbits with contrast showing a mass in the left orbit.

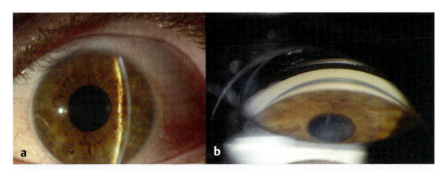

Fig. 6.5 (a) Shallow anterior chamber on slit lamp examination (b) narrow angle on gonioscopy in a patient with recurrent episodes of painful transient monocular visual loss.

result in stretching of the optic nerve and intermittent compression of the nerve or of its blood supply, with resulting transient loss of vision (▶ Fig. 6.4).

Eyes with a narrow anterior chamber angle may have episodes of angle closure glaucoma resolving spontaneously (▶ Fig. 6.5). During such episodes, the intraocular pressure is elevated, and patients complain of painful transient monocular blurry vision with the perception of halos around lights.

Patients with dry eyes often complain of fluctuation of vision, especially while reading.

6.2.2 Patient Evaluation

The clinical history and a detailed ocular examination help determine the mechanism of the TMVL.

Among the first things to ask the patient about are the onset and duration of TMVL. The answers can help determine the cause. For example, retinal emboli produce a very sudden TMVL, lasting from 1 to 4 minutes. TMVL as a result of ocular hypoperfusion would be progressive, at least 5 to 10 minutes, and be precipitated by standing up or looking at bright lights. Venous congestion causes a progressive loss, lasting at least 10 to 20 minutes. TVOs from optic nerve head anomalies are very brief, lasting only a few seconds, and are precipitated by bending over or by Valsalva maneuvers.

Accompanying manifestations helpful in determining the mechanism of TMVL include the following:

- Headache, scalp tenderness, jaw claudication, and diplopia: giant cell arteritis
- Eye or brow pain: intermittent angle closure glaucoma or giant cell arteritis
- Neck pain: cervical carotid artery dissection
- Ipsilateral Horner syndrome: carotid artery dissection
- Simultaneous contralateral hemisensory or motor findings: ipsilateral carotid artery stenosis
- Presyncope: systemic hypotension or a hyperviscosity syndrome
- TMVL when moving the eye: orbital mass
- Blurry vision when reading: dry eyes

The ocular examination can help to rule out local causes of TMVL and detect retinal emboli, retinal ischemia, venous stasis retinopathy, or evidence of optic nerve ischemia.

Eyes with a narrow anterior chamber angle may have episodes of angle closure glaucoma resolving spontaneously (▶ Fig. 6.5). During such episodes, the intraocular pressure is elevated, and patients complain of painful transient monocular blurry vision with the perception of halos around lights.

6.2.3 Vascular TMVL

Vascular TMVL is the most common and perhaps most important ophthalmologic symptom of carotid occlusive disease (see Chapter 20). Patients with vascular TMVL complain of isolated or recurrent episodes of acute, monocular loss of vision that may be partial or complete.

▶ Fig. 6.6 shows the blood supply of the eyes and the orbits. The main blood supply to the eye and orbital contents comes from the ophthalmic artery, a branch of the internal carotid artery (▶ Fig. 6.7). Any vascular disease involving the arteries between the heart and the ophthalmic artery may result in ocular ischemia and visual loss.

The external carotid artery and its branches also contribute to the vascularization of the eye and orbital contents. In cases of internal carotid artery stenosis or occlusion, the entire ocular vascularization may originate from the external carotid artery. In this situation, there may be a steal phenomenon from the eye to the brain, and the flow may be reversed in the ophthalmic artery so that most of the blood flow contributes to the vascularization of the ipsilateral cerebral hemisphere.

Branches of the ophthalmic artery (▶ Fig. 6.8 and ▶ Fig. 6.9) include the central retinal artery to the inner retina; the short posterior ciliary arteries to the choroid and optic nerve; the long posterior ciliary arteries to the ciliary body and iris; and the anterior ciliary arteries, which arise from the vessels of the rectus muscles. Occlusion of

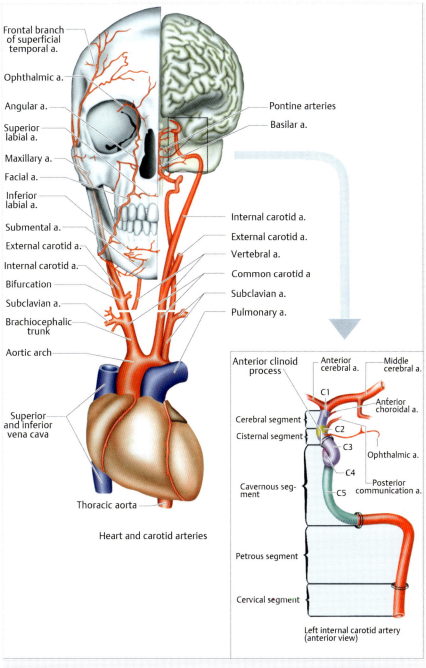

Fig. 6.6 Blood supply of the eyes and orbits. (From Rohkamm R. Color Atlas of Neurology. New York, NY: Thieme; 2004:11. Reprinted by permission.)

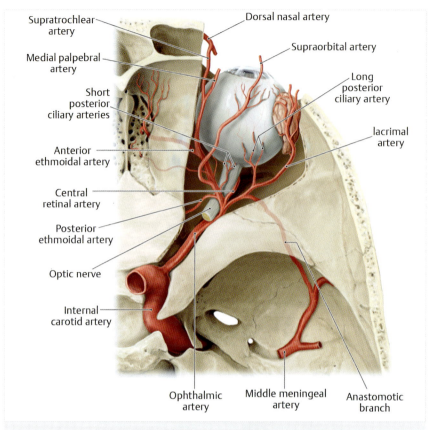

Fig. 6.7 Superior view of the right orbit showing the ophthalmic artery and its branches. (From Schuenke M, Schulte E, Schumacher U, Ross LM, Lamperti ED, Voll M. THIEME Atlas of Anatomy, Head and Neuroanatomy. Stuttgart, Germany: Thieme; 2007. Illustration by Karl Wesker.)

the ophthalmic artery results in complete ocular ischemia, whereas occlusion of the central retinal artery results in retinal ischemia.

Pearls

The external carotid artery is important for collateral circulation for the orbit and for the brain when there is severe occlusive disease of the internal carotid artery (▶ Fig. 6.10 and ▶ Fig. 6.11).

Mechanisms of Vascular TMVL

The mechanisms of vascular TMVL are emboli, hypoperfusion of the eye (hemodynamic TMVL), vasculitis (usually giant cell arteritis), arterial vasospasm (central retinal artery), and venous congestion (central retinal vein).

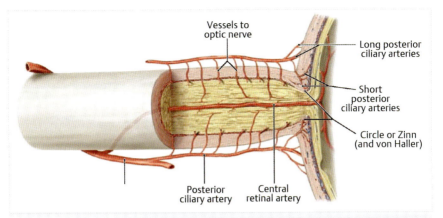

Fig. 6.8 Lateral view of the optic nerve showing the arterial blood supply of the optic nerve. The central retinal artery (first branch of the ophthalmic artery) enters the optic nerve from below about 1 cm behind the eye and courses within it to the retina where it gives off multiple branches. The posterior ciliary arteries give off several small branches that supply the orbital optic nerve. The optic nerve head receives its arterial blood supply from an arterial ring (circle of Zinn) formed by anastomoses among branches from the short posterior ciliary arteries. (From Schuenke M, Schulte E, Schumacher U, Ross LM, Lamperti ED, Voll M. THIEME Atlas of Anatomy, Head and Neuroanatomy. Stuttgart, Germany: Thieme; 2007. Illustration by Karl Wesker.)

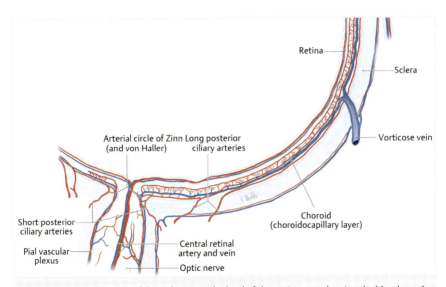

Fig. 6.9 Horizontal section of the right eye at the level of the optic nerve showing the blood supply of the eye. The central retinal artery (for the inner retina) is of relatively large caliber and can be occluded by emboli, which may migrate into its branches (branch retinal arteries). The short posterior ciliary arteries (choroid and optic nerve) are too small to be affected by emboli. (From Schuenke M, Schulte E, Schumacher U, Ross LM, Lamperti ED, Voll M. THIEME Atlas of Anatomy, Head and Neuroanatomy. Stuttgart, Germany: Thieme; 2007. Illustration by Karl Wesker.)

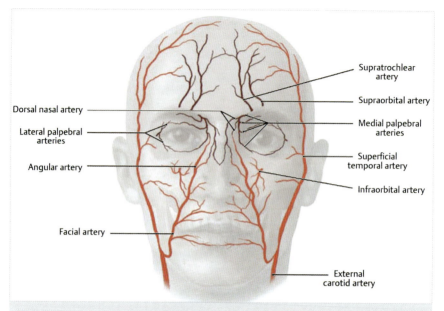

Fig. 6.10 Branches of the external carotid artery. (From Schuenke M, Schulte E, Schumacher U, Ross LM, Lamperti ED, Voll M. THIEME Atlas of Anatomy, Head and Neuroanatomy. Stuttgart, Germany: Thieme; 2007. Illustration by Karl Wesker.)

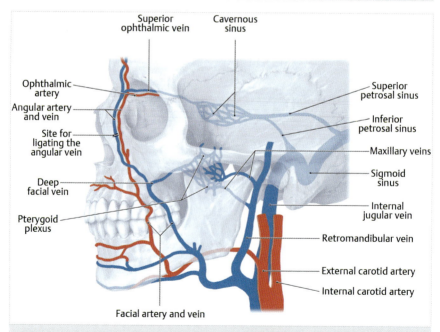

Fig. 6.11 Contribution of the external carotid artery to the blood supply of the orbit. (From Schuenke M, Schulte E, Schumacher U, Ross LM, Lamperti ED, Voll M. THIEME Atlas of Anatomy, Head and Neuroanatomy. Stuttgart, Germany: Thieme; 2007. Illustration by Karl Wesker.)

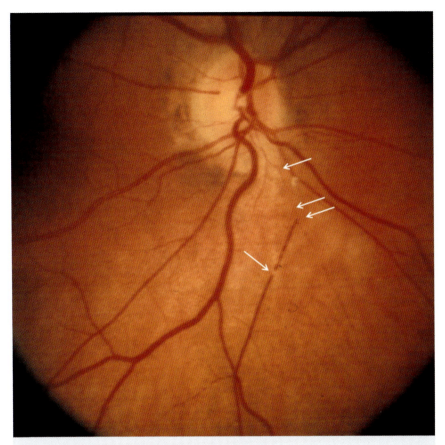

Fig. 6.12 Platelet–fibrin emboli in a retinal artery (*arrows*).

- Emboli into the retinal circulation (▶ Fig. 6.12, ▶ Fig. 6.13, ▶ Fig. 6.14) (central and branch retinal arteries) most often result from lesions of the common or internal carotid arteries that embolize material to the retinal circulation. With emboli, most commonly a black or dark shade spreads across the visual field of the affected eye, disappearing after a few minutes. Occasionally, emboli may be observed ophthalmoscopically as they pass through the retinal arterioles.

Pearls

Emboli (in the central retinal artery or the ophthalmic artery) represent the most common cause of transient or permanent retinal ischemia, which should warrant an immediate workup looking for a source of emboli. Carotid disease is the most common cause of retinal ischemia.

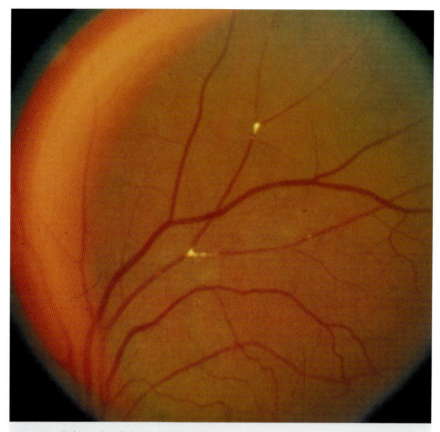

Fig. 6.13 Cholesterol emboli in a retinal artery.

- Hypoperfusion of the eye (▶ Fig. 6.15 and ▶ Fig. 6.16) is seen in severe stenosis of the carotid circulation, which causes TMVL due to retinal or choroidal hypoperfusion. Ocular hypoperfusion may be associated with transient but prolonged visual loss (several minutes to hours) and positive visual phenomena. TMVL is classically induced by situations that either decrease perfusion pressure (e.g., postural change) or increase retinal oxygen demand (e.g., exposure to bright light), or when blood flow is shunted elsewhere systemically (e.g., after eating a meal or during exercise). Venous stasis retinopathy or ischemic ocular syndrome with development of ocular neovascularization may be observed. Revascularization procedures restoring normal ocular perfusion may prevent the development of ocular ischemic syndrome.
- Giant cell arteritis is an important cause of recurrent TMVL in subjects older than age 50. The ocular examination may be normal or may show optic nerve edema, suggesting impending permanent visual loss from arteritic anterior ischemic optic neuropathy. These patients need to be treated with high-dose steroids emergently to prevent permanent visual loss (see Chapter 20).

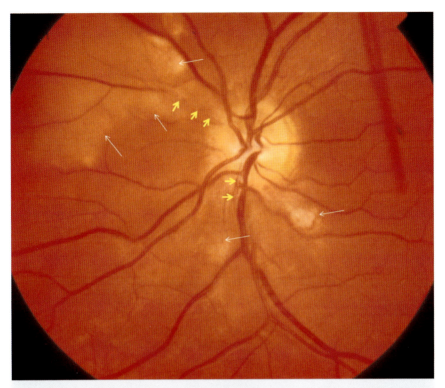

Fig. 6.14 Multiple emboli in retinal arteries (*yellow arrows*) with small retinal infarctions (*white arrows*).

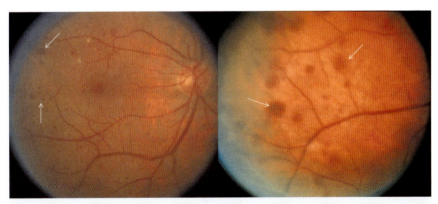

Fig. 6.15 Retinal venous stasis retinopathy from chronic ocular hypoperfusion. Note the multiple dot blot hemorrhages in the midperiphery of the retina (*arrows*).

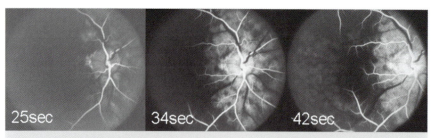

Fig. 6.16 Retinal fluorescein angiography in chronic ocular ischemic syndrome. Choroidal and retinal vascular filling is very delayed because of severe carotid occlusive disease.

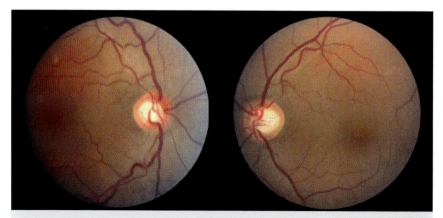

Fig. 6.17 Dilation of the retinal veins in the right eye (left image) secondary to impending central retinal vein occlusion. The patient had recurrent episodes of blurry vision in the right eye, lasting up to 20 minutes. One week later, she developed a central retinal vein occlusion with persistent visual loss. The veins are normal in the left eye (right image).

- Vasospasm of the central retinal artery may produce episodes of isolated, painless, sudden, complete loss of vision in one eye, usually lasting between 30 seconds and 1 minute. Vasospasm most often affects young, healthy people, and its cause is unclear. The prognosis is excellent without subsequent risk of ocular or cerebral infarction. Antiplatelet agents or calcium channel inhibitors are usually prescribed.
- Central retinal vein occlusion (► Fig. 6.17) may be preceded by episodes of transient monocular blurry vision. These episodes last longer than with arterial ischemia, and the visual loss is usually incomplete.

Natural History

The natural history of vascular TMVL varies depending on the age of the patient and on the etiology of the TMVL. Vascular TMVL is clearly a marker of systemic vascular disease and should prompt an immediate evaluation with the help of a stroke neurologist.

Patients with vascular TMVL face a number of risks. Among them are irreversible visual loss (central retinal artery occlusion), which is estimated to be about 1% per year in patients with internal carotid stenosis; and cerebral infarction, whose rate varies depending on the cause of TMVL. TMVL patients and ipsilateral atheromatous internal carotid stenosis $\geq 50\%$ have a risk of infarction of 10% at 3 years, the majority of which occurs within a few days after the episode of TMVL. The risk of cerebral infarction increases with the degree of carotid stenosis. Additionally, the risk of vascular death (myocardial infarction) is estimated to be about 4% per year in patients with TMVL and atheromatous disease.

Patient Evaluation

The patient evaluation varies depending on the clinical presentation and the patient's characteristics (▶ Fig. 6.18). Patients seen on the day of TMVL should be evaluated emergently, and giant cell arteritis should be ruled out in all patients older than age 50.

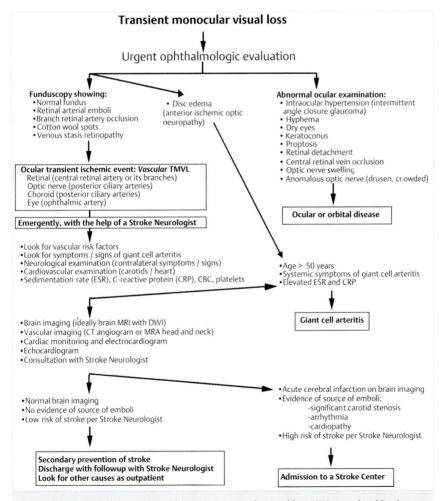

Fig. 6.18 Evaluation of the patient with transient monocular visual loss. CBC, complete blood count; CTA, computed tomographic angiography; DWI, diffusion = weighted imaging; MRA, magnetic resonance angiography; MRI, magnetic resonance imaging; TMVL, transient monocular visual loss.

> **Pearls**
>
> Intermittent choroidal and optic nerve ischemia may produce TMVL in patients with giant cell arteritis. Erythrocyte sedimentation rate (ESR) and C-reactive protein (CRP) should be obtained systematically in all patients older than age 50 with TMVL.

An ocular examination needs to be performed immediately. If a vascular cause is suspected, blood tests including complete blood count, platelets, ESR, and CRP are obtained emergently.

> **Pearls**
>
> Vascular TMVL is a medical emergency similar to cerebral TIAs. The American Heart Association recommends that patients with presumed vascular TMVL undergo the same immediate workup as those with cerebral TIAs, including brain imaging (ideally brain magnetic resonance imaging [MRI] with diffusion-weighted images). It is common to discover asymptomatic cerebral infarctions on brain MRI of patients with isolated TMVL.

6.2.4 Treatment of Transient Monocular Visual Loss

Treatment involves first addressing ocular causes. With vascular TMVL, treatment addresses secondary prevention of ocular and cerebral infarction.

Risk factor management includes the following:

- Blood pressure should be decreased in both hypertensive and nonhypertensive patients.
- Cigarette smoking should be discontinued.
- Coronary artery disease, cardiac arrhythmias, congestive heart failure, and valvular heart disease should be treated appropriately.
- Excessive use of alcohol should be eliminated (limit to one or two drinks a day).
- Treatment of hyperlipidemia is recommended. If a lipid-lowering agent is used, a statin is recommended.
- Fasting blood glucose levels < 126 mg/dL are recommended.
- Physical activity is recommended.
- Long-term antiplatelet agents should be given to every patient who has experienced a noncardioembolic TMVL and has no contraindication (aspirin 50 to 325 mg per day, combination of aspirin 25 mg and extended-release dipyridamole 200 mg twice a day, and clopidogrel 75 mg per day are all acceptable options for initial therapy).
- Long-term anticoagulation (target international normalized ratio: 2.5) should be used for prevention of stroke in patients with atrial fibrillation, with other high-risk cardiac sources of embolism, and in some hypercoagulable states.
- Carotid endarterectomy should be considered shortly after the episode of TMVL in selected high-risk patients who are good surgical candidates with an ipsilateral internal carotid stenosis of 70 to 99%.

7 Retinal Vascular Diseases

Occlusion of the retinal arteries or veins produces retinal ischemia and visual loss. Because the eye and orbit share their blood supply with the brain, retinal vascular disorders are common in neurology.

7.1 Retinal Artery Occlusions

Central retinal and branch retinal artery occlusions produce acute monocular visual loss. Unless the retinal vascular occlusion is secondary to giant cell arteritis or to a carotid dissection, the visual loss is painless.

Permanent visual loss may have been preceded by one or more episodes of transient monocular visual loss.

The visual prognosis is usually poor. These patients are at risk of recurrent ocular or cerebral infarction, and, like patients with cerebral infarctions, they should be evaluated emergently.

7.1.1 Types of Retinal Artery Occlusions

Asymptomatic Cholesterol Retinal Emboli

Asymptomatic retinal emboli (most often cholesterol) are found in 1 to 2% of patients older than age 50 (▶ Fig. 7.1). They should prompt an evaluation for atheromatous vascular risk factors, which need to be aggressively controlled.

Central Retinal Artery Occlusion

Central retinal artery occlusion results in severe monocular visual loss (▶ Fig. 7.2, ▶ Fig. 7.3, ▶ Fig. 7.4). It is associated with retinal edema with a cherry red spot (the fovea appears red by contrast with the surrounding ischemic retina, which is whitish). The retina is very thin at the fovea, and the underlying normally vascularized choroid appears red. The retinal edema develops within a few hours, and the fundus may be almost normal initially. The retinal arteries are usually attenuated, sometimes with emboli. There is a dense relative afferent pupillary defect (RAPD) because the inner retinal layers, including the nerve fiber layer, are affected.

Approximately 30% of patients have a cilioretinal artery, which originates from the posterior ciliary circulation. In cases of central retinal artery occlusion, the retinal territory vascularized by the cilioretinal artery is not affected, and some vision is preserved (▶ Fig. 7.5). If the cilioretinal artery provides the blood supply to the fovea, then the central visual acuity remains good.

Ophthalmic Artery Occlusion

Like central retinal artery occlusion, ophthalmic artery occlusion results in severe monocular visual loss and is associated with a dense RAPD; attenuated retinal arteries, sometimes with emboli; and retinal edema (▶ Fig. 7.6). Unlike central retinal artery occlusion, there is no cherry red spot (the underlying choroid is also ischemic). There is often associated mild disc edema from optic nerve ischemia.

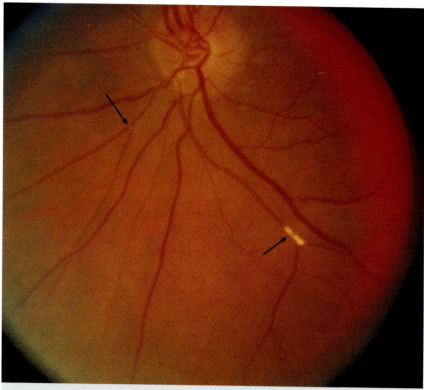

Fig. 7.1 Asymptomatic cholesterol retinal emboli (*arrows*). The emboli are located at arterial bifurcations and are bright.

Ophthalmic artery occlusion is most often related to internal carotid artery disease, with large emboli involving the origin of the ophthalmic artery. Giant cell arteritis should also be considered.

Branch Retinal Artery Occlusion

Branch retinal artery occlusion is characterized by partial monocular visual loss, a moderate RAPD, an attenuated branch retinal artery, usually with one or more emboli, and localized retinal edema (▶ Fig. 7.7, ▶ Fig. 7.8, ▶ Fig. 7.9). There is a corresponding visual field defect (usually superior or inferior altitudinal). This type of occlusion is most often related to emboli in the branch retinal artery. The clinical features of the emboli sometimes allow understanding of the nature and the source of the emboli (▶ Table 7.1). Giant cell arteritis is less likely.

Susac syndrome is a very rare cause of recurrent branch retinal artery occlusions. It is a vasculopathy of unknown cause leading to occlusion of small retinal, cochlear, and cerebral arteries, mostly occurring in young women. It is characterized by the clinical triad of branch retinal artery occlusions, hearing loss, and encephalopathy with focal neurologic signs and psychiatric manifestations.

Recommended tests include ocular examination with retinal fluorescein angiography to look for occlusion of multiple arterial branches, either uni- or bilateral; an

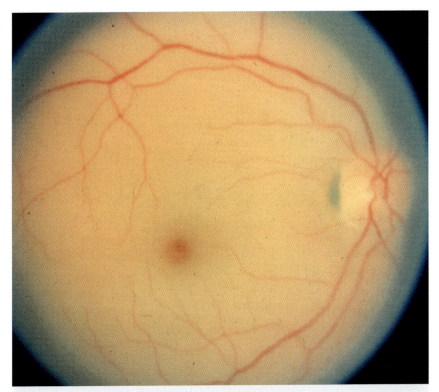

Fig. 7.2 Acute central retinal artery occlusion in the right eye (seen 24 hours after visual loss). The retina is diffusely pale and the fovea appears red (cherry red spot). The arteries are attenuated.

audiogram to determine whether hearing loss is uni- or bilateral; and magnetic resonance imaging (MRI) with gadolinium to check for multiple small enhancing lesions in the white and gray matter of the brain.

Giant Cell Arteritis

Retinal ischemia can be caused by giant cell arteritis (▶ Fig. 7.10). It is usually associated with optic nerve ischemia or choroidal ischemia (see Chapter 20).

> **Pearls**
>
> The association of branch or central retinal artery occlusion with anterior ischemic optic neuropathy is highly suggestive of giant cell arteritis.

7.1.2 Causes and Evaluation of Patients with Acute Retinal Arterial Ischemia

Giant cell arteritis, carotid disease, and other sources of emboli are classic causes of retinal ischemia (see ▶ Table 7.2).

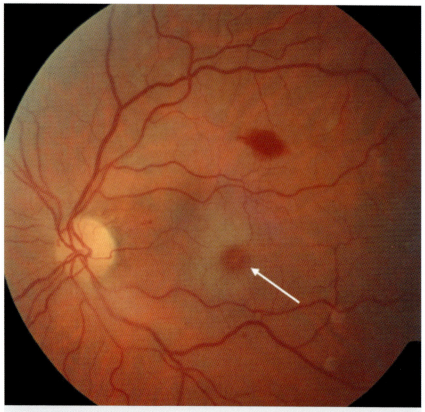

Fig. 7.3 Acute central retinal artery occlusion in the left eye, with a cherry red spot (*arrow*) (seen 3 hours after visual loss). There is a retinal hemorrhage above the macula, but the retina is not edematous yet, and therefore does not appear pale.

7.1.3 Treatment of Acute Retinal Arterial Ischemia

Acute treatment consists of the following:
- Patients seen acutely should be admitted for immediate workup by a stroke neurologist and initiation of secondary prevention.
- Most treatments used have not proven to be effective and are decided on a case-by-case basis.
- Reduce the intraocular pressure (ocular massage, drops).
- Consider thrombolytics for central retinal artery occlusion in selected patients seen within a few hours of visual loss.
- In cases of giant cell arteritis, admit the patient for high-dose intravenous steroids (methylprednisolone 250 mg every 6 hours for 3 or 5 days) followed by oral prednisone (1 mg/kg/d).

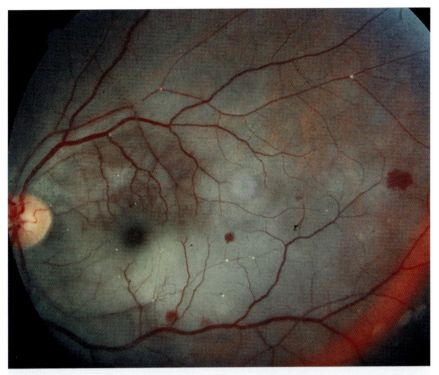

Fig. 7.4 Acute central retinal artery occlusion in the left eye, with multiple retinal emboli (seen at least 10 hours after visual loss). There are scattered retinal hemorrhages.

Secondary prevention of ocular and cerebral infarction is characterized as follows:
- Should be initiated at the time of diagnosis
- Is similar to that recommended for patients with cerebral infarctions and transient visual loss (see Chapter 6)

7.2 Ocular Ischemic Syndrome

Chronic hypoperfusion of the eye results in diffuse ocular ischemia. Ocular ischemia develops in patients with severe stenosis or occlusion of the ipsilateral internal carotid artery and poor collateral circulation. These patients often have low blood flow in the ophthalmic artery. The flow is sometimes reversed in the ophthalmic artery to protect the ipsilateral brain (there is then a steal phenomenon involving the eye) (see Chapter 6, ▶ Fig. 6.15 and ▶ Fig. 6.16).

7.2.1 Features

Venous stasis retinopathy (▶ Fig. 7.11), or hypotensive retinopathy, is the first sign of chronic ocular ischemia. It resembles diabetic retinopathy or central retinal vein

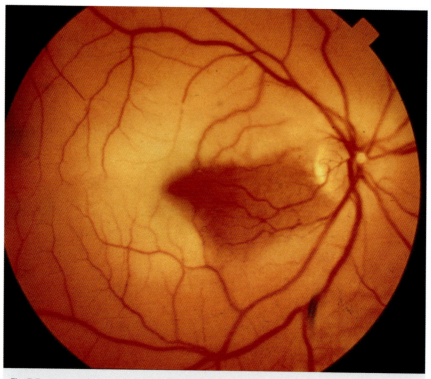

Fig. 7.5 Acute embolic central retinal artery occlusion with cilioretinal sparing in the right eye. The ischemic retina is whitish, whereas the retina is still normal in the territory of the cilioretinal artery.

occlusion and is characterized by a unilateral appearance, dilation and tortuosity of the retinal veins, and blot hemorrhages, mostly in the midperiphery of the retina.

Venous stasis retinopathy is usually asymptomatic. Patients may have episodes of hemodynamic transient monocular visual loss when standing up, after a meal, or with exposure to bright lights.

Other features of ocular ischemic syndrome are dull periocular pain that is present when the patient is standing up (it resolves when the patient is lying down), episcleral arteries that may be dilated (result from collateral circulation to the eye from branches of the external carotid artery), low intraocular pressure, and pseudointraocular inflammation.

Neovascularization may develop involving the retina and the anterior segment. It results in neovascular glaucoma (increased intraocular pressure), atonic iris (dilated and nonreactive pupil), cataract, or corneal edema.

7.2.2 Treatment and Prognosis

At this stage, revascularization of the eye (e.g., by performing a carotid endarterectomy if there is an ipsilateral internal carotid artery stenosis) may result in improvement of the retinopathy. If the eye is not revascularized, ocular ischemic syndrome develops (▶ Fig. 7.12).

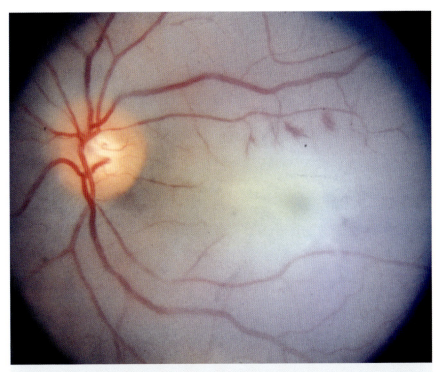

Fig. 7.6 Acute ophthalmic artery occlusion in the left eye. The retina is diffusely pale, and there is no cherry red spot because the choroid is also ischemic. The arteries are very attenuated, and there are a few hemorrhages superiorly.

The prognosis of ocular ischemic syndrome is poor.

Laser panphotocoagulation of the ischemic retina may reduce neovascularization (e.g., as for proliferative diabetic retinopathy). These patients often have ipsilateral internal carotid occlusion, however, and revascularization is not always possible (extra-intracranial bypass procedure is sometimes indicated). Even when revascularization of the eye is performed, the visual prognosis remains poor.

Pearls

Look for giant cell arteritis in the elderly patient with rapidly worsening ocular ischemic syndrome. Giant cell arteritis involves branches of the external carotid artery, which usually supply most of the eye via collateral circulation when there is an internal carotid occlusion. Any disorder affecting branches of the external carotid artery (e.g., giant cell arteritis) will compromise the collateral circulation and may precipitate acute ocular ischemia.

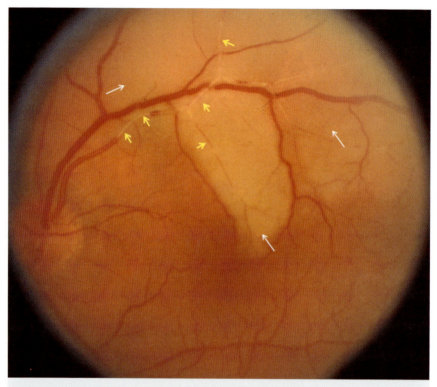

Fig. 7.7 Acute superior branch retinal artery occlusion in the left eye. Platelet fibrin emboli are seen in numerous arteries (*yellow arrows*). The ischemic retina is edematous and appears pale (*white arrows*).

7.3 Retinal Vein Occlusion

7.3.1 Features

Central and branch retinal vein occlusions (▶ Fig. 7.13, ▶ Fig. 7.14, ▶ Fig. 7.15) produce subacute monocular visual loss. The loss of vision is often progressive over a few days and is secondary largely to macular edema and macular ischemia. Relatively prolonged (up to 30 minutes) episodes of transient monocular visual loss may occur before permanent visual loss (see Chapter 6, ▶ Fig. 6.17).

7.3.2 Types of Retinal Vein Occlusions

Acute Central Retinal Vein Occlusion

Acute central retinal vein occlusion is characterized by painless monocular loss of vision over a few hours or a few days; dilated, tortuous veins; retinal hemorrhages; and retinal and optic nerve edema. Retinal ischemia and cotton wool spots suggest an ischemic form. A RAPD is seen if there is extensive retinal ischemia (poor prognosis). Acute

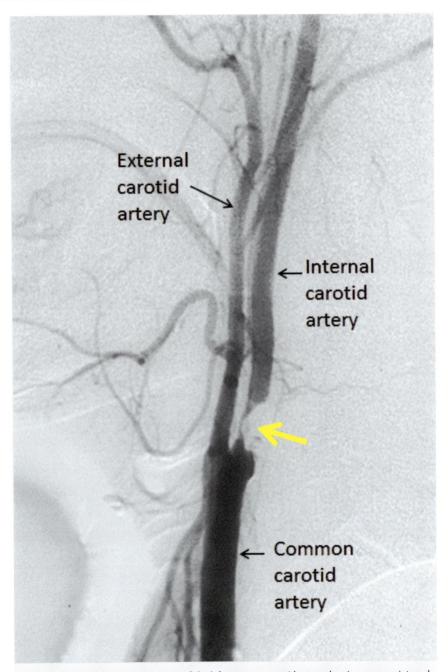

Fig. 7.8 Selective catheter angiogram of the left common carotid artery showing a severe internal carotid artery stenosis (*yellow arrow*) in a patient with a branch retinal artery occlusion.

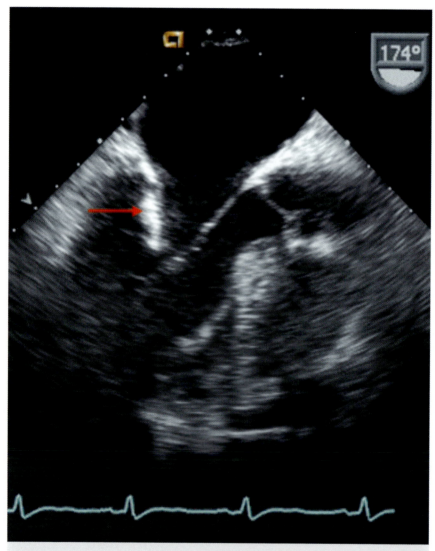

Fig. 7.9 Transesophageal echocardiogram showing a mass on the mitral valve (*arrow*) in a patient with recurrent episodes of transient monocular visual loss in both eyes, followed 2 weeks later by a central retinal artery occlusion in the right eye and a branch retinal artery occlusion in the left eye.

central retinal vein occlusion may present with isolated optic nerve edema (▶ Fig. 7.16). These patients are often mistaken as having an acute optic neuropathy, such as anterior ischemic optic neuropathy.

The usual presence of retinal hemorrhages distant from the swollen optic nerve suggests central retinal vein occlusion. Fluorescein angiography is useful to differentiate vein occlusion from other causes of disc edema.

Table 7.1 Characteristics of retinal emboli

Retinal emboli	Funduscopic appearance	Source of emboli
Cholesterol (Hollenhorst plaque)	Yellow, refractile emboli (multiple in 70% of cases); appear wider than the arteriole; often located at an arteriole bifurcation	Ipsilateral internal carotid artery or aortic arch atheroma
Platelet–fibrin	White, gray emboli, pale, not refractile, often multiple; usually seen distally within the small retinal arterioles	Thrombus (carotid or aortic arch atheroma), cardiac thrombus, cardiac prosthesis
Calcium	White, large emboli, usually isolated; located in the proximal segment of the central retinal artery or its branches	Calcified cardiac valve or calcified atheromatous plaque
Talc	Multiple, yellow emboli; refractile	Intravenous drugs
Fat	Multiple whitish spots, hemorrhages, cotton wool spots	Long bone fractures
Neoplasm	White, gray emboli, often multiple	Cardiac myxoma
Infectious	Multiple white spots (Roth spots)	Bacterial endocarditis, candidemia

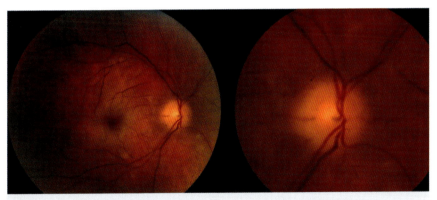

Fig. 7.10 Acute central retinal artery occlusion and anterior ischemic optic neuropathy in the right eye of a 78-year-old woman in the setting of giant cell arteritis. Visual acuity is light perception only, and there is a dense right relative afferent pupillary defect. The arteries are attenuated, and there is a cherry red spot. There is also pallid disc edema (closer view on the right), suggesting associated anterior ischemic optic neuropathy.

Table 7.2 Causes and evaluation of patients with acute retinal arterial ischemia[a]

Causes	Tests to obtain
Giant cell arteritis	CBC, platelets, ESR, CRP Consider fluorescein angiogram Temporal artery biopsy if high suspicion
Associated (silent) cerebral infarction	Brain MRI with diffusion-weighted images (DWI) or head CT
Carotid disease (ipsilateral): • Atheroma • Occlusion by thrombus or cardiac embolus • Dissection • Fibromuscular dysplasia • Vasculitis (Takayasu) • Tumor, external compression	Carotid ultrasound (with transcranial Doppler evaluating ophthalmic artery and intracranial circulation) or CT angiogram or MRA of head and neck
Aortic arch atheroma	Transesophageal echocardiogram CT angiogram of the aortic arch or MRA of the aortic arch
Cardiac source of emboli	Electrocardiogram; cardiac monitoring Transthoracic ± transesophageal echo-cardiogram Holter monitoring if indicated
Hypercoagulable disorder • Thrombophilia • Acquired	Blood tests looking for hypercoagulable states and causes of hyperviscosity, including thrombophilia, antiphospholipid antibody syndrome, hyperhomocysteinemia, sickle cell disease, monoclonal gammopathy, cancer, infection, and disseminated intravascular coagulation

Abbreviations: CBC, complete blood count; CRP, C-reactive protein; CT, computed tomography; ESR, erythrocyte sedimentation rate; MRI, magnetic resonance imaging; MRA, magnetic resonance angiography.
[a]The causes of acute retinal artery occlusions and appropriate tests are organized from the most urgent or common to the least likely.

▶ Table 7.3 lists the causes of acute retinal vein ischemia, with suggested tests.

Acute Branch Retinal Vein Occlusion and Hemiretinal Vein Occlusion

Both acute branch retinal vein occlusion and hemiretinal vein occlusion are characterized by painless monocular loss of vision over a few hours or a few days; dilated, tortuous veins; and retinal hemorrhages with edema in the territory of the occluded vein (see ▶ Fig. 7.14 and ▶ Fig. 7.15).

7.3.3 Natural History and Patient Evaluation

Most retinal vein occlusions occur in patients older than age 50 who have vascular risk factors. In these cases, vascular risk factors need to be aggressively controlled, but very little workup is obtained. Blood tests looking for hypercoagulable states are obtained only in patients in whom there is a high suspicion of hypercoagulability (recurrent

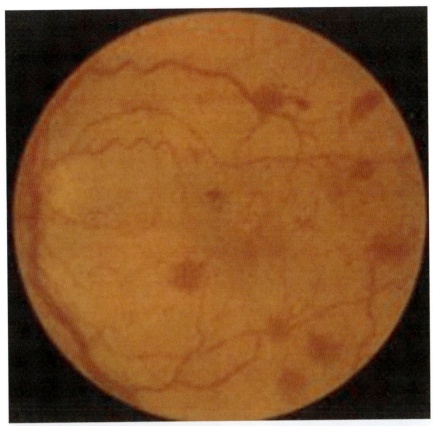

Fig. 7.11 Venous stasis retinopathy in a patient with internal carotid occlusion. The veins are dilated and tortuous. There are multiple large dot-blot hemorrhages in the midperiphery of the retina.

retinal vein occlusions, bilateral retinal vein occlusion, young patients, and/or a personal or familial history of vein occlusions) (see Chapter 20).

Orbital imaging is obtained only in patients with clinical evidence of orbital syndrome, cavernous sinus syndrome, or optic neuropathy.

7.3.4 Prognosis and Treatment

The visual prognosis is mostly based on the type of vein occlusion (ischemic form or not). When visual loss is mostly related to macular edema, vision usually improves over time. When the macula is ischemic (there is a RAPD in the affected eye), the visual prognosis is poor.

In most cases, the hemorrhages and retinal edema resolve spontaneously over a few weeks or months. In nonischemic central retinal vein occlusion, the visual prognosis is good, and visual function improves when macular edema resolves. Ischemic forms have a high risk of ocular neovascularization and permanent visual loss. Various treatments, such as decreasing intraocular pressure, retinal laser, intravitreal injections of steroids,

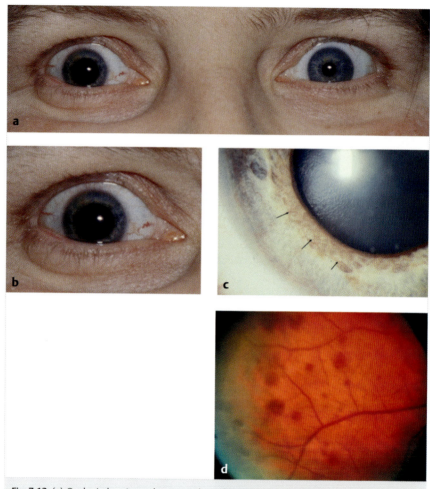

Fig. 7.12 (a) Ocular ischemic syndrome on the right. The episcleral arteries are dilated, and the pupil is spontaneously dilated and not reactive. There is visual loss and pain over the right eye. (b) Close view of the right eye. Note the dilated episcleral arteries. (c) Neovascularization of the iris (arrows show the neovessels) with mild cataract. The neovessels invade the angle and result in increased intraocular pressure (neovascular glaucoma). (d) Venous stasis retinopathy with blot hemorrhages in the midperiphery of the retina.

and anti-vascular endothelial growth factor (VEGF) drugs, are offered by retinal specialists.

Shunt vessels may develop after a central retinal vein occlusion (▶ Fig. 7.17). It is common to observe these dilated vessels during a routine ocular examination. An optic nerve sheath meningioma needs to be ruled out by an MRI scan of the orbits with contrast and fat suppression.

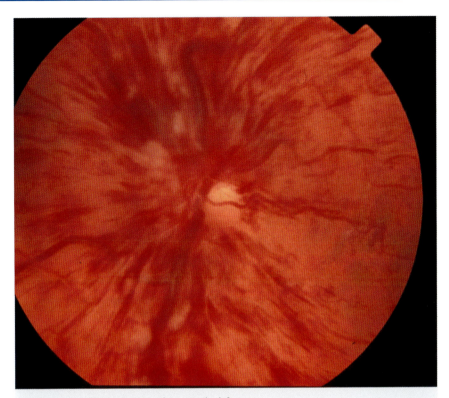

Fig. 7.13 Central retinal vein occlusion in the left eye.

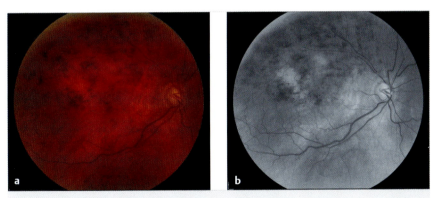

Fig. 7.14 (a) Superior branch retinal vein occlusion in the right eye. (b) Fluorescein angiogram showing delayed filling of the vein.

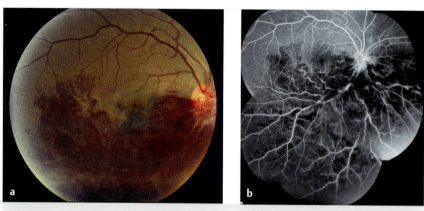

Fig. 7.15 (a) Acute inferior hemiretinal vein occlusion with segmental disc edema and retinal hemorrhages. (b) Composite photograph a few weeks later showing diffuse retinal hypoperfusion on a fluorescein angiogram (ischemic form).

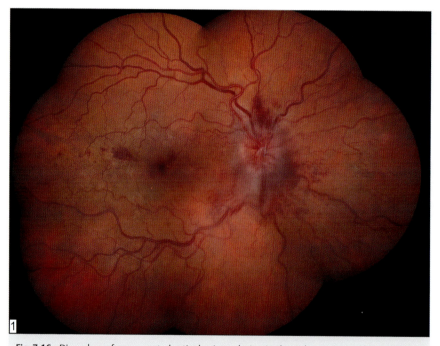

Fig. 7.16 Disc edema from a central retinal vein occlusion in the right eye. Note the macular hemorrhages and the hemorrhages temporal to the macula.

Table 7.3 Causes of acute retinal vein ischemia with suggested tests

Causes	Tests to obtain
Local arteriolosclerosis Compression of the vein by an atherosclerotic, rigid artery	Look for vascular risk factors Blood pressure, lipid profile
Hypercoagulable disorder • Thrombophilia • Acquired	Blood tests looking for hypercoagulable states and causes of hyperviscosity, including thrombophilia, antiphospholipid antibody syndrome, hyperhomocysteinemia, sickle cell disease, monoclonal gammopathy, cancer, infection, and disseminated intravascular coagulation
Compression of the optic nerve or veins in the orbit by: • Orbital mass • Optic nerve sheath meningioma	Orbital imaging
Venous congestion caused by: • Carotid cavernous fistula • Cavernous sinus thrombosis • Severe papilledema	Brain and orbital imaging

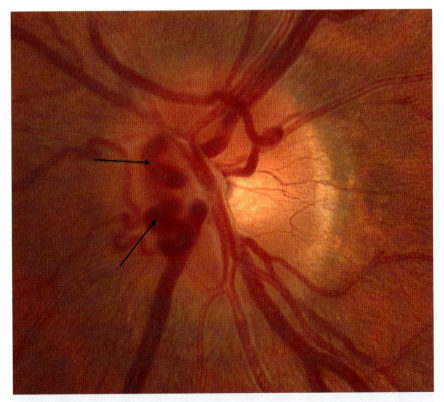

Fig. 7.17 Shunt vessels (*arrows*) over the optic nerve months after a central retinal vein occlusion.

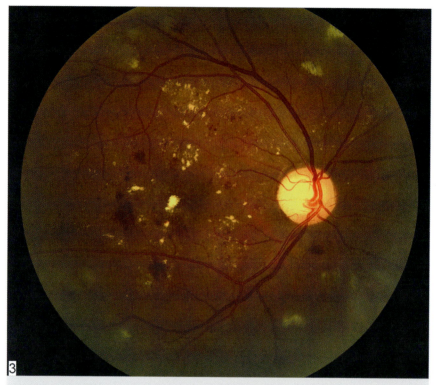

Fig. 7.18 Nonproliferative diabetic retinopathy (right eye). There are retinal exudates and hemorrhages with cotton wool spots. There is no neovascularization.

7.4 Diabetic Retinopathy

Diabetic retinopathy (▶ Fig. 7.18, ▶ Fig. 7.19, ▶ Fig. 7.20) is a common cause of visual loss. Macular edema and retinal ischemia can result in severe visual loss. The ischemia is diffuse, often involves the macula (responsible for central visual loss), and is ultimately complicated by neovascularization of the eye (proliferative diabetic retinopathy).

The neovascularization in proliferative diabetic retinopathy is responsible for hemorrhages and traction retinal detachment. Destruction of the peripheral retina with laser (panphotocoagulation) decreases the neovascularization but also results in night blindness and constriction of the visual field.

7.5 Hypertensive Retinopathy

Retinal vascular changes occur as a result of chronically elevated arterial blood pressure, usually bilaterally. Hypertensive retinopathy (▶ Fig. 7.21, ▶ Fig. 7.22, ▶ Fig. 7.23) is associated with a higher risk of cardiovascular disease, including coronary artery disease and stroke. It is a marker of poorly controlled arterial hypertension.

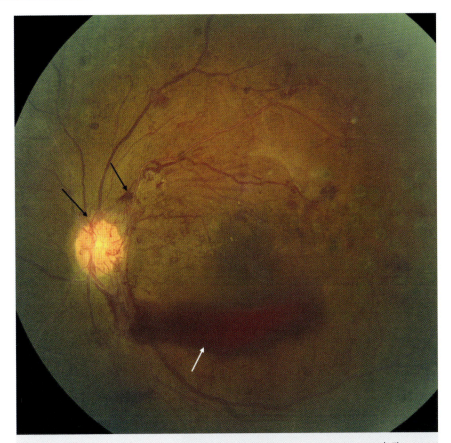

Fig. 7.19 Proliferative diabetic retinopathy (left eye). The arteries are very attenuated. There are retinal hemorrhages as well as a large subhyaloid hemorrhage (*white arrow*). The black arrows show neovascularization on the retina and the optic nerve.

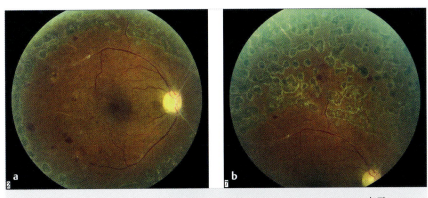

Fig. 7.20 (**a**) Severe diabetic retinopathy (right eye). The arteries are very attenuated. There are retinal exudates and hemorrhages. There are scars from panretinal laser photocoagulation in the midperiphery. The optic nerve is pale. (**b**) Severe diabetic retinopathy (superior retina of the right eye). The scars are sequelae from treatment with panretinal laser photocoagulation.

169

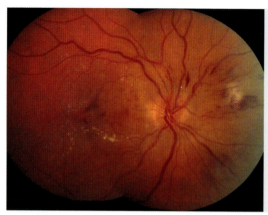

Fig. 7.21 Hypertensive retinopathy with macular edema and visual loss. There are yellow exudates and flame hemorrhages. The arteries are attenuated.

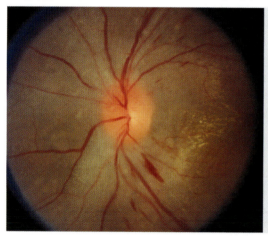

Fig. 7.22 Moderate hypertensive retinopathy. There are yellow exudates and flame hemorrhages. The arteries are attenuated.

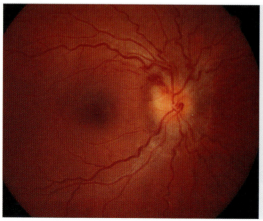

Fig. 7.23 Isolated optic nerve edema from acute hypertensive retinopathy. Note the unusual absence of retinal hemorrhages or retinal exudates.

7.5.1 Features

The following are key features of hypertensive retinopathy:
• Bilateral retinal vascular changes (may be asymmetric)
• Narrowing and irregularity of retinal arteries
• Arteriovenous nicking (narrowing of retinal veins at arteriovenous crossing sites)
• Retinal hemorrhages
• Microaneurysms
• Cotton wool spots

Moderate chronic hypertensive retinopathy is usually asymptomatic. Visual loss may occur as a result of macular exudates, macular edema, and chronic retinal ischemia.

Pearls

The blood pressure needs to be measured in all patients with bilateral optic nerve edema. Acutely elevated systemic arterial blood pressure may present with bilateral optic nerve edema and headaches. Retinal changes may be absent.

Acute hypertensive retinopathy (▶ Fig. 7.24 and ▶ Fig. 7.25) represents retinal and choroidal vascular changes occurring as a result of acutely elevated systemic arterial blood pressure.

Key features of acute hypertensive retinopathy are as follows:
• Retinal arteriolar spasm
• Retinal hemorrhages
• Cotton wool spots
• Retinal exudates
• Serous retinal detachment
• Optic nerve edema

Acute hypertensive retinopathy is often complicated by permanent visual loss from choroidal ischemia, retinal pigment epithelium changes, and ischemic optic

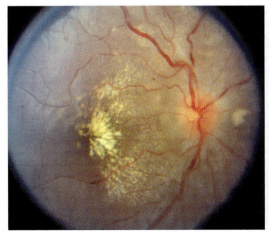

Fig. 7.24 Severe acute hypertensive retinopathy. Note the optic nerve edema and the macular exudates responsible for severe visual loss.

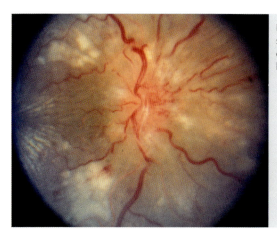

Fig. 7.25 Severe acute hypertensive retinopathy. Note the severe optic nerve edema and numerous large cotton wool spots.

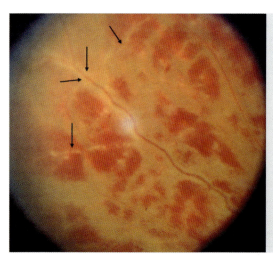

Fig. 7.26 Retinal vasculitis. Note the numerous retinal hemorrhages and the vascular sheathing (*black arrows*).

neuropathy. Other complications are bilateral visual loss from cerebral blindness (reversible posterior leukoencephalopathy), intracranial hemorrhages, and renal failure.

7.6 Retinal Vasculitis

Vasculitis of the retinal vasculature (▶ Fig. 7.26 and ▶ Fig. 7.27) can involve the arteries, the veins, or both, and may result in visual loss. As for cerebral vasculitis, the term *retinal vasculitis* implies that there is inflammation in or around the vessel wall. It therefore should be reserved for those disorders definitely secondary to inflammation. For example, Susac syndrome is associated with retinal vasculopathy, not vasculitis—there is no inflammation despite the fluorescein angiographic vascular leakage.

Causes of retinal vasculitis are numerous and include all classic causes of cerebral and systemic vasculitides (see Chapter 20). Recognition of whether the vasculitis involves the arteries or the veins, and associated ocular findings, is helpful.

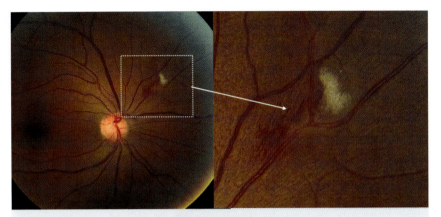

Fig. 7.27 Localized retinal vasculitis. Note the narrowing of the artery with sheathing, hemorrhage, and cotton wool spot (retinal ischemia).

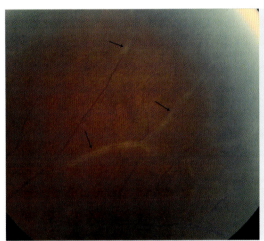

Fig. 7.28 Retinal sheathing in multiple sclerosis. Note the vascular sheathing (*black arrows*) seen in the retinal periphery.

For example, retinal vasculitis from Behçet syndrome involves the veins, is usually extensive, and is classically associated with anterior chamber inflammation. Periphlebitis associated with multiple sclerosis involves only the veins, affects the peripheral retina, and is asymptomatic. The involved vessels are attenuated (appear small), with sheathing (whitish line along the vessels), and are sometimes occluded (▶ Fig. 7.28). There are retinal hemorrhages and cotton wool spots secondary to retinal ischemia. Fluorescein angiography demonstrates occlusion of the small vessels and leakage of fluorescein (▶ Fig. 7.29).

Retinal vasculitis may be localized and mild. Finding vascular sheathing in an area of retinal ischemia is highly suggestive of vasculitis.

The following classic systemic disorders are associated with retinal vasculitis:

- Infections
  - Syphilis
  - Cytomegalovirus (▶ Fig. 7.30)

- ○ Toxoplasmosis
- ○ Cat scratch disease
- ○ Herpes simplex and herpes zoster (► Fig. 7.31)
- Inflammatory disorders
  - ○ Sarcoidosis
  - ○ Systemic lupus erythematosus
  - ○ Behçet syndrome
  - ○ Multiple sclerosis (peripheral periphlebitis) (see ► Fig. 7.28)

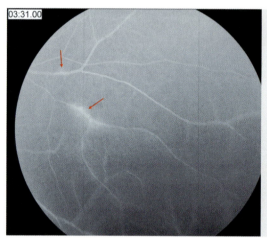

Fig. 7.29 Fluorescein angiogram in retinal vasculitis. Note the leakage of the fluorescein (*arrows*).

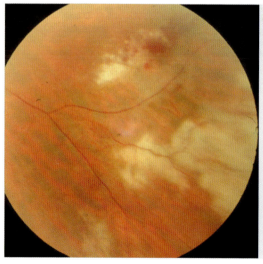

Fig. 7.30 Cytomegalovirus retinitis in a patient with human immuno-deficiency virus. Note the white and hemorrhagic retinal lesions associated with vascular sheathing.

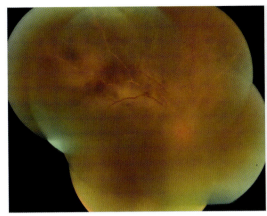

Fig. 7.31 Acute retinal necrosis from herpes zoster. Note the extensive retinal vasculitis (ghost vessels) with ocular inflammation blocking the view. The retina is necrotic and pale with hemorrhages.

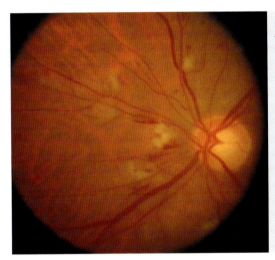

Fig. 7.32 Radiation retinopathy with retinal hemorrhages and cotton wool spots.

7.7 Radiation Retinopathy

Radiation retinopathy is a chronic progressive retinal vasculopathy induced by radiation and responsible for progressive, painless visual loss (▶ Fig. 7.32).

Radiation retinopathy may be unilateral or bilateral, depending on the type of radiation. It develops months or years after radiotherapy and is more common in patients with underlying retinal vascular disease (e.g., hypertension or diabetes).

Key findings include the following:
- Retinal hemorrhages
- Retinal microaneurysms
- Retinal exudates
- Cotton wool spots
- Macular edema

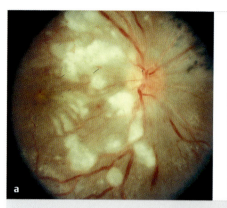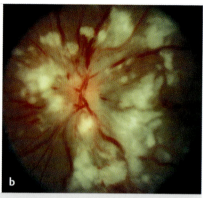

Fig. 7.33 Bilateral Purtscher retinopathy in a patient with acute pancreatitis. (a) Right eye (b) Left eye.

Complications of radiation retinopathy include retinal ischemia, retinal neovascularization, vitreous hemorrhage, traction retinal detachment, neovascularization of the anterior segment, and optic atrophy.

7.8 Purtscher Retinopathy

The chief feature of Purtscher retinopathy is bilateral peripapillary retinal infarctions with numerous cotton wool spots (▶ Fig. 7.33). This type of retinopathy classically occurs after trauma, acute pancreatic disorders, and amniotic fluid embolism.

7.9 Retinal Vascular Tortuosity

Retinal vascular tortuosity (▶ Fig. 7.34) is bilateral, involving the arteries and veins. It is usually asymptomatic and can be discovered during a routine funduscopic examination. It is rarely associated with retinal hemorrhages and cerebral leukoencephalopathy and may be familial.

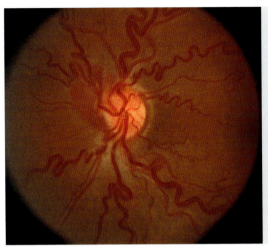

Fig. 7.34 Congenital Retinal vascular tortuosity.

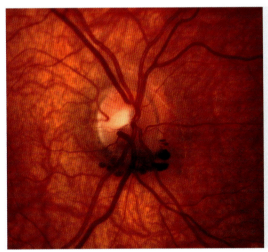

Fig. 7.35 "Cluster of grapes" appearance of cavernous hemangiomas at the edge of the disc in a patient with multiple intracranial cavernomas.

7.10 Retinal Vascular Malformations

Retinal vascular malformations are usually found during a routine fundus examination (▶ Fig. 7.35 and ▶ Fig. 7.36).

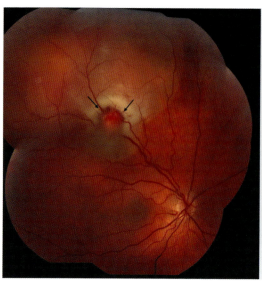

Fig. 7.36 Retinal hemangioma (*arrows*) in a patient with von Hippel–Lindau disease. These hemangiomas may leak and generate retinal exudates. They can mimic optic nerve swelling when located near the optic nerve.

8 Optic Neuropathies

Disorders of the optic nerve are called optic neuropathies. Optic neuropathies associated acutely with a normal optic nerve are referred to as *posterior or retrobulbar optic neuropathies*. Those with optic nerve head swelling are *anterior optic neuropathies*. In almost all cases, the optic nerve becomes pale (optic atrophy) 4 to 6 weeks after the onset of visual loss, even when vision recovers (▶ Fig. 8.1 and ▶ Fig. 8.2).

8.1 Diagnosis

The diagnosis of optic neuropathy is based on clinical examination, checking for the following:
- Visual loss
- Impaired color vision
- Abnormal visual field
- Relative afferent pupillary defect (RAPD) in all unilateral or asymmetric optic neuropathies (▶ Fig. 8.3)
- Optic nerve head appearance
  - Acutely: normal or swollen
  - Late (after 4–6 weeks): pale

Electrophysiologic testing is most often unnecessary. However, visual evoked responses and electroretinography are useful when the diagnosis is unclear (e.g., in cases with bilateral visual loss and no RAPD and when there is concern for a retinal disease rather than optic neuropathy). Patients with optic neuropathies have abnormal visual evoked responses. The P100 latency is delayed, and the amplitude is decreased (▶ Fig. 8.4).

8.1.1 Localization of the Lesion

The optic nerve may be affected in the orbit, at the level of the optic canal, or in its intracranial portion. In the orbit, the optic neuropathy may be isolated. The presence of associated symptoms or signs such as diplopia, ptosis, and proptosis suggests a process involving more than just the optic nerve, such as inflammation, infection, or neoplasm (▶ Fig. 8.5 and ▶ Fig. 8.6).

> **Pearls**
>
> A painful orbital apex syndrome in a diabetic patient is highly suggestive of mucormycosis infection.

Neurovascular structures enter and exit the orbit through the optic canal and the superior orbital fissure. In the optic canal, the optic nerve exits the orbit, and the ophthalmic artery enters the orbit. In the superior orbital fissure, the superior ophthalmic vein exits the orbit, and cranial nerves III (superior and inferior branches), IV, V1 (lacrimal, frontal, and nasociliary nerves), and VI enter the orbit (▶ Fig. 8.7).

An optic neuropathy may result from a lesion involving the intracranial portion of the optic nerve. When the lesion is close to the optic chiasm, visual field testing demonstrates a junctional scotoma (▶ Fig. 8.8).

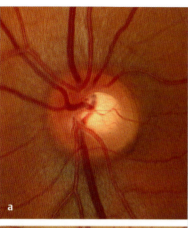

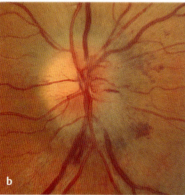

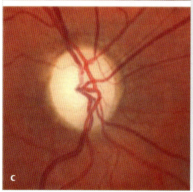

Fig. 8.1 (a) Normal left optic nerve appearance in posterior optic neuropathy (onset < 6 weeks). (b) Right optic nerve head swelling (edema) in anterior optic neuropathy. (c) Right optic nerve pallor in chronic optic neuropathy (> 6 weeks).

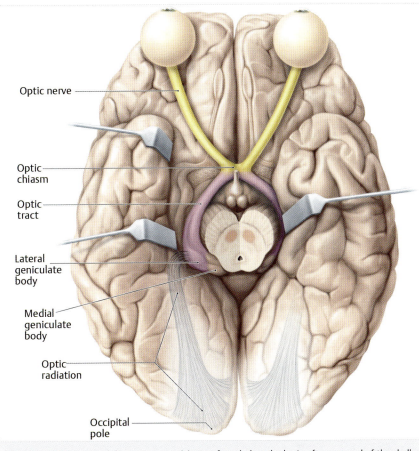

Fig. 8.2 a–d Anatomy of the optic nerve. (**a**) View from below the brain after removal of the skull. (*continued*)

Optic nerve

Optic chiasm

Optic tract

Lateral geniculate body

Medial geniculate body

Optic radiation

Occipital pole

8.2 Types of Optic Neuropathies (▶ Table 8.1)

The following lists the main types of optic neuropathies, with subcategories:

- Inflammatory (optic neuritis)
  - Idiopathic demyelinating optic neuritis (associated with multiple sclerosis)
  - Neuromyelitis optica (NMO; Devic disease)
  - Acute disseminated encephalomyelitis
  - Systemic infections
  - Systemic inflammatory diseases (e.g., sarcoidosis)
- Vascular (ischemic optic neuropathy)
  - Anterior/posterior
  - Arteritic/nonarteritic
- Compressive/infiltrative
  - Neoplastic
  - Non-neoplastic

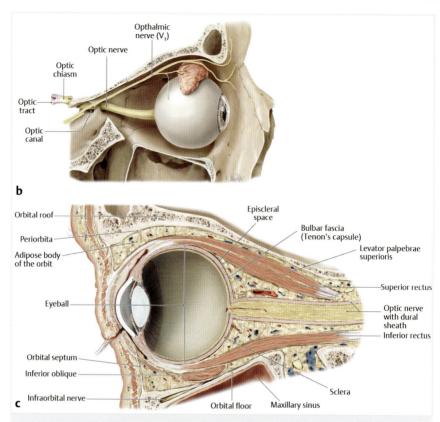

Fig. 8.2 (*continued*) (**b**) View from the side after removal of the lateral orbital wall. (**c**) Sagittal cut of the orbit. The optic nerve sheath (made of meninges) covers the optic nerve in the orbit. Note the relationship with the orbital fat and the extraocular muscles. (*continued*)

- Hereditary
- Toxic/nutritional
- Traumatic
- Raised intracranial pressure (papilledema)
- Glaucomatous
- Anomalous optic nerve
  - Congenitally anomalous
  - Drusen

Optic neuropathies and maculopathies have overlapping presentations. Both cause central visual loss and dyschromatopsia. Many chronic maculopathies are associated with mild optic nerve pallor. When the macula appears normal, it may be difficult to differentiate an optic neuropathy from a maculopathy (▶ Table 8.2). Autofluorescence imaging of the macula (see ▶ Fig. 4.5) and spectral optical coherence tomography (OCT) (see ▶ Fig. 4.12) are very helpful in distinguishing optic neuropathies from maculopathies when the macula appears normal on funduscopic examination.

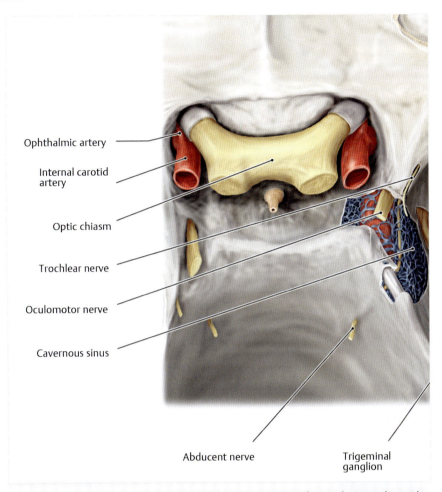

Ophthalmic artery

Internal carotid artery

Optic chiasm

Trochlear nerve

Oculomotor nerve

Cavernous sinus

Abducent nerve

Trigeminal ganglion

Fig. 8.2 (*continued*) (**d**) Intracranial portion of the optic nerve. It is close to the internal carotid artery and the origin of the ophthalmic artery. The pituitary gland is below. (**a,b**) From Schuenke M, Schulte E, Schumacher U, Ross LM, Lamperti ED, Voll M. THIEME Atlas of Anatomy, Head and Neuroanatomy. Stuttgart, Germany: Thieme; 2007. Illustration by Markus Voll. (**c,d**) From Schuenke M, Schulte E, Schumacher U, Ross LM, Lamperti ED, Voll M. THIEME Atlas of Anatomy, Head and Neuroanatomy. Stuttgart, Germany: Thieme; 2007. Illustration by Karl Wesker.

8.3 Patient Evaluation

The following clinical characteristics are particularly helpful in determining the mechanism of the optic neuropathy:

- Mode of onset of visual loss
  - Acute (ischemic and inflammatory neuropathies)
  - Progressive (compressive or toxic optic neuropathies)
- Color vision (often relatively spared in ischemic optic neuropathies and usually very abnormal in inflammatory optic neuropathies)

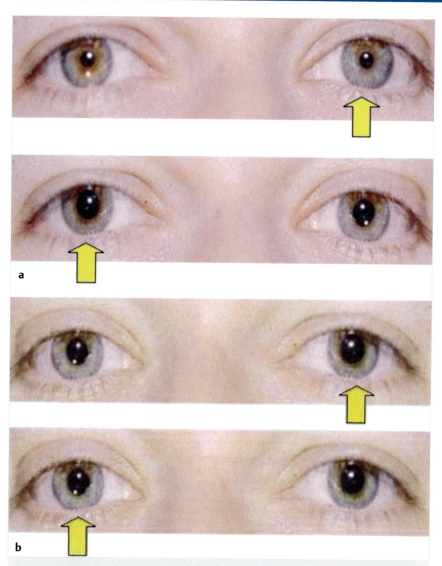

Fig. 8.3 (a) Right relative afferent pupillary defect (RAPD) from a right optic neuropathy. When the light is shone in the left eye, both pupils constrict briskly; both pupils dilate when the light is shone in the right eye. (b) Pupillary reaction in bilateral and symmetric optic neuropathies. There is no RAPD, but both pupils are sluggish in response to light stimulation.

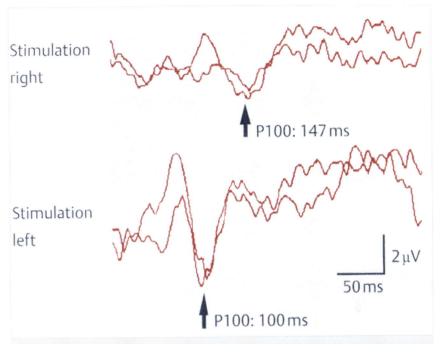

Stimulation right

P100: 147 ms

Stimulation left

2 µV

50 ms

P100: 100 ms

Fig. 8.4 Visual evoked responses (abnormal in the right eye with optic neuritis; normal in the left eye).

- The presence of pain with eye movements (highly suggestive of an inflammatory mechanism)
- Funduscopic appearance (variable in inflammatory optic neuropathies, reveals a swollen optic nerve in all cases of anterior ischemic optic neuropathy, and shows a sometimes cupped optic nerve in compressive and hereditary optic neuropathies)
- Associated retinal changes in neuroretinitis

Evaluating the patient with suspected optic neuropathy includes the following:
1. Confirm the diagnosis of optic neuropathy by clinical examination.
2. Look for associated symptoms and signs.
3. Try to localize the optic nerve lesion (anterior, posterior in the orbit, orbital apex, or intracranial).
4. Determine the presumed etiologic diagnosis.
5. Obtain ancillary testing, such as imaging and laboratory workup, to confirm the diagnosis prior to initiating treatment.

Recommended tests include the following:
- Magnetic resonance imaging (MRI) of the brain and orbits with gadolinium (orbital images should be with fat suppression)
- Blood tests
  - Blood tests will vary, based on the presumed diagnosis.

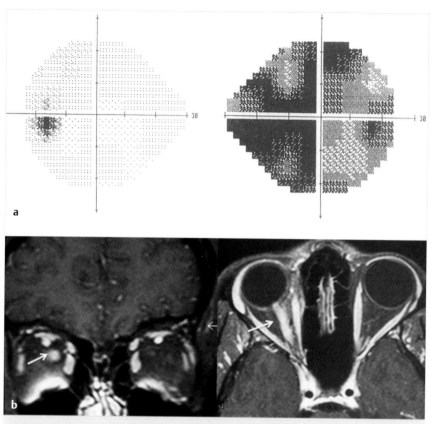

Fig. 8.5 (a) Isolated right inflammatory optic neuropathy. There is a large central scotoma seen as diffuse depression on a 24–2 Humphrey visual field test. (b) Coronal and axial T1-weighted magnetic resonance imaging with fat suppression and contrast showing enhancement of the orbital portion of the right optic nerve (*arrow*).

○ Helpful tests include those for syphilis, sarcoidosis (angiotensin-converting enzyme [ACE]), cat scratch disease (*Bartonella* antibodies), Lyme disease, human immunodeficiency virus (HIV), inflammatory biologic syndrome (complete blood count [CBC], C-reactive protein [CRP], and erythrocyte sedimentation rate [ESR]), autoantibodies for autoimmune diseases (antinuclear antibodies [ANAs] and antineutrophil cytoplasmic antibodies [ANCAs]), and vitamin B12 and folate (bilateral and progressive painless optic neuropathies), as well as genetic testing for Leber hereditary optic neuropathy (severe unilateral or bilateral optic neuropathies) and for dominant optic atrophy (bilateral and progressive painless optic neuropathies).
- Cerebrospinal fluid (CSF) (lumbar puncture)
  ○ Helpful in cases of bilateral optic neuropathies, or when an infectious, systemic inflammatory, or neoplastic cause is suspected

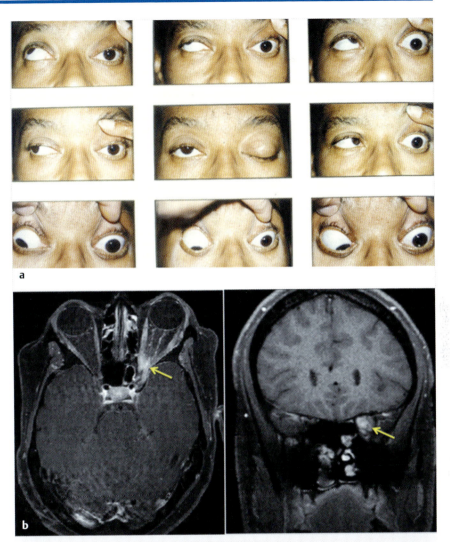

Fig. 8.6 (a) Left orbital apex syndrome. There is visual loss in the left eye from an optic neuropathy, with associated pain (V1), ptosis, and ophthalmoplegia from left third, fourth, and fifth nerve palsies. (b) Axial and coronal T1-weighted magnetic resonance imaging with fat suppression and contrast showing left optic nerve enhancement at the level of the orbital apex. Note the adjacent sphenoid sinusitis. The patient is diabetic. A sphenoid biopsy confirmed the diagnosis of mucormycosis infection (*arrow*).

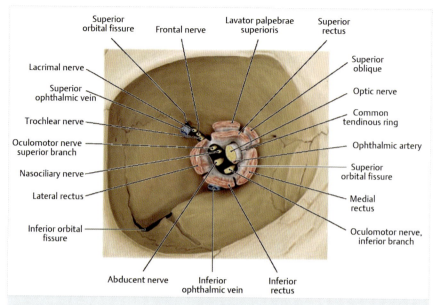

Fig. 8.7 Posterior view of the right orbit. (From Schuenke M, Schulte E, Schumacher U, Ross LM, Lamperti ED, Voll M. THIEME Atlas of Anatomy, Head and Neuroanatomy. Stuttgart, Germany: Thieme; 2007. Illustration by Karl Wesker.)

8.4 Inflammatory Optic Neuropathy (Optic Neuritis)

Inflammation of the optic nerve is called *optic neuritis*. There are several different types of optic neuritis.

8.4.1 Characteristics

Optic neuritis is characterized by subacute, painful loss of central vision that may progress for 7 to 10 days (visual acuity varies from a mild reduction to severe loss); pain that is usually exacerbated by eye movement and may precede or coincide with visual loss; and abnormal color vision that is usually impaired out of proportion to visual acuity.

Optic nerve appearance varies depending on which part of the optic nerve is inflamed. The term *retrobulbar optic neuritis* is used when the optic nerve appears normal in the acute phase. The terms *anterior optic neuritis* and *papillitis* are used when there is optic disc swelling. In both cases, temporal pallor of the disc develops 4 to 6 weeks after visual loss.

Optic nerve enhancement is often seen on orbital MRI.

8.4.2 Causes

There are multiple causes of optic neuritis, including infectious diseases, such as syphilis and cat scratch disease, and noninfectious inflammation, such as sarcoidosis. However, in most cases, optic neuritis remains idiopathic or is associated with multiple sclerosis. Optic neuritis may also be associated with other primary demyelinating diseases, such as NMO (Devic disease) and acute disseminated encephalomyelitis (ADEM).

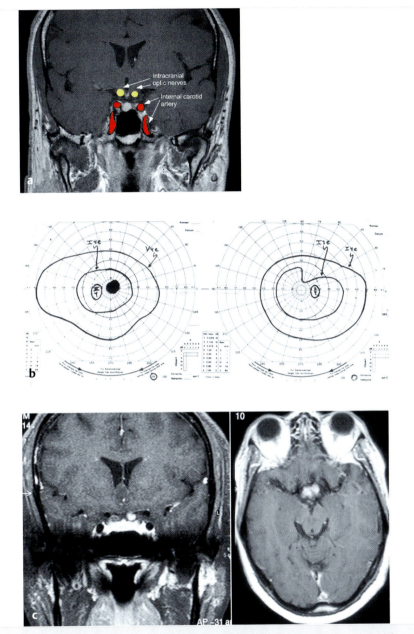

Fig. 8.8 (a) Intracranial portion of the optic nerves. (b) Goldmann visual fields showing a left central scotoma from a left optic neuropathy. There is a superior temporal defect respecting the vertical meridian in the right eye, suggesting a lesion of the posterior left optic nerve encroaching upon the chiasm (junctional scotoma). (c) Coronal and axial T1-weighted magnetic resonance imaging with contrast showing left optic nerve and chiasmal enhancement (*arrows*). The patient has neurosarcoidosis.

Table 8.1 Clinical characteristics of common optic neuropathies

	Optic neuritis	AION	Compressive/infiltrative	Toxic/nutritional	Hereditary	Papilledema
Age of patients	Younger	Older (>age 50)	Age 30–40: meningioma Childhood: glioma	Any age	Younger	Any age
Laterality	Unilateral	Unilateral	Unilateral	Bilateral	Bilateral	Bilateral
Visual loss	Rapidly progressive; acuity rarely spared	Acute; acuity variable	Progressive	Slowly progressive	Subacute (LHON); progressive (DOA)	Acuity preserved until late
Pain	Orbital pain frequent with eye movements	Pain infrequent (except in GCA)	Absent	Absent	Absent	Headache (raised ICP)
Color vision	Abnormal	Variably spared	Abnormal	Affected early	Abnormal	Preserved until late
Visual field	Central defect	Altitudinal defect	Variable	Cecocentral scotoma	Cecocentral scotoma	Peripheral constriction
Optic disc Acute	Normal (two thirds) or disc edema (one third)	Disc edema, ± segmental; small cup-to-disc ratio	Variable	Normal or hyperemic	Pseudoedema in LHON	Disc edema
Late	Temporal pallor	Segmental pallor	Pale	Pale, cupped	Pale	Pale swelling
Visual prognosis	Good	Variable; 15% risk for the other eye within 5 years	Variable	May improve	Poor	Reversible if treated early
Systemic diseases	Risk of development of multiple sclerosis	HTN (51%), DM (24%) GCA to be ruled out	Neurofibromatosis malignancy	Poor nutrition, peripheral neuropathy	Mitochondrial diseases, DIDMOAD syndrome	Any cause of raised ICP

Abbreviations: AION, anterior ischemic optic neuropathy; DIDMOAD, diabetes insipidus, diabetes mellitus, optic atrophy, and deafness; DM, diabetes mellitus; DOA, dominant optic atrophy; GCA, giant cell arteritis; HTN, hypertension; ICP, intracranial pressure; LHON, Leber hereditary optic neuropathy.

Table 8.2 Differentiation of optic nerve disease from macular disease

	Optic nerve disease	Macular disease
Visual acuity	Variable	Variable
Color vision	Very reduced	Mildly reduced
Amsler grid	Scotoma	Metamorphopsia
Visual field	Variable	Central scotoma or diffuse depression
Pupils	RAPD if optic neuropathy is unilateral or asymmetric	No RAPD, unless the entire macula is affected
Photostress recovery	Normal	Delayed
Visual evoked responses	Abnormal	Normal or mildly abnormal
ERG	Normal	Abnormal (full-field ERG often normal; multifocal ERG is usually abnormal)

Abbreviations: ERG, electroretinogram; RAPD, relative afferent pupillary defect.

8.4.3 Patient Evaluation

Evaluation of the patient includes checking for these characteristics:
- Cat exposure
- Recent travel
- Tick bite
- Immunosuppression
- Associated systemic symptoms and signs, including fever, lymphadenopathy, weight loss, skin lesions, cough, and arthralgias
- Associated neurologic symptoms and signs, including focal neurologic signs; a history of vertigo, diplopia, numbness, Lhermitte sign, or Uhthoff phenomenon; headaches; and meningismus
- Associated ocular findings, including intraocular inflammation and retinitis

The cause of optic neuritis is often suspected after the history and clinical examination. Ancillary tests are obtained to confirm a presumed diagnosis.

Ancillary tests vary based on the foregoing evaluation and include the following:
- MRI of the brain and orbits with contrast (confirms optic nerve enhancement and looks for demyelinating disease in the brain)
- Chest radiograph (looking for sarcoidosis)
- Blood tests (vary based on presumed diagnosis): CBC, platelets, angiotensin-converting enzyme (ACE) level, and syphilis testing
- Lumbar puncture: performed when an infectious cause or underlying systemic inflammatory disease is suspected; should always be obtained when the optic neuritis is bilateral and is obtained in most cases of optic neuritis in children
- MRI of the spine with contrast if neurologic signs suggest spinal cord disease or if NMO is suspected
- NMO antibodies: obtained in the serum of patients with bilateral optic neuritis, recurrent optic neuritis, severe optic neuritis with poor visual recovery, or when there is a spinal cord lesion or symptoms suggesting transverse myelitis

8.4.4 Classification

1. Optic neuritis associated with demyelinating disease
   - Idiopathic optic neuritis
   - Optic neuritis as a manifestation of any of the following:
     - Multiple sclerosis
     - NMO (Devic disease)
     - ADEM
2. Optic neuritis associated with infectious diseases
   - Bacterial infections: syphilis, cat scratch disease (*Bartonella henselae*), Lyme disease, any bacterial meningitis, *Mycoplasma pneumoniae*, tuberculosis, Whipple disease (syphilis and cat scratch disease are the most common causes)
   - Viral infections: herpes zoster, herpes simplex, HIV, Epstein–Barr virus, coxsackie virus, adenovirus, cytomegalovirus, hepatitis A and B virus, measles, mumps, rubella virus (herpes zoster is the most common cause)
   - Parasitic infections: toxoplasmosis, cysticercosis, toxocariasis, intraocular nematode infection (toxoplasmosis is the most common cause)
   - Fungal infections: cryptococcosis, aspergillosis, mucormycosis, histoplasmosis (cryptococcosis is the most common cause)
3. Post-vaccination optic neuritis
   - Hepatitis B virus; rabies virus; tetanus toxoid; variola virus; combined smallpox, tetanus, and diphtheria vaccine; combined measles, mumps, and rubella vaccine; influenza vaccine; bacille Calmette-Guérin (BCG)
4. Optic neuritis associated with other inflammatory disorders
   - Sarcoidosis
   - Systemic lupus erythematosus
   - Sjögren syndrome
   - Polyarteritis nodosa
   - Wegener granulomatosis
   - Inflammatory bowel disease
   - Behçet syndrome
   - Bee and wasp stings
5. Isolated recurrent optic neuritis (autoimmune optic neuritis)

8.4.5 Idiopathic Demyelinating Optic Neuritis

Idiopathic demyelinating optic neuritis is the most common acute optic neuropathy in persons under the age of 45. It is also the most common cause of optic neuritis and often the presenting sign of multiple sclerosis.

Characteristics

Idiopathic demyelinating optic neuritis is more prevalent in young women than men (3:1). It is unilateral (occasionally bilateral) and is characterized by acute to subacute onset (usually rapidly progressive over a few days), decreased visual acuity (variable) and color vision (usually pronounced), pain with eye movements (in > 90% of cases), and exacerbation with heat or exercise (Uhthoff phenomenon).

There is a strong association between optic neuritis and multiple sclerosis. Most patients with multiple sclerosis eventually have visual loss from optic neuritis. Many patients with acute isolated optic neuritis eventually develop multiple sclerosis.

Patient Evaluation

Examination should include the following:
- RAPD (if unilateral or asymmetric)
- Funduscopy:
  - Normal (two thirds of cases) or swollen (one third of cases) optic nerve head
  - Normal macula and retina (no exudates, no hemorrhages)
  - Optic disc pallor (only if at least 4–6 weeks after onset or if previous episode of optic neuritis)
- Visual field test:
  - Often central scotoma (diffuse depression on Humphrey visual field test)

In > 90% of cases, spontaneous improvement is seen within several weeks; the absence of improvement should raise concern for another diagnosis. Risk of multiple sclerosis (▶ Fig. 8.9) should also be assessed.

In > 90% of patients with typical acute idiopathic demyelinating optic neuritis, visual acuity improves spontaneously to at least 20/40 at 6 months. The diagnosis should be reconsidered when the visual acuity does not improve.

Association between Idiopathic Demyelinating Optic Neuritis and Multiple Sclerosis

Patients diagnosed with idiopathic demyelinating optic neuritis are at high risk of subsequent development of multiple sclerosis after an isolated attack of idiopathic optic neuritis (as high as 74% at 15 years). Initial MRI helps stratify the risk of multiple sclerosis (as per the Optic Neuritis Treatment Trial):
- The overall risk of multiple sclerosis at 15 years is 50%.
- If the brain MRI is normal, the 15 year risk of multiple sclerosis is 23%.
- If the brain MRI shows one T2-weighted ovoid > 3 mm in diameter, highly suggestive of multiple sclerosis, the 15 year risk of multiple sclerosis is 56%.
- If the brain MRI shows at least six T2-weighted white matter lesions suggestive of multiple sclerosis, the 15 year risk of multiple sclerosis is 74%.

Lumbar puncture may detect oligoclonal bands in the CSF of patients with idiopathic demyelinating optic neuritis. However, it provides additional information only when the brain MRI is normal (an abnormal brain MRI is the strongest predictor of multiple sclerosis in a patient with optic neuritis).

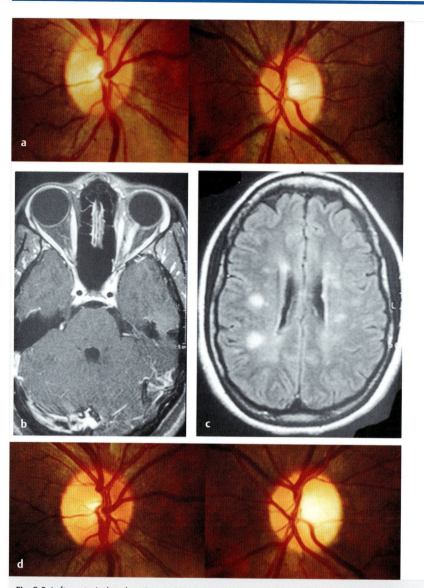

Fig. 8.9 Left acute isolated optic neuritis in a young woman. (**a**) Initial fundus showing normal optic nerves. Visual acuity is 20/200 in the left eye, and there is a left relative afferent pupillary defect (RAPD) and a central scotoma. (**b**) Axial T1-weighted magnetic resonance imaging (MRI) of the orbits with contrast and fat suppression (performed at initial presentation) showing left optic nerve enhancement. (**c**) Axial fluid-attenuated inversion recovery (FLAIR) MRI of the brain showing multiple hypersignals in the white matter, mostly periventricular, highly suggestive of multiple sclerosis. (**d**) Two months later, the left optic nerve has developed temporal pallor. Visual acuity has recovered to 20/25, and the visual field is full.

To determine the prognosis for multiple sclerosis in patients with typical acute isolated optic neuritis, the only test definitely indicated is an MRI scan of the brain with contrast. Other tests are sometimes obtained (vary with patient characteristics and centers), for example, MRI of the orbits with contrast and fat suppression, lumbar puncture for CSF oligoclonal bands, blood tests (syphilis testing and ACE level for sarcoidosis), NMO antibodies, and chest radiograph.

The spontaneous visual prognosis is good without treatment.

Treatment of idiopathic acute optic neuritis should consider the following:

- Intravenous methylprednisolone (250 mg, every 6 hours for 3 days) followed by oral prednisone (1 mg/kg/d for 11 days, then tapered off over 3 days):
  - Hastens the rate of visual recovery by about 2 weeks but does not change the final extent of visual recovery
  - May help alleviate the pain
  - Delays neurologic symptoms and signs from multiple sclerosis for 2 years but does not change the risk of multiple sclerosis after 2 years
- Oral prednisone (1 mg/kg/d) should *not* be prescribed:
  - No beneficial effect on recovery of vision or risk of multiple sclerosis
  - Doubles the risk of recurrent optic neuritis (in the Optic Neuritis Treatment Trial)
- Disease-modifying agents decrease the risk of subsequent neurologic symptoms and signs related to multiple sclerosis and should be considered in selected high-risk patients (those with typical idiopathic optic neuritis and white matter lesions highly suggestive of demyelinating disease on brain MRI).

Pearls

Treatment with intravenous methylprednisolone hastens visual recovery, but it does not change the long-term prognosis of patients with acute isolated optic neuritis.

In the Optic Neuritis Treatment Trial, treatment with oral prednisone 1 mg/kg/d alone doubled the risk of recurrent optic neuritis and should not be prescribed to patients with acute isolated optic neuritis.

8.4.6 Neuromyelitis Optica (Devic Disease)

NMO, also known as Devic disease, is the association of acute or subacute severe visual loss in one or both eyes caused by acute optic neuritis. Transverse myelopathy precedes or follows visual loss. NMO is diagnosed with an abnormal cervical spine MRI scan (long T2-weighted hypersignal over more than three segments) and a brain MRI scan that is typically normal or shows T2-weighted hypersignals not typical of multiple sclerosis (not involving the periventricular region and not scattered in the white matter). Positive NMO immunoglobulin G (IgG) antibodies are also a major criterion for the diagnosis of NMO.

The prognosis is usually poor, with permanent, severe visual loss and paraplegia. Treatment usually consists of high-dose intravenous steroids followed by a slow taper of oral prednisone and long-term immunosuppressive therapy. Plasmapheresis is sometimes performed in cases with acute symptoms (▶ Fig. 8.10).

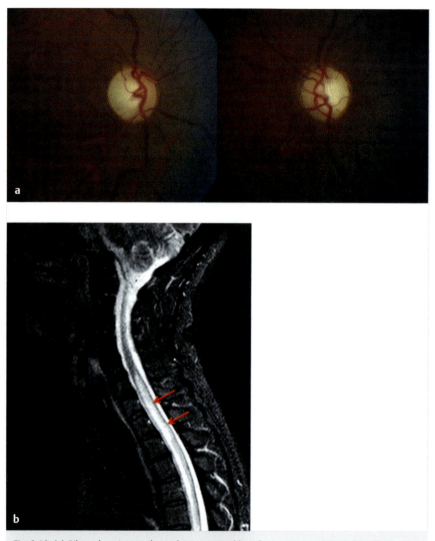

Fig. 8.10 (a) Bilateral optic atrophy and severe visual loss from neuromyelitis optica. (b) Sagittal T2-weighted cervical spine magnetic resonance imaging showing an extensive hypersignal consistent with myelitis (*arrows*). The patient is paraplegic.

8.4.7 Acute Disseminated Encephalomyelitis

ADEM or subacute encephalomyelitis occurs during the course of various infections, most often as a postinfectious or autoimmune response. It is particularly common in children, but it may occur at any age.

The clinical symptoms and MRI changes may mimic multiple sclerosis; however, unlike multiple sclerosis, which is a relapsing-remitting disorder, patients usually have only one episode of ADEM. Unilateral or bilateral optic neuritis (often with disc edema) may develop during the course of ADEM.

8.4.8 Other Causes of Optic Neuritis

Less commonly, inflammatory optic neuritis is not associated with a primary demyelinating process in the optic nerve or the central nervous system (CNS). Instead, the condition develops in the setting, or as the presenting manifestation, of a systemic infection or a systemic inflammatory disease.

Systemic symptoms and signs, patients' characteristics, and associated ocular findings such as neuroretinitis should direct the subsequent workup.

Syphilitic Optic Neuritis

Optic neuritis is common in secondary and tertiary syphilis. It is usually associated with lymphocytic meningitis and is a sign of neurosyphilis. Raised intracranial pressure with papilledema is common with syphilitic lymphocytic meningitis. Testing for syphilis (rapid plasma reagin [RPR] and fluorescent treponemal antibody absorption [FTA-ABS]) should be considered in patients with optic neuritis. When blood tests are positive, a lumbar puncture (with opening pressure, CSF analysis, and Venereal Disease Research Laboratories [VDRL] testing) and HIV testing are mandatory. Syphilitic optic neuritis is treated like neurosyphilis. The visual prognosis is usually good (▶ Fig. 8.11).

Optic Neuritis in Patients with HIV

Optic neuritis is a not uncommon cause of visual loss in patients infected with HIV (see Chapter 20). Syphilis is the most common cause of optic neuritis in patients with HIV.

Most opportunistic infections invading the CNS can produce an optic neuritis. Infections by cytomegalovirus, toxoplasmosis, and cryptococcus are the most classic causes.

A lumbar puncture should always be performed, and CSF should be evaluated for all causes of infections and malignancies (e.g., lymphoma) common in patients with HIV (▶ Fig. 8.12).

Sarcoid Optic Neuritis

Sarcoid optic neuritis may be isolated, or it may develop in a patient with neurosarcoidosis (see discussion in Chapter 20). The lumbar puncture often shows abnormal CSF (lymphocytic meningitis), and the MRI scan typically demonstrates intense gadolinium enhancement of the affected optic nerve. There is sometimes associated meningeal enhancement.

Workup (general examination, ACE level, chest radiograph, chest computed tomography [CT], gallium scan, or fluorodeoxyglucose positron-emission tomography [FDG-PET] scan) may suggest systemic sarcoidosis. Biopsy of a lesion (usually skin lesion, lymph node, pulmonary lesion, or lacrimal gland) confirms the diagnosis of sarcoidosis.

In sarcoidosis, the optic neuritis may result from lymphocytic meningitis present in neurosarcoidosis. Uni- or bilateral optic nerve edema may be present if there is raised intracranial pressure. Optic neuritis may also result from granulomatous infiltration of the optic nerve head associated with elevation of the optic nerve. Retinal lesions (infiltrates, vasculitis) and vitreous cells are common in this setting. Another cause is granulomatous infiltration of the intracranial portion of the optic nerve and the chiasm.

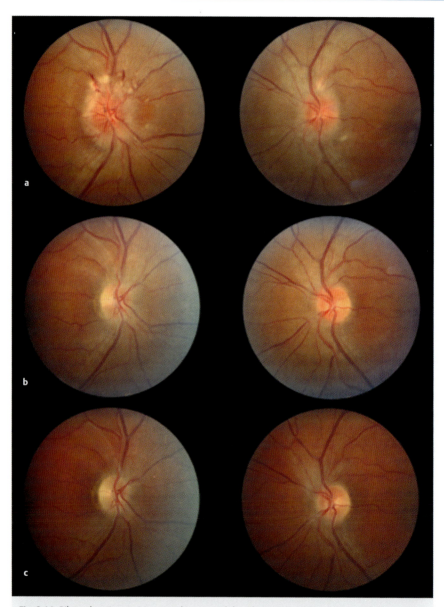

Fig. 8.11 Bilateral optic neuritis secondary to syphilis. There is visual loss in the right eye with a right relative afferent pupillary defect (RAPD) and a central scotoma. The patient was found to be positive for human immunodeficiency virus (HIV) at the time of visual loss. (**a**) The right optic nerve is very swollen, and there are yellow exudates and a few peripapillary hemorrhages. Note the mild swelling and exudates of the left optic nerve. (**b**) After treatment with intravenous penicillin, a few weeks later, the swelling is improved in both eyes. (**c**) Three months after treatment, the optic nerve swelling has completely resolved, and there is mild temporal pallor of the right optic nerve. The visual function is normal in both eyes.

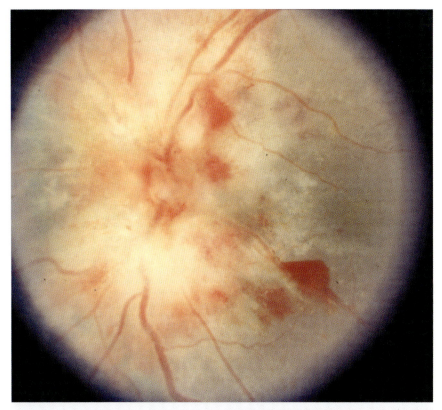

Fig. 8.12 Left optic neuritis secondary to cytomegalovirus in a patient with acquired immunodeficiency syndrome (AIDS). The optic nerve head is not visible. Note the diffuse white infiltrates and hemorrhages. The vessels are abnormal from vasculitis.

In most cases, the optic neuropathy responds well to corticosteroids and may be steroid-dependent, requiring long-term treatment with an immunosuppressive agent (▶ Fig. 8.13).

Neuroretinitis

Neuroretinitis associates inflammation of the optic nerve head with retinal lesions. It is characterized ophthalmoscopically by optic disc swelling associated with a macular star figure composed of lipid. The retinal abnormalities typically appear days to weeks after the onset of visual loss.

This form of optic neuritis is *not* caused by demyelination and occurs most often in the setting of cat scratch disease or in association with other systemic infectious diseases, such as Lyme disease and syphilis, as well as with sarcoidosis. These patients are not at subsequent risk for the development of multiple sclerosis (▶ Fig. 8.14 and ▶ Fig. 8.15).

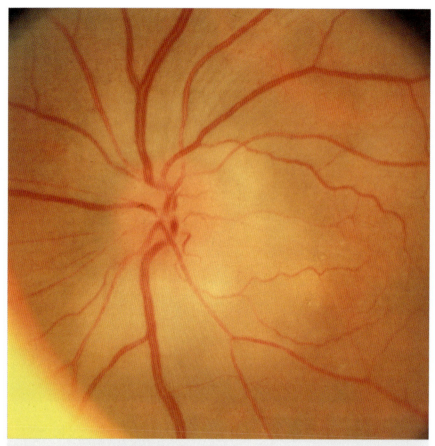

Fig. 8.13 Left optic neuritis secondary to sarcoidosis. The left optic nerve head is elevated inferiorly (granuloma). Note the yellow infiltrate elevating the vessels.

Optic Neuritis in Children

As in adults, optic neuritis is often the first sign of multiple sclerosis in children. Infectious causes are also common. Bilateral optic neuritis is also more common in children than in adults. Children with acute optic neuritis are usually evaluated and treated similarly to adults.

8.5 Ischemic Optic Neuropathies

Ischemic optic neuropathies are the most common acute optic neuropathies in patients over 50 years of age; they can rarely occur in younger patients, in whom they must be differentiated from other causes of optic neuropathies such as optic neuritis. The term *ischemic optic neuropathy* is used to refer to all presumed ischemic causes of optic neuropathy.

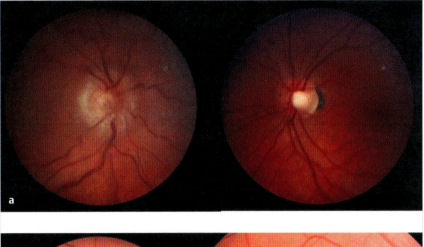

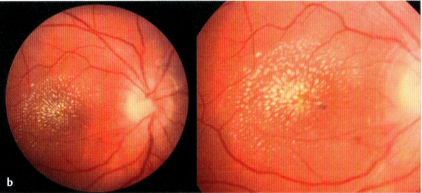

Fig. 8.14 (a) Neuroretinitis in the right eye, 1 week after visual loss. The right optic nerve is swollen, and there is some peripapillary edema. (b) Neuroretinitis with macular star, 2 weeks later (same patient). There are exudates involving the macula (shaped like a star because they are located in the outer plexiform layer).

8.5.1 Clinical Anatomy

The posterior ciliary arteries provide the blood supply to the optic nerve (short posterior ciliary arteries to the optic nerve head and long posterior ciliary arteries to the retrobulbar optic nerve). They originate from the ophthalmic artery. These are small arteries that may be affected by several local disorders, such as atherosclerosis and vasculitis. Emboli do not usually reach these arteries (▶ Fig. 8.16).

Because of the anatomy of the posterior ciliary arteries, optic nerve ischemia often results in superior (more often) or inferior segmental optic nerve atrophy. There is pallor affecting only the superior or inferior half of the optic nerve. This explains why altitudinal defects are common with ischemic optic neuropathies. Superior segmental optic atrophy results in an inferior altitudinal defect (▶ Fig. 8.17).

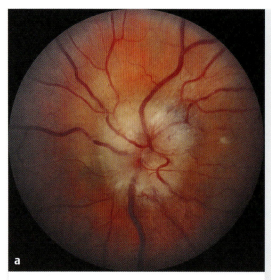

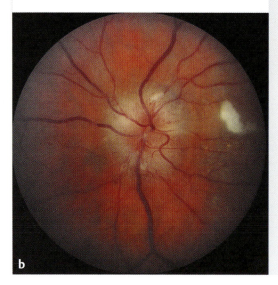

Fig. 8.15 (a) Left optic neuritis with neuroretinitis related to cat scratch disease. A few days after visual loss, the optic nerve is swollen, and there are whitish exudates. (b) Same patient, 2 weeks later. The optic nerve head edema has spontaneously improved, but the retinal lesions have increased, and a macular star is developing.

Pearls

Although ischemic optic neuropathies are considered the equivalent of a "stroke of the optic nerve," they cannot be directly compared with cerebral infarctions. The causes and mechanisms of ischemic optic neuropathies are different, and the workup of a patient with an ischemic optic neuropathy is not the same as that for patients with a retinal or cerebral infarction.

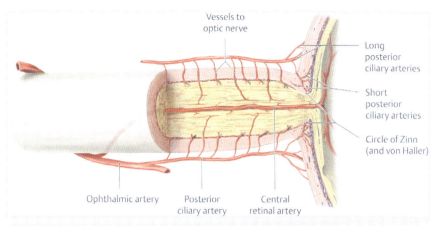

Fig. 8.16 Blood supply to the optic nerve. (From Schuenke M, Schulte E, Schumacher U, Ross LM, Lamperti ED, Voll M. THIEME Atlas of Anatomy, Head and Neuroanatomy. Stuttgart, Germany: Thieme; 2007. Illustration by Karl Wesker.)

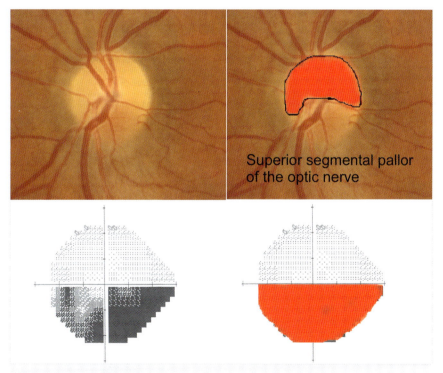

Fig. 8.17 Superior segmental optic nerve pallor corresponding to an inferior altitudinal defect on the Humphrey visual field.

8.5.2 Classification

Ischemic optic neuropathies include *anterior ischemic optic neuropathy* (AION), which is always associated with disc edema, and *posterior ischemic optic neuropathy* (PION), when the optic nerve appears normal acutely. AION is much more common than PION, accounting for 90% of cases of optic nerve ischemia.

Ischemic optic neuropathies are categorized as *nonarteritic ischemic optic neuropathy* and *arteritic ischemic optic neuropathy* (usually in the setting of giant cell arteritis). Patients with giant cell arteritis and ischemic optic neuropathy are in danger of catastrophic, irreversible, bilateral total blindness that may be prevented by prompt treatment with corticosteroid therapy.

Pearls

Nonarteritic AION typically occurs in the setting of a disc-at-risk (small crowded optic nerve with a small cup-to-disc ratio) (▶ Fig. 8.18). The absence of a disc-at-risk in a patient with AION should suggest giant cell arteritis or another underlying disorder.

In a patient with suspected ischemic optic neuropathy, the first step should always be to consider giant cell arteritis.

It is essential to correctly diagnose patients with ischemic optic neuropathies. Indeed, inflammatory optic neuritis is often overdiagnosed in patients with acute optic neuropathy, especially in patients younger than 50. A brain MRI scan is usually obtained in

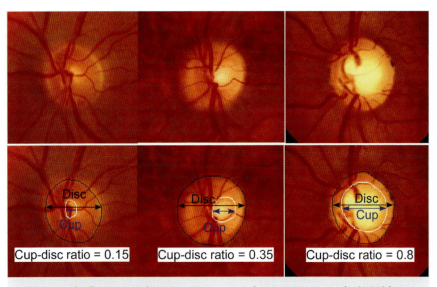

Fig. 8.18 Nearly all patients with nonarteritic anterior ischemic optic neuropathy (AION) have a crowded optic nerve with a small cup-to-disc ratio (also called disc-at-risk). The cup-to-disc ratio is measured during funduscopic examination by estimating the ratio between the central cup diameter and the entire disc diameter. Small cups are congenital and physiologic (left photos). Most people have a cup-to-disc ratio between 0.2 and 0.5 (middle photos). A large cup-to-disc ratio (right photos) is suspicious for glaucoma.

Table 8.3 Clinical characteristics of nonarteritic and arteritic AION compared with those of inflammatory optic neuritis

	Optic neuritis	Nonarteritic AION	Arteritic AION
Age of patients	Younger (<age 45)	Older (>age 50)	Elderly (mostly >age 65)
Laterality	Unilateral	Unilateral	Uni- or bilateral
Visual loss	Rapidly progressive Acuity rarely spared	Acute Acuity variable	Acute Severe visual loss
Pain	Orbital pain frequent with eye movement	Pain infrequent	Pain common
Color vision	Commonly abnormal	Commonly spared if acuity good	Commonly abnormal
Visual field	Central defect	Altitudinal defect	Any defect (severe)
Optic disc: Acute	Normal (two thirds) or disc edema (one third)	Disc edema, small cup-to-disc ratio	Disc edema, pallid Retinal infarction
Optic disc: Late	Temporal pallor	Segmental pallor	Diffuse pallor
Visual prognosis	Good	Variable 15% risk for the other eye within 5 years	Poor risk for the other eye within 10 days
Systemic diseases	Risk of development of multiple sclerosis	HTN, diabetes, GCA to be ruled out	GCA

Abbreviations: AION, anterior ischemic optic neuropathy; GCA, giant cell arteritis; HTN, hypertension.

these patients, who may be found to have one hyperintensity on the T2-weighted images. This inappropriately prompts a diagnosis of optic neuritis and presumed multiple sclerosis with dramatic consequences for the patient's life and treatment. In addition, when ischemic optic neuropathy is missed, then giant cell arteritis may also be overlooked (▶ Table 8.3).

8.5.3 Nonarteritic Anterior Ischemic Optic Neuropathy

Characteristics

Nonarteritic AION (▶ Fig. 8.19) is most common in Caucasians older than age 50. It is characterized by acute, painless monocular loss of vision that may progress over several hours or days. There is a RAPD and optic disc swelling, frequently with peripapillary hemorrhages. Gradually over weeks the optic disc develops pallor, and the edema resolves. Occasionally, disc swelling may be seen prior to visual loss (incipient AION). The typical visual field defect is altitudinal or arcuate, especially inferiorly. Acutely, some patients develop "luxury perfusion" of the ischemic optic nerve head, seen as dilated capillaries on the disc edema, or adjacent to the optic nerve pallor (▶ Fig. 8.20).

Diabetic papillopathy is believed to be an atypical form of AION that usually occurs in young patients with insulin-dependent diabetes. It is distinguished from typical nonarteritic AION by the slight degree (or even absence) of visual loss, the frequency of bilateral involvement (50%), the long duration of disc edema, and the good visual outcome (▶ Fig. 8.21).

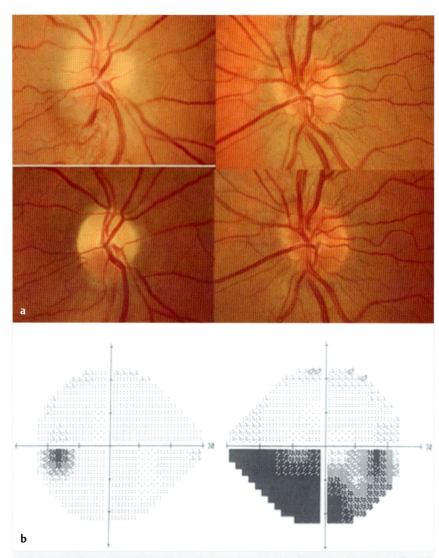

Fig. 8.19 (a) Right nonarteritic anterior ischemic optic neuropathy (AION) in the setting of a crowded optic nerve (disc-at-risk seen in the fellow eye). (Top) At the time of visual loss, there is disc edema with small peripapillary hemorrhages. (Bottom) Two months later, the disc edema has resolved, and there is segmental superior atrophy of the optic nerve (the top of the nerve is pale). (b) Corresponding Humphrey visual field. The left eye is normal. In the right eye, there is an inferior altitudinal defect.

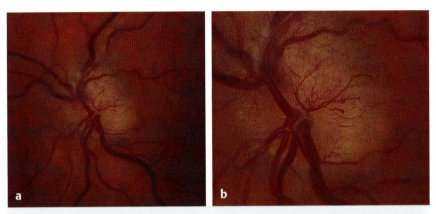

Fig. 8.20 (a, b) "Luxury perfusion" in anterior ischemic optic neuropathy (AION).

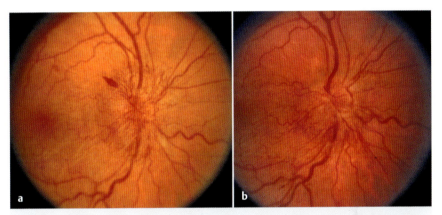

Fig. 8.21 (a) Diabetic papillopathy in a patient with type 2 diabetes mellitus and nonproliferative diabetic retinopathy. There is no visual loss, and the right optic nerve remained chronically swollen for at least 6 months. (b) The second photograph of the same optic nerve was taken 6 months later and shows persistent disc edema with dilated capillaries.

Causes

Although nonarteritic AION results from vascular occlusive disease of small vessels supplying the anterior portion of the optic nerve, its exact cause remains unclear. Anatomical factors such as a congenitally small and crowded optic nerve head with a small cup-to-disc ratio (so-called disc-at-risk) may mechanically contribute to the vascular event. As a disease of the small vessels, nonarteritic AION is not associated with ipsilateral internal carotid artery stenosis, and embolic AION is extremely rare.

Risk Factors

Proposed risk factors for nonarteritic AION include the following:
- Small, crowded disc (disc-at-risk) (see ▶ Fig. 8.18)
- Other abnormalities localized to the disc
  - Optic nerve head drusen
  - Anomalous disc
  - Severe papilledema
- Severe hypotension
  - Operative (▶ Fig. 8.22)
  - Systemic massive hemorrhage
  - Cardiac arrest
  - Renal dialysis
- Severe anemia
- Hypercoagulable disorders
- Radiation optic neuropathy
- Acute intraocular hypertension (during ocular surgery, after an intravitreal injection of steroids, or during an attack of angle-closure glaucoma)
- Vascular risk factors for atherosclerosis are commonly found in AION patients.

Pearls

Nonarteritic AION is not an embolic disorder. Evaluation of the internal carotid artery is not indicated in isolated, typical AION. There is no definite increased risk of cerebrovascular disease in the population of patients with AION, but vascular risk factors are common and should be controlled.

In rare cases, AION may occur in a patient with optic nerve head drusen or papilledema. The drusen or the papilledema makes the optic nerve head more crowded and may "choke" the optic nerve head, which becomes ischemic (▶ Fig. 8.23). Medications, such as amiodarone, may induce an optic neuropathy often indistinguishable from AION.

Natural History

Up to 50% of patients retain visual acuity of 20/60 or better. Recurrences in the same eye are rare (< 5%). Subsequent involvement of the fellow eye is about 15% at 5 years in patients with a disc-at-risk.

Treatment

There is no established treatment for nonarteritic AION. The clinician's primary role is to exclude giant cell arteritis, control vascular risk factors, treat anemia, and prevent hypotension (e.g., in the setting of dialysis).

8.5.4 Nonarteritic Posterior Ischemic Optic Neuropathy

Characteristics

Nonarteritic PION (▶ Fig. 8.24) is characterized by acute, painless monocular loss of vision that may progress over several hours or days. There is a RAPD. The optic disc is

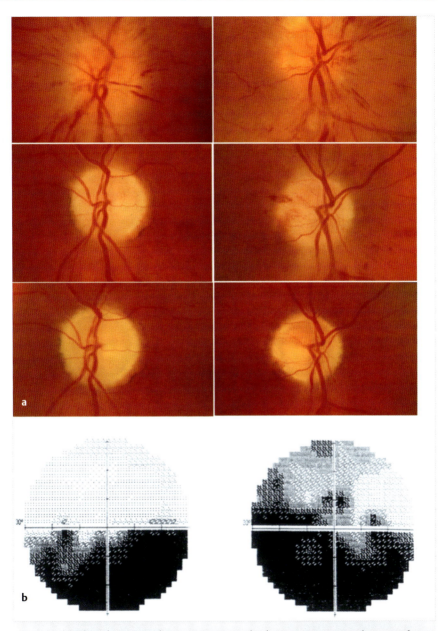

Fig. 8.22 (a) Bilateral anterior ischemic optic neuropathy during coronary artery bypass graft. (Top) Bilateral optic nerve edema with splinter hemorrhages. (Middle) One month later, most hemorrhages have resolved, and the edema is improved. (Bottom) Two months later, there is bilateral optic atrophy. The visual function did not improve. (b) Humphrey visual field test 2 months after visual loss. There is diffuse depression in the right eye (on the right) and an inferior altitudinal defect in the left eye (on the left). Visual acuity is 20/400 in the right eye and 20/40 in the left eye.

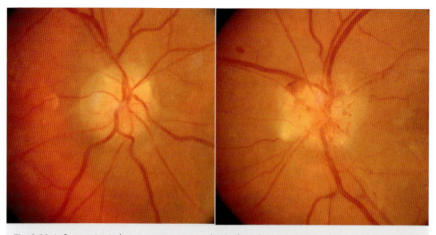

Fig. 8.23 Left anterior ischemic optic neuropathy (right-side image) in a patient with optic nerve head drusen. The drusen are seen in both eyes. There is disc edema with small hemorrhages in the left eye.

normal, initially. Gradually, over 4 to 6 weeks, the optic disc develops pallor. The typical visual field defect is altitudinal or arcuate, especially inferiorly.

Diagnosis and Causes

Nonarteritic PION is extremely rare and may occur during lengthy spinal and cardiac surgery or in patients with acute systemic hypotension. It is usually a diagnosis of exclusion made only after compression of the posterior optic nerve is ruled out by a good-quality MRI scan of the orbits with contrast, along with an extensive systemic workup looking for an underlying systemic inflammatory disorder. Non operative PION in patients older than age 50 is usually indicative of giant cell arteritis.

Risk Factors

Presumed risk factors for nonarteritic PION include the following:
- Operative
  - Spine (prone; long duration)
  - Coronary artery bypass
- Severe hypotension
  - Systemic hemorrhage
  - Cardiac arrest
  - Renal dialysis
- Severe anemia
- Hypercoagulable disorders
- Radiation optic neuropathy

8.5.5 Radiation Optic Neuropathy

Radiation optic neuropathy is a subacute optic neuropathy in patients previously treated with radiation therapy to the brain, skull base, or orbit. It is most common in

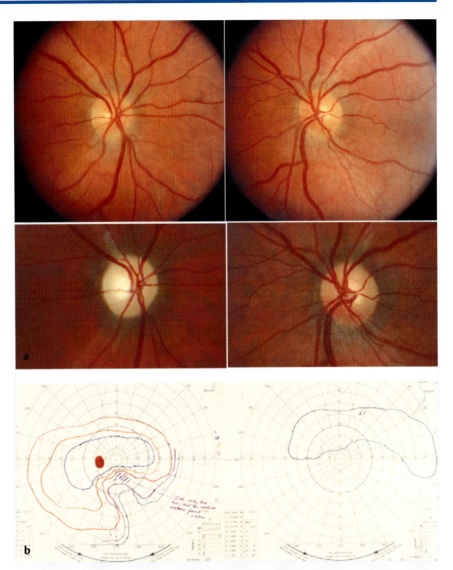

Fig. 8.24 (a) Bilateral posterior ischemic optic neuropathy (PION) during spinal surgery. The patient underwent uneventful prolonged multilevel spinal fusion in the prone position. He awoke with severe visual loss in the right eye and mild visual loss in the left eye. The fundus was normal acutely (top), and pupils were sluggish in response to light, suggesting bilateral PION. Two months later (bottom), there is bilateral optic nerve pallor worse on the right. (b) Goldmann visual fields obtained 2 months after visual loss in the same patient showing a remaining superior island of vision in the right eye and an incomplete altitudinal defect in the left eye. Visual acuity is count fingers in the right eye and 20/25 in the left eye.

patients with skull base tumors or with pituitary tumors and craniopharyngiomas (in whom radiation was administered close to the optic nerve or chiasm). It is thought to be an ischemic disorder of the optic nerve from radiation-induced vasculopathy.

Radiation optic neuropathy may develop a few months to years after radiation. It is characterized by rapidly progressive, painless loss of vision that is most often posterior (no disc edema). MRI shows marked enhancement of the affected optic nerve. The prognosis is poor, and there is currently no treatment with proven benefit (steroids and hyperbaric oxygen are sometimes tried, with only anecdotal success).

8.5.6 Arteritic Anterior and Posterior Ischemic Optic Neuropathy

AION is the most common ophthalmic manifestation of giant cell arteritis, and giant cell arteritis is the most common cause of PION (see Chapter 20).

> **Pearls**
>
> Suspect and rule out giant cell arteritis in all patients older than age 50 presenting with an ischemic optic neuropathy (ION).

Characteristics

Arteritic ischemic optic neuropathy is most often seen in older Caucasian patients, typically in their 70 s and 80 s. It is usually associated with systemic symptoms, such as headache, scalp tenderness, jaw claudication, polymyalgia rheumatica, fatigue, and weight loss. However, visual loss can be the only manifestation of the disease (so-called occult forms of giant cell arteritis).

Visual loss in arteritic ION is usually severe, with acuities reduced to no light perception, light perception only, or hand motion. It is often bilateral and can be associated with a concurrent retinal or choroidal infarction. Visual loss may be preceded by recurrent episodes of transient monocular visual loss or transient diplopia.

Diagnosis

Elevation of erythrocyte sedimentation rate (ESR) and C-reactive protein (CRP) is highly suggestive of the disease. The diagnosis is proven by finding granulomatous inflammation with giant cells and disruption of the internal elastic lamina on biopsy of a superficial temporal artery. In the absence of treatment, vision deteriorates, and there is a high risk of involvement of the second eye within days or weeks.

In arteritic AION, the visual loss is profound. The optic nerve appears pale, even acutely, at the time of visual loss. The peripapillary retina is often pallid, suggesting associated choroidal and retinal ischemia. Cotton wool spots are common and indicate diffuse ocular ischemia when associated with AION (▶ Fig. 8.25).

Causes

Causes of arteritic AION and PION are giant cell arteritis and systemic vasculitis other than giant cell arteritis, such as systemic lupus erythematosus, periarteritis nodosa, and Churg–Strauss syndrome.

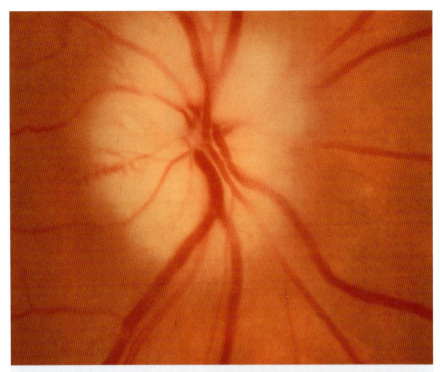

Fig. 8.25 Arteritic anterior ischemic optic neuropathy with pallid swelling at the time of visual loss.

Treatment

Arteritic AION and PION require emergency treatment to prevent complete blindness. Systemic corticosteroid therapy should be instituted immediately upon presumed diagnosis and should not be delayed awaiting results of the temporal artery biopsy (see Chapter 20).

8.6 Compressive and Infiltrative Optic Neuropathies

Various lesions may compress or infiltrate the intraorbital, intracranial, or prechiasmal optic nerves. Anterior or large intraorbital lesions often produce optic disc swelling (▶ Fig. 8.26), whereas intracranial, intracanalicular, and posterior orbital compressive lesions typically do not produce disc swelling.

8.6.1 Characteristics

The clinical presentation varies based on the type and location of the mass:
- Progressive unilateral optic neuropathy (progressive visual loss with abnormal color vision, visual field defect, and optic disc pallor or disc edema)
- Intracranial lesions in the region of the chiasm that may produce vision loss in both eyes (bilateral optic neuropathies, bitemporal hemianopia, junctional scotoma)

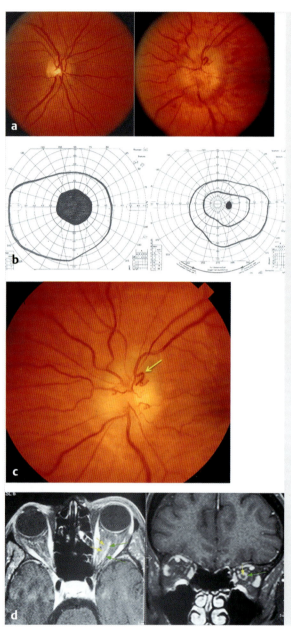

Fig. 8.26 (a) Left optic nerve sheath meningioma (on the right) with optic disc edema. (b) Left central scotoma on Goldmann visual fields (on the left). (c) A few months later, the left optic nerve is pale with residual mild disc edema and more obvious optociliary shunt vessels (*arrow*). (d) T1-weighted axial (left) and coronal (right) magnetic resonance imaging of the orbits with fat suppression and with contrast showing the left optic nerve sheath meningioma. There is enhancement of the optic nerve sheath (*green arrow*), whereas the optic nerve itself (*yellow arrow*) does not enhance.

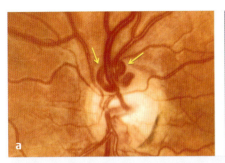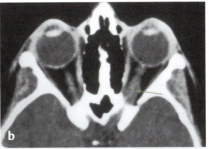

Fig. 8.27 (a) Left optic nerve sheath meningioma. The optic nerve is pale temporally, and there are optociliary shunt vessels superiorly (*arrows*). (b) Axial computed tomography of the orbits with contrast showing a left optic nerve sheath meningioma (*arrow*).

- Usually, no pain with eye movements
- Headache if raised intracranial pressure (large tumor, hydrocephalus) or involvement of branches of the trigeminal nerve (cavernous sinus)
- Proptosis and diplopia common in orbital lesions
- Cranial nerve palsies common in lesions extending into the cavernous sinus

Optociliary shunt vessels may develop as a result of optic nerve compression (▶ Fig. 8.26 and ▶ Fig. 8.27).

The optic nerve may also be compressed or infiltrated by neoplasm (▶ Fig. 8.28, ▶ Fig. 8.29, ▶ Fig. 8.30, ▶ Fig. 8.31, ▶ Fig. 8.32, ▶ Fig. 8.33, ▶ Fig. 8.34, ▶ Fig. 8.35) or by an inflammatory process, such as orbital inflammatory pseudotumor or thyroid eye disease (see ▶ Fig. 8.31).

Cupping of the optic nerves is not uncommon in chronic compression. There is pallor of the remaining rim, unlike in glaucomatous nerve cupping, in which the cups are large with retained pink rims (▶ Fig. 8.30).

8.6.2 Causes

Causes of compressive optic neuropathy include the following:
- Neoplastic
  - Optic nerve sheath meningioma
  - Intraorbital tumor (hemangioma, lymphangioma, metastasis, etc.)
  - Sphenoid meningioma
  - Pituitary tumor
  - Craniopharyngioma
- Non-neoplastic
  - Thyroid eye disease
  - Orbital pseudotumor
  - Orbital hemorrhage
  - Paget disease
  - Fibrous dysplasia
  - Ophthalmic artery aneurysm
  - Ectatic internal carotid artery

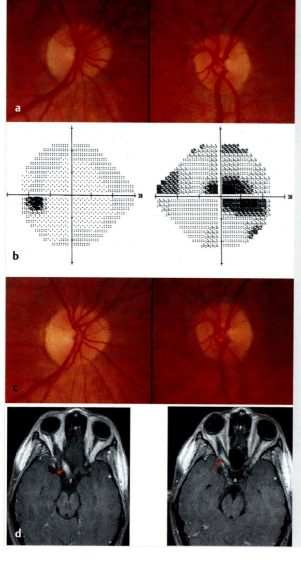

Fig. 8.28 (a) Pilocytic astrocytoma involving the right optic nerve with rapidly progressive painless right optic neuropathy. A few weeks after visual loss, the right optic nerve is only very mildly pale. (b) Humphrey visual fields showing a central scotoma in the right eye. (c) More pronounced right optic nerve pallor 2 months later (on the left). (d) Axial T1-weighted magnetic resonance imaging of the orbits with contrast. The right optic nerve is enlarged and is enhancing in its intraorbital and intracranial portions (*arrows*).

Causes of infiltrative optic neuropathy (▶ Table 8.4):

- Neoplastic
  - Optic nerve glioma
  - Metastatic carcinoma
  - Nasopharyngeal carcinoma and other contiguous tumors
  - Lymphoma
  - Leukemia
  - Meningeal carcinomatosis
- Non-neoplastic
  - Sarcoidosis

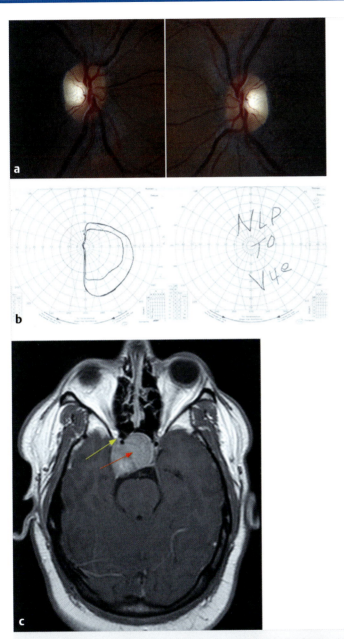

Fig. 8.29 (a) Bilateral progressive visual loss with optic nerve pallor from optic nerve compression. The right eye (on the left) is "no light perception," and the left eye (on the right) sees 20/80. (b) Goldmann visual field showing no response in the right eye and a dense temporal defect respecting the vertical meridian in the left eye, suggesting a lesion of the chiasm and right optic nerve. (c) Large pituitary tumor (*red arrow*) compressing the right optic nerve (*yellow arrow*) and the chiasm.

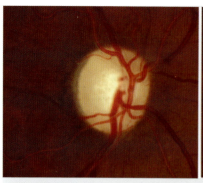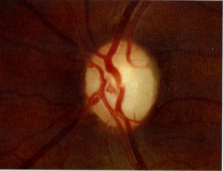

Fig. 8.30 Bilateral optic atrophy and large cup-to-disc ratio in compressive optic neuropathies from a craniopharyngioma.

Pearls

The diagnosis of compressive optic neuropathy is confirmed by imaging. However, tumors compressing the anterior visual pathways may be missed on routine brain CT or MRI. Dedicated views of the orbits, the sella turcica, or the cavernous sinus are necessary and should be obtained based on clinical suspicion. MRI with contrast is preferred.

8.6.3 Diagnosis

In most cases, a presumed diagnosis of compressive or infiltrative optic neuropathy is made based on clinical presentation and neuroimaging. A biopsy is the only way to obtain a definite diagnosis, but it is rarely possible in optic nerve tumors or optic nerve sheath meningiomas because optic nerve biopsy usually results in permanent visual loss. In many of these cases, treatment is based on the presumed diagnosis.

Optic nerve sheath meningiomas arise from the dural sheath of the intraorbital optic nerve. This tumor occurs mostly in middle-aged women who present with unilateral, painless, progressive loss of vision in one eye. Episodes of transient monocular visual loss are common. The optic disc is often already pale at the time of diagnosis, and it may be swollen. There may be optociliary shunt vessels on the optic disc (dilated veins resulting from chronic central retinal vein compression) (see ▶ Fig. 8.26 and ▶ Fig. 8.27). Imaging often misses optic nerve sheath meningiomas, which can be difficult to visualize, especially if there are no dedicated orbital images with fat suppression and contrast. Without treatment, the vision deteriorates, and the tumor may even extend intracranially through the optic canal. However, its progression is very slow, and treatment is based on the amount of visual loss and the size of the tumor. Prognosis is mostly based on the type and location of the tumor, as well as the duration of visual loss. Vision often improves (at least partially) after treatment.

Pilocytic astrocytoma and optic nerve glioma are more common and more benign in children than in adults (see ▶ Fig. 8.28). Pituitary tumors are the most common cause of compressive optic neuropathy (see ▶ Fig. 8.29).

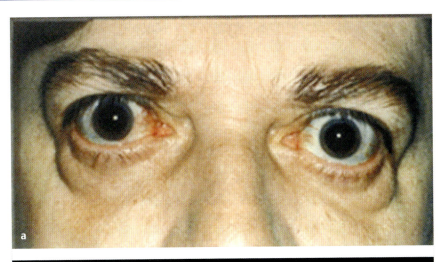

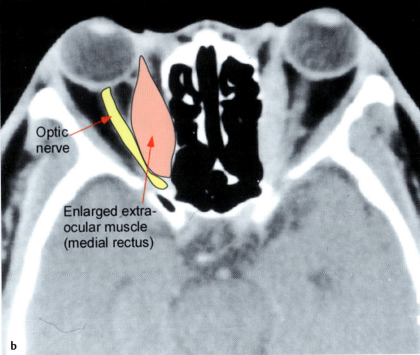

Fig. 8.31 (a) Thyroid eye disease responsible for bilateral optic neuropathies. There is periorbital edema, proptosis, and lid retraction. (b) Compression of the right optic nerve by an enlarged medial rectus muscle secondary to thyroid eye disease.

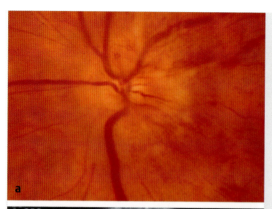

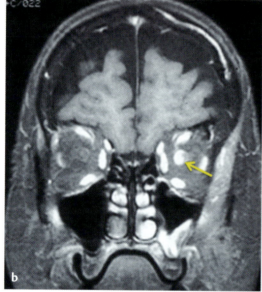

Fig. 8.32 (a) Left optic neuropathy from breast cancer. There is disc edema, with small flame hemorrhages. (b) Coronal T1-weighted magnetic resonance imaging of the orbits with fat suppression and contrast showing enhancement of the left optic nerve (*arrow*).

8.7 Hereditary Optic Neuropathies

Hereditary optic neuropathies usually produce bilateral painless optic neuropathies and permanent visual loss. They should be suspected in any case of optic neuropathy of unknown cause, even in patients without a family history of visual loss. The most common cause of hereditary optic neuropathy is dominant optic atrophy, which is often overlooked and misdiagnosed as glaucoma in adults. Hereditary optic neuropathies may present at any age, although they are most common in children and young adults. The optic neuropathy may occur in isolation or may be part of a systemic metabolic or neurologic degenerative disorder. There is no treatment for these optic neuropathies.

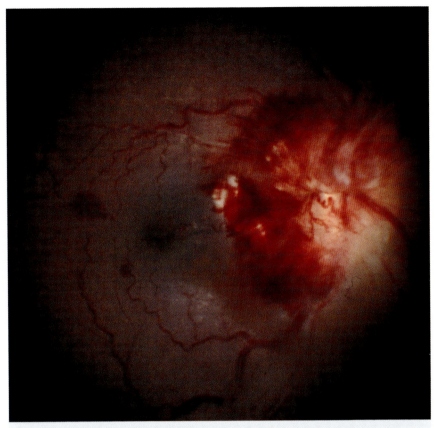

Fig. 8.33 Metastasis (breast cancer) to the optic nerve head. The nerve is elevated, and there are infiltrates in addition to hemorrhages.

8.7.1 Classification of Hereditary Optic Neuropathies

Monosymptomatic Hereditary Optic Neuropathies

There are two types of monosymptomatic hereditary optic neuropathies:
- Leber hereditary optic neuropathy (LHON)
- Dominant (or Kjer) optic atrophy

Hereditary Optic Atrophy with Other Neurologic or Systemic Signs

The main types of hereditary optic atrophy with other neurologic or systemic signs include the following:
- Wolfram/diabetes insipidus, diabetes mellitus, optic atrophy, and deafness (DIDMOAD) syndrome
- Autosomal dominant optic atrophy and deafness
- Autosomal dominant optic atrophy with associated deafness and other neurologic signs
- Behr syndrome

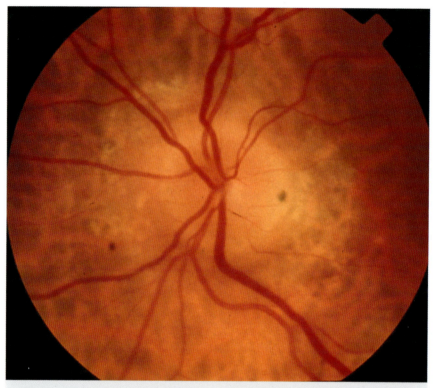

Fig. 8.34 Lymphoma involving the left optic nerve and adjacent choroid. The nerve is elevated, and the choroid appears whitish.

Optic Neuropathy as a Manifestation of Hereditary Degenerative or Developmental Diseases

Hereditary degenerative or developmental diseases associated with optic neuropathy include the following:

- Hereditary ataxias
  - Friedreich ataxia
  - Spinocerebellar ataxias
- Hereditary polyneuropathies
  - Charcot–Marie–Tooth disease
  - Familial dysautonomia (Riley–Day syndrome)
- Hereditary spastic paraplegias
- Hereditary muscular dystrophies
- Storage diseases and cerebral degenerations of childhood
- Mitochondrial diseases of childhood
  - Leigh syndrome
  - Mitochondrial myopathy, encephalopathy, lactic acidosis, and stroke-like episodes (MELAS) syndrome
  - Myoclonic epilepsy and ragged red fibers (MERFF) syndrome
  - Chronic progressive external ophthalmoplegia (CPEO)/Kearns–Sayre syndrome

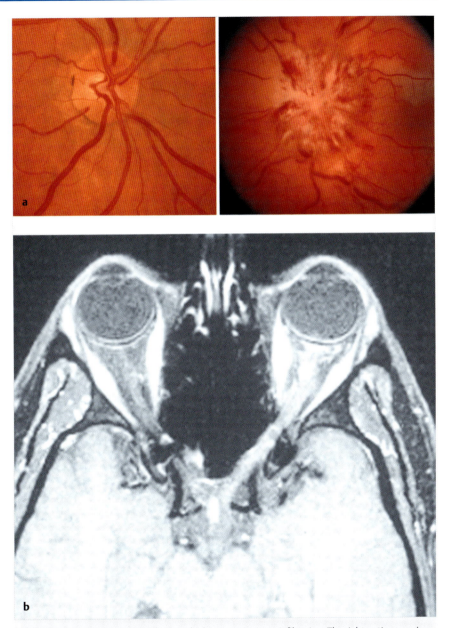

Fig. 8.35 (a) Left optic neuropathy from leukemic optic nerve infiltration. The right optic nerve (on the left) is normal, and the left optic nerve (on the right) is edematous. There are infiltrates and hemorrhages. (b) Axial T1-weighted magnetic resonance imaging of the orbits with contrast and fat suppression showing diffuse enhancement of the left optic nerve from leukemic infiltration.

Table 8.4 Common neoplasms affecting the optic nerves and the chiasm

	Risk group	Clinical features	Imaging	Prognosis	Management
Optic nerve sheath meningioma	Adults Women > men	Slowly progressive monocular visual loss Disc edema with optociliary shunt vessels	Enlargement and enhancement of optic nerve sheath (tram-track sign)	Very slow progression in adults (more aggressive in children)	Based on vision Radiotherapy if vision loss or progression Surgery if intracranial extension or complete vision loss
Optic nerve glioma/ pilocytic astrocytoma	< age 10 Girls = boys Neurofibromatosis type 1 in 30%	Progressive visual loss Proptosis Strabismus nystagmus in young children	Fusiform enlargement of optic nerve; often involves chiasm	Slow progression in children; may be malignant and rapidly progressive in adults	Radiotherapy or chemotherapy if progression Surgery if complete vision loss
Sphenoid wing meningioma	Adults Women > men	Slowly progressive monocular visual loss	Enhancing mass adjacent to the sphenoid wing Calcification on CT	Very slow progression Good visual prognosis if early decompression	Based on tumor size and vision Surgery and radiotherapy
Pituitary tumor	Adults Women = men	Progressive bitemporal visual field defect Progressive mono- or binocular visual loss Endocrine dysfunction	Enhancing sellar mass	Slow progression Good visual prognosis if early decompression Recurrence common	Based on hormonal secretion, tumor size, and vision Endocrine treatment, surgery, radiotherapy

Table 8.4 (continued)

	Risk group	Clinical features	Imaging	Prognosis	Management
Craniopharyngioma	< age 20 age 50–70 Women = men	Progressive bitemporal or homonymous visual field defect Progressive mono- or binocular visual loss Headache, hydrocephalus Papilledema Endocrine dysfunction	Enhancing suprasellar mass with cystic component	Poor visual prognosis Recurrence common	Based on tumor size and vision Endocrine supplementation, surgery, radiotherapy Cyst aspiration CSF shunting often necessary
Germinoma	< Age 30 Women = men	Progressive bitemporal visual field defect Progressive mono- or binocular visual loss Endocrine dysfunction	Enhancing and infiltrating suprasellar mass	Recurrence common	Based on tumor size and vision Endocrine supplementation, surgery, radiotherapy
Metastasis	Rare Young: leukemia and lymphoma Older: breast	Rapidly progressive mono- or binocular visual loss Papilledema (raised ICP) Headaches	Enhancing, infiltrating mass	Poor prognosis	Based on type of cancer, location of tumor Surgery, radiotherapy, chemotherapy

Abbreviations: CSF, cerebrospinal fluid; CT, computed tomography; ICP, intracranial pressure.

8.7.2 Leber Hereditary Optic Neuropathy

LHON (▶ Fig. 8.36) is a maternally inherited mitochondrial disease due to mitochondrial DNA point mutations; that is, the mutation is transmitted by the mother. All children inherit the mutation, but only women (even if unaffected phenotypically) pass it on to the next generation. Men cannot transmit the disease to their children. LHON is a bilateral sequential or simultaneous optic neuropathy that occurs predominantly in otherwise healthy young men, but may affect any gender at any age. Visual acuity typically deteriorates permanently to levels of 20/200 or worse, and visual fields show central or cecocentral defects.

During the acute phase of visual loss, the funduscopic appearance may be normal, or there may be hyperemia and apparent swelling of the optic disc with dilation and tortuosity of the retinal vasculature. Ultimately, the patient will develop optic nerve pallor.

In LHON, the visual loss is most often isolated. It may be associated with cardiac conduction abnormalities, minor neurologic abnormalities, or disease clinically indistinguishable from multiple sclerosis.

Diagnosis is confirmed by genetic analysis (blood test): screening for three primary mutations in the mitochondrial DNA (positions 11778, 14484, and 3460). Not all subjects with the mutation will develop visual loss (about 20–50% of men and about 4–32% of women). The 11778 mutation is the most common.

Some spontaneous recovery of vision may occur in up to 70% of patients with LHON and the 14484 mutation, but in only 4 to 20% of patients with the 11778 mutation.

Pearls

Patients diagnosed with a mitochondrial disorder such as Leber hereditary optic neuropathy should be screened with electrocardiography looking for cardiac conduction abnormalities.

8.7.3 Autosomal Dominant Optic Atrophy (Kjer Disease)

Autosomal dominant optic atrophy (DOA), or Kjer disease, affects both men and women, and 50% of offspring have the mutation (▶ Fig. 8.37). It is characterized by symmetrical, insidious onset of visual loss in the first decade of life. Visual acuity loss is often moderate, and diagnosis is usually delayed (patients lose approximately one line of vision per decade on the Snellen visual acuity chart). Visual loss is variable even within families and ranges from subtle to 20/200. Color vision is abnormal. Visual fields show cecocentral scotomas. There is bilateral temporal pallor of both optic nerves, which often appear cupped. Other neurologic abnormalities are uncommon, but there may be hearing loss in some families and even progressive neurologic dysfunction, including CPEO. The disease is genetically heterogeneous and has been linked to chromosome 3 (most commonly) and chromosome 18. The gene product is a protein necessary for mitochondrial function, making DOA also a "mitochondrial disease," although transmitted via nuclear genes. Genetic screening is available in selected laboratories.

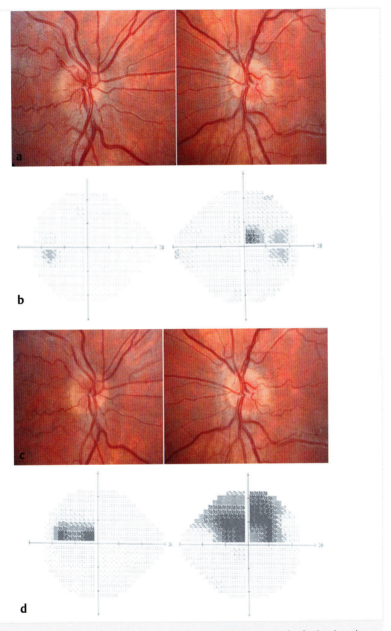

Fig. 8.36 (a) Acute visual loss in the right eye of a 12-year-old boy as a result of Leber hereditary optic neuropathy. The right optic nerve (on the left) is hyperemic with telangiectasias. There is no true disc edema. (b) Humphrey visual fields showing a cecocentral scotoma in the right eye. The left eye is normal. (c) One month later, there is acute visual loss in the left eye of the same boy. Visual acuity is now 20/400 in each eye. (d) Humphrey visual fields showing a new cecocentral scotoma in the left eye. The defect is worse in the right eye.

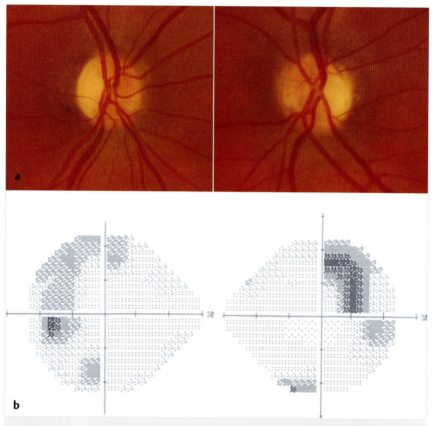

Fig. 8.37 (a) Bilateral optic neuropathies from dominant optic atrophy. Both optic nerves are pale temporally. (b) Humphrey visual fields showing bilateral visual field defects in dominant optic atrophy. The visual field defects mimic a bitemporal hemianopia.

8.8 Toxic and Nutritional Optic Neuropathies

Toxic and nutritional optic neuropathies generally have similar clinical features and may even coexist in the same patient.

8.8.1 Features

Characteristic clinical features include progressive, symmetrical central visual loss; reduced perception of color; and cecocentral scotomas. Acutely, the optic nerve may be normal or may appear slightly swollen. Temporal optic disc pallor is seen at least 6 weeks after the onset of visual loss.

8.8.2 Causes

Causation in many cases is likely multifactorial. In humans, definitively proven cases of optic nerve damage caused by a single recognized toxic agent or a deficiency in a single identified nutrient are rare. In some cases, discontinuation of the agent or vitamin supplementation may result in improvement of visual function. However, visual loss is often irreversible.

Among the suspected toxins linked to optic neuropathies are methanol, ethylene glycol, cobalt, lead, zinc, organic solvents, toluene, tobacco (usually, cigars), ethambutol, amiodarone, linezolid, and disulfiram. Nutritional causes include vitamin B_{12}, folate, and copper deficiencies. Several of the leading types of toxic and nutritional optic neuropathies are described in the following section.

8.8.3 Types

Methanol

Methanol ingestion is the most widely recognized cause of toxic optic neuropathy. It is also most often accidental (mistaken for or added to ethyl alcohol). Methanol-related optic neuropathy is acute, and the optic nerves are usually swollen.

Visual loss from bilateral optic neuropathies is associated with headaches and nausea. Worse visual loss, abdominal pain, respiratory distress, confusion, and, ultimately, coma, and death happen 18 to 48 hours after ingestion. Metabolic acidosis is one of the hallmarks of methanol ingestion.

Ethylene Glycol

Ethylene glycol is the active ingredient in automobile antifreeze. It may be consumed accidentally or in a suicide attempt. It is very toxic to the optic nerves. Symptoms and signs resemble those of methanol intoxication, except for renal insufficiency, which is common with ethylene glycol.

Ethambutol

Ethambutol, an antimycobacterial drug used to treat tuberculosis, is the medication most often implicated in toxic optic neuropathy (▶ Fig. 8.38). Toxicity is usually dose related (develops in patients taking the drugs for a few months—usually at least 2 months, with a mean of 7 months).

Bitemporal visual field defects may reflect early involvement of the chiasm, and color vision is affected early. Visual loss is bilateral and slowly progressive. Visual function may improve after discontinuation of the drug.

Amiodarone

Although it is still debated, there is good evidence that sequential bilateral optic neuropathies may develop in patients treated with amiodarone, an antiarrhythmic agent. Toxicity is dose related and usually occurs in patients who have been treated with it for a few months. It is classically associated with disc edema resembling nonarteritic anterior ischemic optic neuropathy (▶ Fig. 8.39). Visual loss may be subacute or slowly progressive. Visual function may improve after discontinuation of the medication (which can be done only after consulting with the patient's cardiologist).

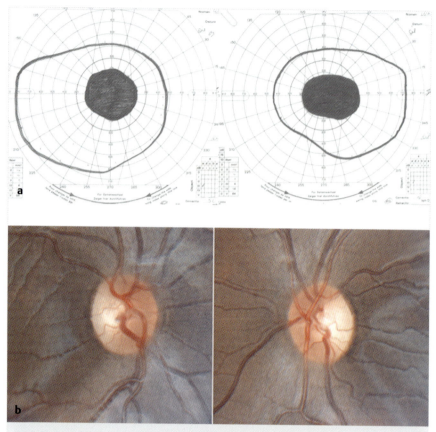

Fig. 8.38 (a) Goldmann visual field showing bilateral cecocentral scotoma in a patient treated with ethambutol for tuberculosis. (b) Bilateral temporal pallor of the optic nerves from ethambutol toxicity.

Pearls

The diagnosis of toxic optic neuropathy is usually a diagnosis of exclusion. Workup ruling out other causes of bilateral optic neuropathies, such as compression, vitamin B_{12} deficiency, and hereditary optic neuropathies, should always be obtained.

Vitamin B_{12} Deficiency

Severe vitamin B_{12} deficiency (usually from impaired absorption) may produce bilateral, slowly progressive optic neuropathies (▶ Fig. 8.40). The optic neuropathies are often the first sign of vitamin B_{12} deficiency and may precede the anemia and other neurologic symptoms and signs.

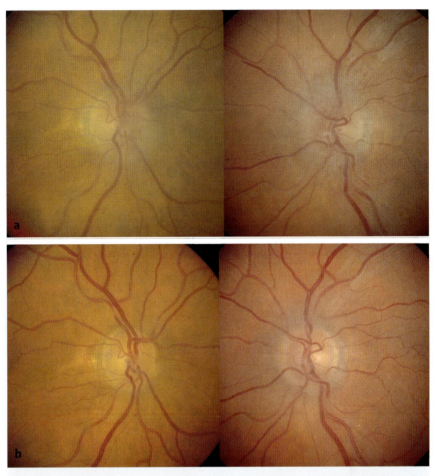

Fig. 8.39 (**a**) Bilateral disc edema (worse in the left eye) in a patient treated with amiodarone for atrial fibrillation who developed visual loss in his left eye. (**b**) One month after discontinuing the amiodarone, the disc edema has resolved and his visual function has improved.

Copper Deficiency

Chronic copper deficiency is very rare and can cause many hematological manifestations, such as myelodysplasia, anemia, leukopenia, and neutropenia, as well as ataxia, peripheral neuropathy, and bilateral optic neuropathies.

Pearls

Always check vitamin B_{12} and copper levels in patients with progressive bilateral visual loss and bilateral optic atrophy.

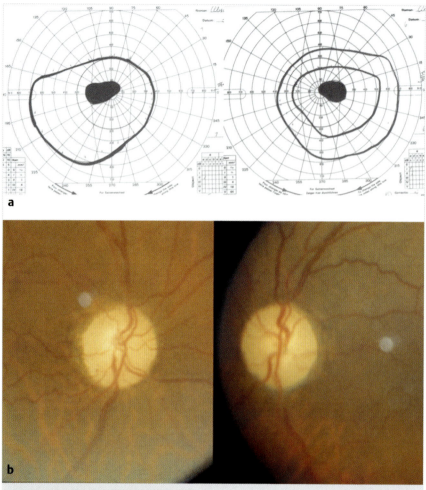

Fig. 8.40 (a) Goldmann visual fields showing bilateral cecocentral scotomas from vitamin B$_{12}$ deficiency. (b) Bilateral optic atrophy.

8.9 Traumatic Optic Neuropathy

Traumatic optic neuropathy is an uncommon but potentially devastating complication of head injury. It should always be suspected in any patient with evidence of optic nerve dysfunction (e.g., otherwise unexplained decreased visual acuity, RAPD, or dyschromatopsia) following head trauma. Because of associated neurologic deficits and other traumatic injuries, the diagnosis is often delayed. However, systematic examination of the pupils in the emergency room (looking for a RAPD) should allow early diagnosis, even in unresponsive patients.

8.9.1 Mechanism

The optic nerve may be injured directly by an orbital foreign body or by a bone fragment in case of orbital fracture (*direct traumatic optic neuropathy*; ▶ Fig. 8.41), or indirectly, as a result of concussive forces to the head, particularly the forehead (*indirect traumatic optic neuropathy*; ▶ Fig. 8.42). The latter causes both a mechanical and an ischemic insult to the optic nerve, likely at the level of the optic canal.

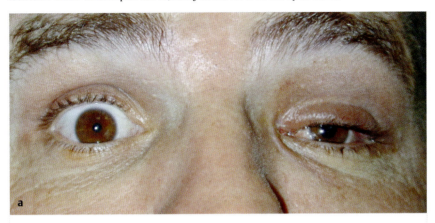

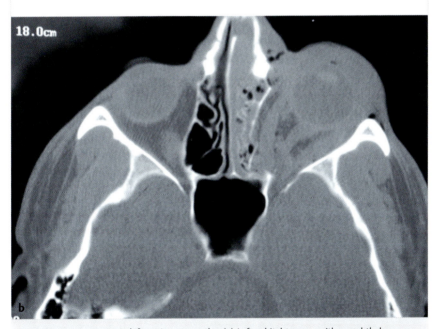

Fig. 8.41 Direct traumatic left optic neuropathy. (a) Left orbital trauma with enophthalmos, impaired motility in the left eye, and profound left visual loss. There is a left relative afferent pupillary defect, and the fundus is normal. (b) Computed tomographic scan of the brain and orbits without contrast (bone window) showing an extensive fracture of the left medial wall of the orbit, involving the optic canal.

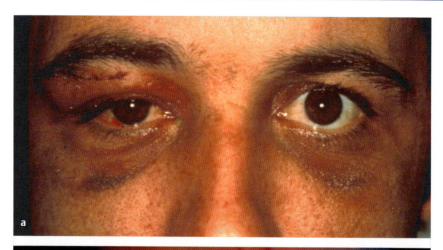

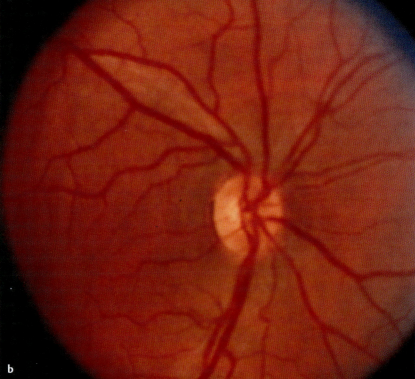

Fig. 8.42 Indirect traumatic right optic neuropathy. (a) Facial trauma with bilateral periorbital ecchymosis and indirect traumatic optic neuropathy. There is visual loss in the right eye, and pupil examination shows a right relative afferent pupillary defect. The fundus is normal. The computed tomographic scan of the brain and orbits is normal. There is no fracture and no orbital foreign body. (b) Mild optic nerve pallor 6 weeks later.

8.9.2 Treatment

Direct traumatic optic neuropathies usually require emergent surgical treatment to decompress the optic nerve and treat the fracture.

The management of indirect traumatic optic neuropathy is controversial. Although visual loss may be devastating and permanent, vision may also recover spontaneously. There is no indication for surgical decompression of the injured optic nerve, and corticosteroids (even very high doses) are not helpful and may even be harmful when administered more than 8 hours after injury. In addition, the use of corticosteroids should be avoided in patients with systemic traumatic injuries and traumatic brain injury who are at risk for infectious complications.

> **Pearls**
>
> Check the visual acuity and the pupils of all trauma patients. If abnormal, request an ophthalmology consultation. Obtain a CT scan of the brain and orbits without contrast and with bone windows.

8.10 Glaucomatous Optic Neuropathy

Chronic open-angle glaucoma is the most common cause of nonacute progressive bilateral optic neuropathy. This disorder is characterized by slowly progressive peripheral visual field loss, elevated intraocular pressures (the normal range is 8–21 mm Hg), and cupping of the optic disc. The diagnosis of open-angle glaucoma generally requires documentation of all three findings.

Because the visual field defects primarily involve the nasal periphery, central visual acuity is preserved until very late in the course of the disease (▶ Fig. 8.43).

> **Pearls**
>
> Low-tension glaucoma is a rare type of glaucoma in which patients with normal intraocular pressure develop a glaucomatous optic neuropathy. It is a diagnosis of exclusion, and other causes of optic neuropathies, particularly compressive, need to be ruled out by neuroimaging.

8.11 Optic Nerve Anomalies

8.11.1 Optic Nerve Head Drusen

Drusen are small, calcific concretions present in the optic nerve of 1 to 2% of the population (▶ Fig. 8.44). Autosomal dominant transmission is suspected in most cases.

Optic nerve head drusen are usually bilateral, but they may be asymmetric. They may be visible on fundus examination in teenagers and in adults (often buried in younger children) and may slowly increase over time. They are often asymptomatic

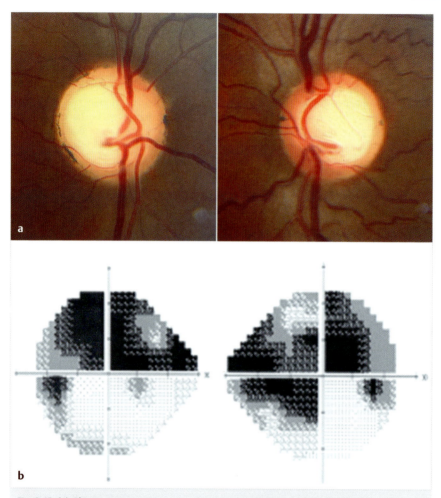

Fig. 8.43 (a) Glaucomatous optic neuropathies. A vertically enlarged cup with nasal displacement of the vessels and the absence of pallor of the retained rim of neural tissue are highly suggestive of glaucoma. (b) Humphrey visual fields showing bilateral nasal defects and constriction from glaucoma. Central visual acuity and color vision are normal until late in the course of the disease.

and discovered during routine fundus examination. Some patients have brief episodes of transient visual obscurations.

The drusen may mimic disc edema when they are buried in the optic nerve head. They may result in peripheral visual field defects, which may worsen slowly over time (optic nerve head drusen usually do not produce central visual loss).

The diagnosis is easy when the drusen are superficial and seen on funduscopic examination. Buried drusen can be seen with autofluorescence imaging of the optic nerves, OCT, B-scan ultrasonography and CT scan of the orbits showing calcifications in the optic nerve heads (see ▶ Fig. 8.44).

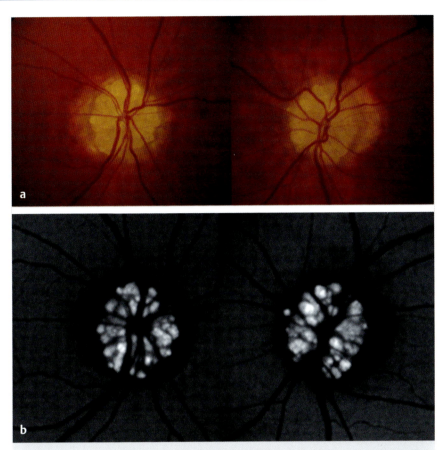

Fig. 8.44 a–e (**a**) Bilateral optic nerve head drusen. Geode-like calcifications are seen at the level of the optic nerve heads. They raise the vessels and may be responsible for small infarctions or axonal compression, resulting in visual field defects. (**b**) Bilateral optic nerve head drusen seen in autofluorescence in the same patient (red-free photo taken by the camera used for fluorescein angiography). (*continued*)

Complications are rare and include acute visual loss from anterior ischemic optic neuropathy (crowded optic nerve head) and acute visual loss from peripapillary choroidal neovascular membrane. There is no treatment for optic nerve head drusen.

Pearls

Incidentally found optic nerve drusen are common and are usually asymptomatic. Symptomatic patients should undergo an evaluation for other causes of optic neuropathies because, in some cases, the optic nerve drusen are a red herring.

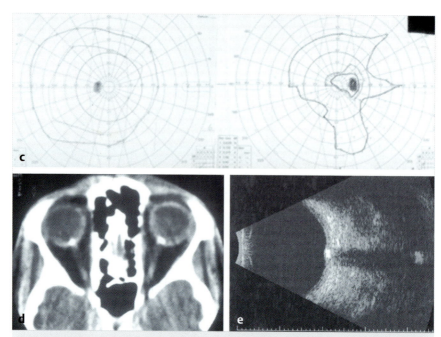

Fig. 8.44 (*continued*) (**c**) Goldmann visual field test showing a constricted visual field in the right eye of a patient with optic nerve drusen. (**d**) Computed tomography of the orbits without contrast showing bilateral optic nerve drusen (calcifications seen as hyperdensities at the level of the optic nerve heads). (**e**) Ultrasound (B-scan) of the eye demonstrating calcified optic nerve head drusen.

8.11.2 Congenital Disc Anomalies

Congenital disc anomalies may be isolated or associated with systemic disorders or malformations. The level of visual loss associated with congenital disc anomalies varies from minimal visual dysfunction to total blindness.

In childhood, the most common presentation of unilateral disc anomaly is strabismus, whereas those with bilateral disc anomalies more frequently present with poor vision or nystagmus. Some may also be diagnosed during adulthood on a routine funduscopic examination.

Optic Nerve Hypoplasia

Optic nerve hypoplasia (▶ Fig. 8.45) is the most common congenital optic nerve anomaly. It is characterized by a small optic nerve (reduced diameter), sometimes with peripapillary halo (double ring sign), and may be unilateral or bilateral.

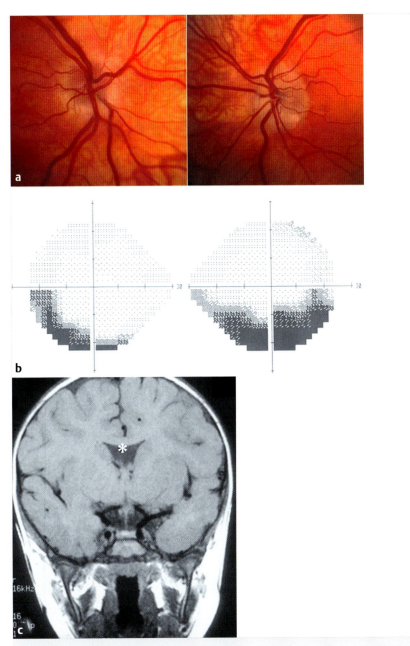

Fig. 8.45 (a) Bilateral optic nerve head hypoplasia, worse in the right eye (left image), in a young adult whose mother was diabetic. (b) Humphrey visual fields showing bilateral inferior defects corresponding to the more pronounced hypoplasia of the superior half of the discs. (c) Coronal T1-weighted brain magnetic resonance imaging showing the absence of septum pellucidum (*) in a patient with septo-optic dysplasia and bilateral optic nerve hypoplasia.

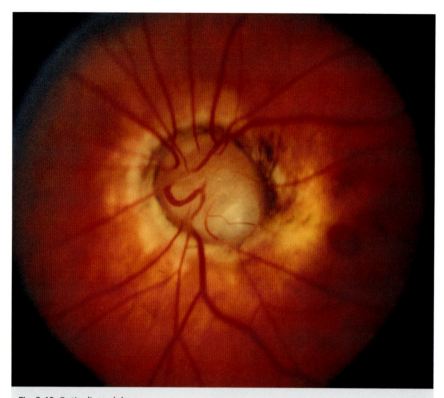

Fig. 8.46 Optic disc coloboma.

Classic systemic and teratogenic associations with optic nerve hypoplasia include the following:
- Midline developmental abnormalities
  - Septo-optic dysplasia (de Morsier syndrome): absent septum pellucidum, thin corpus callosum, hypopituitarism with pituitary ectopia
- Albinism, aniridia, Duane syndrome, and numerous other congenital ocular syndromes
- Maternal diabetes
- Fetal alcohol syndrome
- Drugs or substances taken by the mother during pregnancy, such as phenytoin, quinine, phencyclidine hydrochloride (PCP), lysergic acid diethylamide (LSD), and alcohol

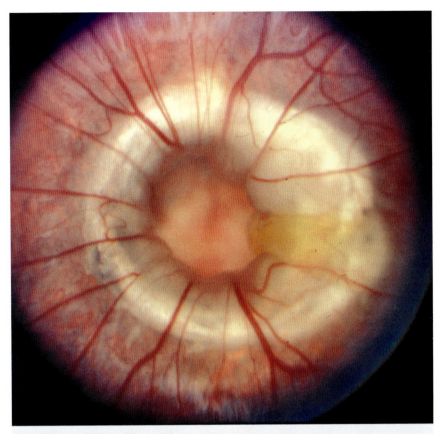

Fig. 8.47 Morning glory disc anomaly.

Optic Disc Coloboma

Optic disc coloboma is faulty closure of the embryonic fetal fissure of the optic stalk and cup. It is isolated or associated with coloboma of the iris, retina, and choroid. A rare association with forebrain abnormalities (basal encephalocele) warrants routine neuro-imaging of patients with colobomas. Characteristic features of the optic disc coloboma (▶ Fig. 8.46) include excavation within the optic disc, asymmetric defect, vision varying based on size and location of the coloboma within the disc, and minimal peripapillary pigmentary changes. Retinal vasculature is normal.

Morning Glory Disc Anomaly

The mechanism behind "morning glory" disc anomaly is debated, but it results at least partially from faulty closure of the embryonic fetal fissure of the optic stalk and cup. Its association with transsphenoidal basal encephaloceles warrants routine neuroimaging of patients with such anomalies. Characteristic features of morning glory disc anomaly (▶ Fig. 8.47) include congenital funnel-shaped excavation of the posterior pole of the

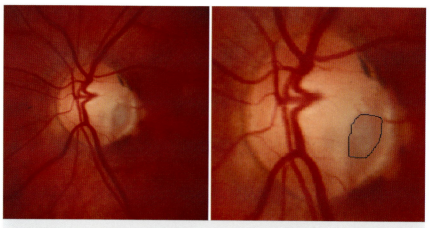

Fig. 8.48 Pit of the inferotemporal edge of the left optic nerve (outlined in enlarged image on the right).

fundus (the optic disc lies within the excavation), severe peripapillary pigmentary changes, and anomalous straightening of the retinal vasculature.

Optic Pit

Optic pit (▶ Fig. 8.48) results from faulty closure of the embryonic fetal fissure of the optic stalk and cup (same as coloboma, which is a more severe variant). It is characterized by a small excavation of the neuroretinal rim of the optic disc and usually involves the inferotemporal portion of the optic nerve. The missing area is often associated with an arcuate visual field defect. Optic pit may be associated with serous detachment of the macula, causing decreased visual acuity.

Tilted Disc Anomaly

Tilted disc anomaly (▶ Fig. 8.49) arises when the optic nerve enters the sclera at an oblique angle. It is common in high myopes and often results in relative bitemporal visual field defects that do not respect the vertical meridian.

Myelinated Nerve Fibers

The optic nerve fibers behind the lamina cribrosa are normally myelinated. Usually, myelin does not enter the eye. Intraocular myelination of retinal nerve fibers is seen in < 1% of the population (▶ Fig. 8.50). Visual field defects are seen only with extensive intraocular myelination, usually in the form of an enlarged blind spot when the myelination surrounds the optic disc.

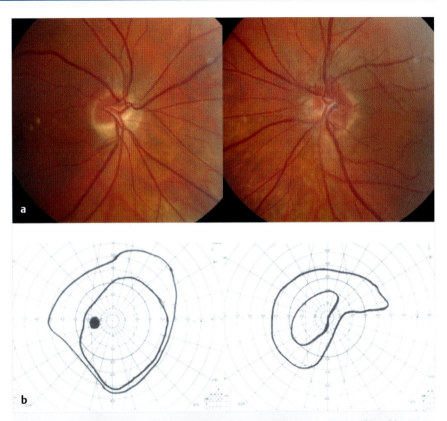

Fig. 8.49 (a) Tilted optic nerves (worse on the right) in a highly myopic patient. (b) Goldmann visual fields showing a bitemporal visual field defect that does not respect the vertical meridian.

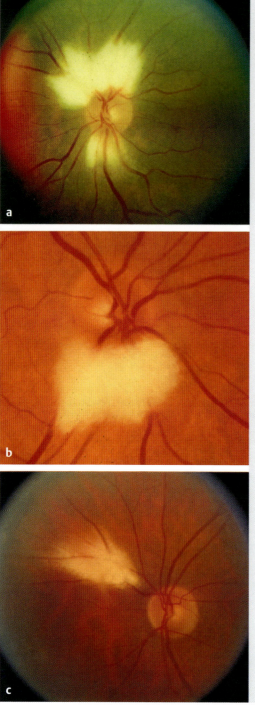

Fig. 8.50 (a) Myelinated nerve fibers. (b) Myelinated nerve fibers below the optic nerve. (c) Myelinated nerve fibers distant from the disc.

9 Disc Edema

Edema of the optic nerve head, or *disc edema*, is a nonspecific term describing localized swelling anterior to the lamina cribrosa (▶ Fig. 9.1).

9.1 Mechanisms of Optic Nerve Edema

Mechanisms of optic nerve edema include the following:
1. Local optic nerve injury, such as from inflammation (anterior optic neuritis or papillitis), ischemia (anterior ischemic optic neuropathy), fluctuations in intraocular pressure (high, as in acute glaucoma, or low, as in ocular hypotony), and toxicity
2. Blockage of retrograde axonal transport from optic nerve compression (optic nerve tumor or orbital mass) and raised intracranial pressure (papilledema)

9.2 Differentiating True Disc Edema from Pseudoedema

Differentiating true optic nerve head edema from pseudoedema is essential (▶ Table 9.1, ▶ Fig. 9.2 and ▶ Fig. 9.3). In most cases, pseudoedema appearance results from a congenital anomaly of the optic nerve and does not require any workup, whereas true disc edema is associated with numerous concerning disorders.

9.3 Differential Diagnosis of Disc Edema

Disc elevation without true swelling:
- Optic disc anomalies
  - Myelinated nerve fibers (▶ Fig. 8.50 and ▶ Fig. 9.4)
  - Drusen (▶ Fig. 8.44 and ▶ Fig. 9.5)
  - Tilted disc (▶ Fig. 8.49)
  - Crowded disc
- Optic disc infiltration
- Leber hereditary optic neuropathy

True disc swelling:
- Elevated intracranial pressure (papilledema) (▶ Fig. 9.6)
- Inflammatory optic neuropathy (▶ Fig. 9.7)
  - Demyelinating
  - Sarcoidosis or other inflammatory diseases
  - Infectious
- Neuroretinitis
- Vascular optic neuropathy
  - Anterior ischemic optic neuropathy (▶ Fig. 9.8)
    – Nonarteritic
    – Arteritic
  - Diabetic papillopathy
  - Central retinal vein occlusion (▶ Fig. 9.9)
  - Carotid-cavernous fistula
  - Malignant systemic hypertension (▶ Fig. 9.10)

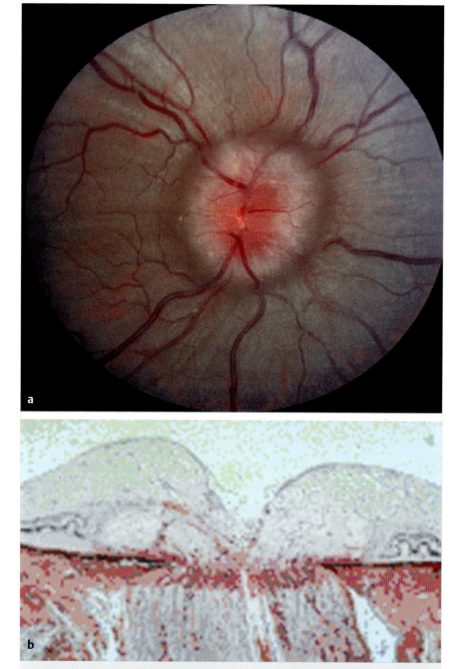

Fig. 9.1 (a) Optic nerve swelling in the right eye. The disc margins are blurry, and there is no central cup. (b) Sagittal section of a swollen optic nerve.

Table 9.1 Characteristics of true disc edema versus pseudoedema

True disc edema (▶ Fig. 9.2)	Pseudoedema (▶ Fig. 9.3)
Elevated optic nerve	Elevated optic nerve
Margins blurry	Sharp margins
Vessels obscured	Vessels not obscured
Venous dilation and tortuosity	Absence of central cup
Peripapillary hemorrhages and exudates	Anomalous retinal vasculature (arterial branching)
Leakage on fluorescein angiogram	No leakage on fluorescein angiogram

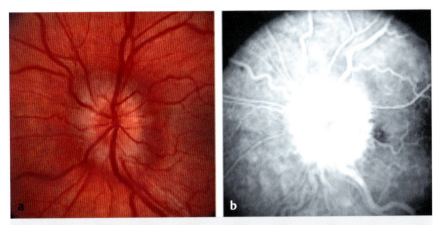

Fig. 9.2 (a) True disc edema with (b) leakage on fluorescein angiography (late phase).

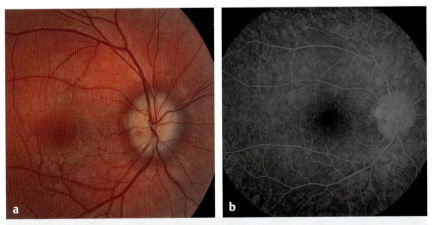

Fig. 9.3 (a) Pseudoedema with (b) no leakage on fluorescein angiography (there is late staining only).

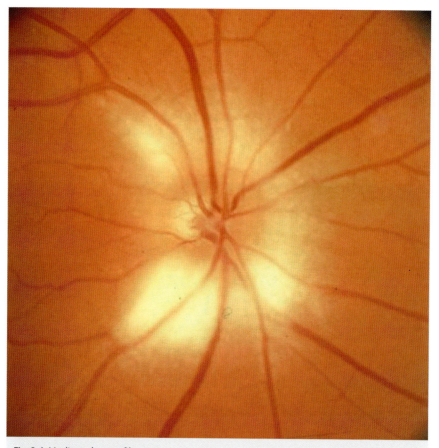

Fig. 9.4 Myelinated nerve fibers.

- Compressive optic neuropathy
  - Neoplastic
    - Meningioma (▶ Fig. 9.11)
    - Hemangioma
    - Lymphangioma
  - Non-neoplastic
    - Thyroid ophthalmopathy
    - Orbital inflammatory pseudotumor
- Infiltrative optic neuropathy
  - Neoplastic
    - Leukemia
    - Lymphoma
    - Glioma
  - Non-neoplastic
    - Sarcoidosis

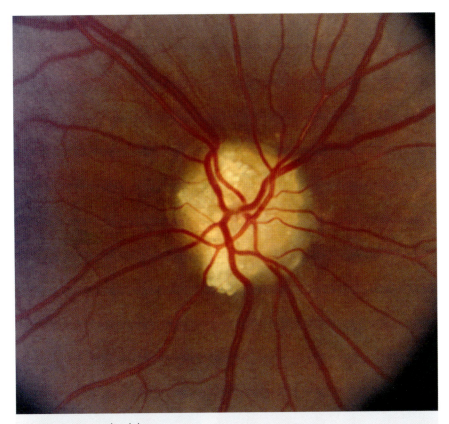

Fig. 9.5 Optic nerve head drusen.

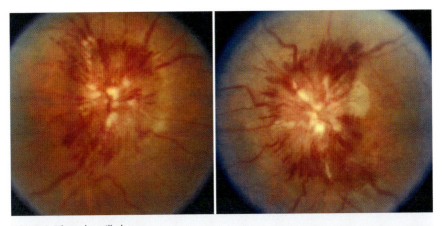

Fig. 9.6 Bilateral papilledema.

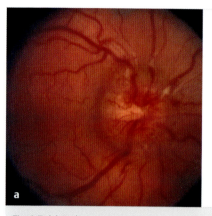
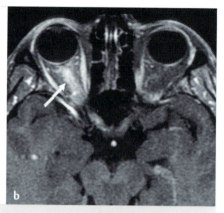

Fig. 9.7 (a) Right anterior optic neuritis with moderate disc edema. (b) Axial T1-weighted magnetic resonance imaging of the orbits with contrast and fat suppression, showing enhancement of the right optic nerve (*arrow*).

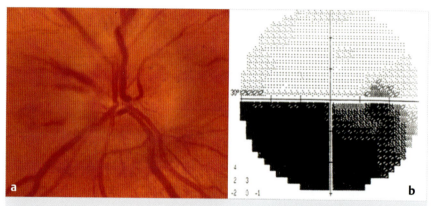

Fig. 9.8 (a) Right anterior ischemic optic neuropathy with mild disc edema and a few peripapillary hemorrhages. (b) Corresponding inferior altitudinal visual field defect on a 30–2 Humphrey visual field test.

- Toxic
- Metabolic/nutritional deficiencies
- Traumatic optic neuropathy
- Intraocular hypotony (low intraocular pressure)

9.4 Evaluation of the Patient with Disc Edema

Once optic disc edema is confirmed, it should be determined whether it is related to an optic nerve disorder (optic neuropathy) or to raised intracranial pressure. *Papilledema* is the term used to describe optic disc edema resulting from raised intracranial pressure (▶ Fig. 9.12). All other optic disc edema is termed disc edema or swollen optic

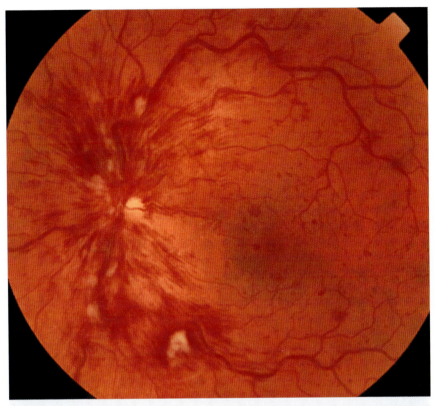

Fig. 9.9 Central retinal vein occlusion with disc edema and numerous retinal hemorrhages distant from the swollen optic nerve.

nerve. ▶ Table 9.2 compares the characteristics of disc edema from anterior optic neuropathy with those from raised intracranial pressure.

The mechanisms responsible for raised intracranial pressure and papilledema are as follows:

- Hydrocephalus (▶ Fig. 9.13)
- Intracranial mass
  - Tumor, abscess (▶ Fig. 9.14)
  - Intracerebral hemorrhage
  - Subdural/epidural hemorrhage
  - Large vascular malformation
- Meningeal process
  - Infectious
  - Inflammatory
  - Neoplastic
- Increased venous pressure
- Cerebral venous thrombosis
- Idiopathic intracranial hypertension

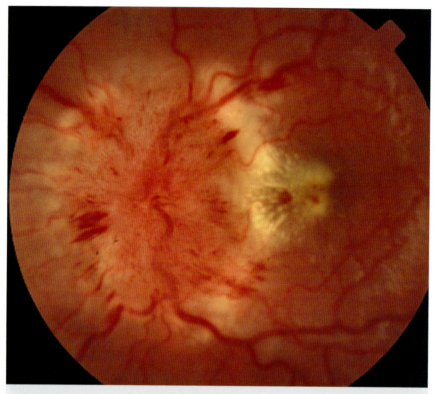

Fig. 9.10 Malignant systemic hypertension with severe disc edema, retinal hemorrhages, and retinal exudates.

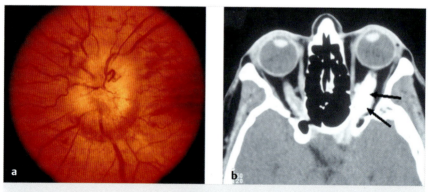

Fig. 9.11 (a) Left optic nerve sheath meningioma with disc edema and shunt vessels. (b) Axial computed tomography of the orbits with contrast showing enhancement along the left optic nerve (*arrows*).

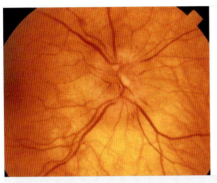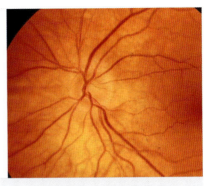

Fig. 9.12 Bilateral asymmetric (right eye worse than left) mild papilledema from raised intracranial pressure.

Most disorders producing raised intracranial pressure are life-threatening emergencies. The finding of papilledema should prompt an immediate workup, ideally in a specialized center with up-to-date neuroimaging, as well as neurologic and ophthalmological consultations.

The workup should include the following:

- Looking for an underlying neurologic process
- Careful evaluation of the visual function (visual acuity and formal visual field testing), as papilledema can result in permanent visual loss from secondary optic atrophy
- Checking blood pressure (severe systemic hypertension or malignant hypertension may produce bilateral disc edema that mimics papilledema)

Pearls

Although papilledema is a reliable sign of raised intracranial pressure, the absence of disc edema does not rule out raised intracranial pressure in a patient presenting with headache.

Table 9.2 Characteristics of disc edema from anterior optic neuropathy versus those from raised intracranial pressure

Optic neuropathy with disc edema	Papilledema (raised ICP)
Decreased visual acuity	Normal visual acuity (until late)
Decreased color vision	Normal color vision
Central, arcuate, or altitudinal visual field defect	Enlarged blind spot, nasal defects, constriction of visual fields
Disc edema more often unilateral	Disc edema almost always bilateral
Often isolated (or associated with symptoms or signs related to underlying disease)	Other symptoms and signs of raised ICP (headache, nausea, diplopia from sixth nerve palsies, pulsatile tinnitus, transient visual obscurations)
	Focal neurologic symptoms if focal intracranial process

Abbreviation: ICP, intracranial pressure.

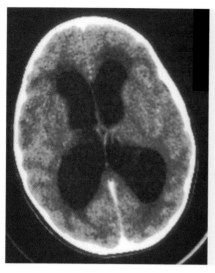

Fig. 9.13 Axial head computed tomography without contrast showing obstructive hydrocephalus (dilated ventricles).

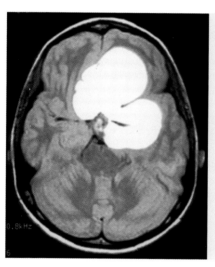

Fig. 9.14 Axial fluid-attenuated inversion recovery magnetic resonance imaging of the brain showing a large brain tumor with mass effect responsible for raised intracranial pressure.

Increased venous pressure produces symptoms and signs of raised intracranial pressure, including papilledema.

The causes of increased venous pressure include all of the causes of decreased venous return (▶ Fig. 9.15):

- Right cardiac insufficiency
- Pulmonary hypertension
- Sleep apnea syndrome
- Superior vena cava syndrome
- Jugular vein occlusion
- Dural fistula
- Cerebral venous stenosis
- Cerebral venous thrombosis

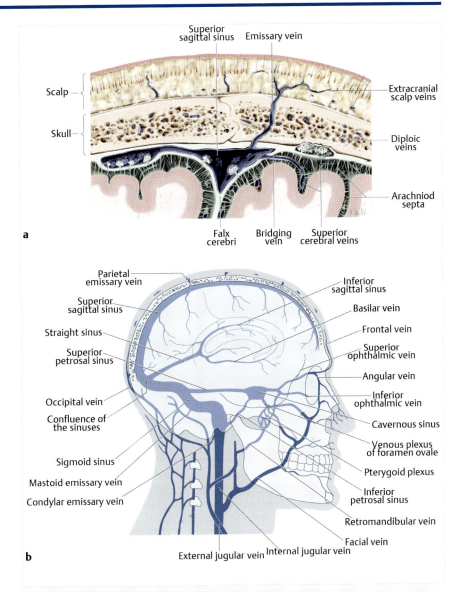

Fig. 9.15 (a) Drainage of the cerebrospinal fluid (CSF) into the intracranial venous sinuses. The CSF is passively resorbed across the Paccioni granulations (most are within the superior sagittal sinus). In cases of venous hypertension or venous thrombosis, the CSF resorption decreases, and the CSF pressure increases. (b) Anatomy of the intracranial venous system. ([a] From Schuenke M, Schulte E, Schumacher U, Ross LM, Lamperti ED, Voll M. THIEME Atlas of Anatomy, Head and Neuroanatomy. Stuttgart, Germany: Thieme; 2007. Illustration by Karl Wesker.) ([b] From Schuenke M, Schulte E, Schumacher U, Ross LM, Lamperti ED, Voll M. THIEME Atlas of Anatomy, Head and Neuroanatomy. Stuttgart, Germany: Thieme; 2007. Illustration by Markus Voll.)

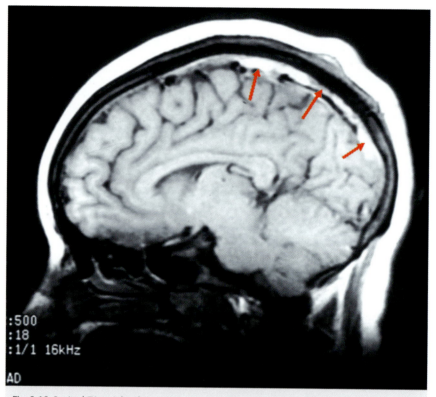

Fig. 9.16 Sagittal T1-weighted magnetic resonance imaging without contrast showing a hyperintense superior sagittal sinus (*arrows*) from cerebral venous thrombosis.

Cerebral venous thrombosis is a classic cause of raised intracranial pressure (▶ Fig. 9.16; see also Chapter 20). Patients may present with isolated raised intracranial pressure, thereby mimicking idiopathic intracranial hypertension. Early recognition may prevent a devastating stroke and visual loss from chronic papilledema.

When evaluating a patient with presumed papilledema (raised intracranial pressure), neuroimaging needs to be obtained emergently to rule out an intracranial process (▶ Fig. 9.17). Magnetic resonance imaging (MRI) with contrast of the brain is the ideal test and is the most sensitive to detect intracranial masses, infiltrative and meningeal processes, and cerebral venous thrombosis. Computed tomography (CT) without contrast, which is often the test of choice in the emergency room, is in most cases not helpful in these patients, unless it is followed by brain MRI. Indeed, the CT is helpful to detect intracranial hemorrhages, hydrocephalus, and large mass lesions, but it does not rule out any of the other intracranial lesions. Patients with a normal head CT should be investigated further with brain MRI (see Chapter 4). A normal brain MRI scan in the setting of papilledema suggests a meningeal process, venous hypertension, or idiopathic intracranial hypertension as the cause of raised intracranial pressure. A lumbar puncture with measurement of the cerebrospinal fluid (CSF) opening pressure and CSF analysis should always be performed.

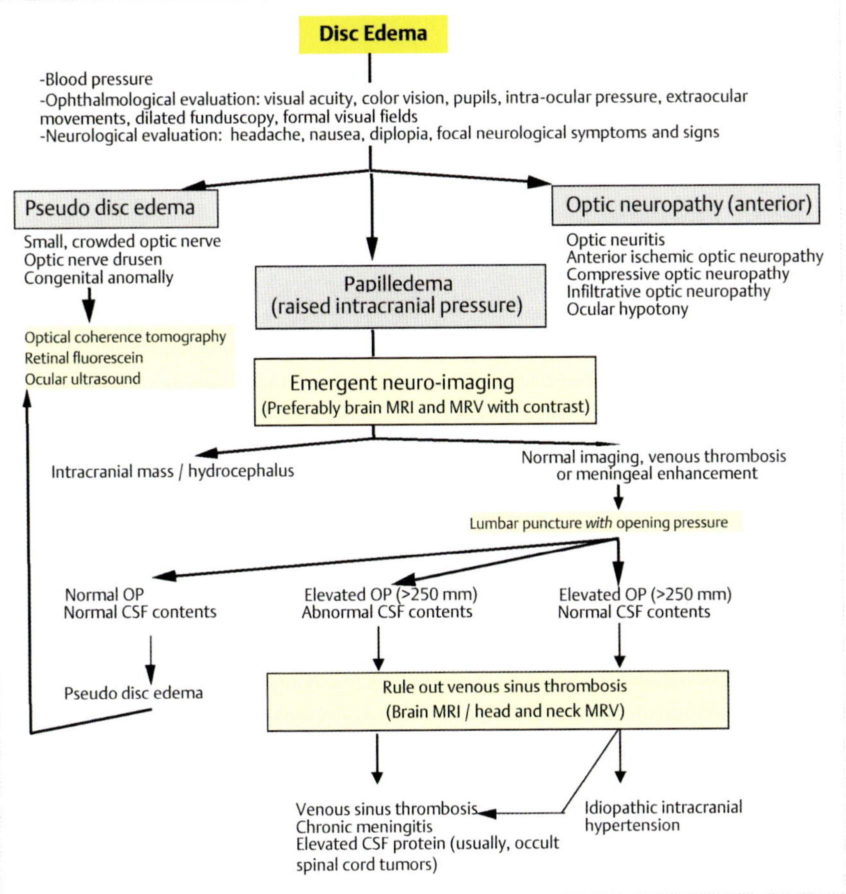

Fig. 9.17 Diagram illustrating the diagnosis of disc edema. OP, opening pressure; CSF, cerebrospinal fluid.

9.5 Classification and Progression of Papilledema

Patients with papilledema often have no visual symptoms initially. They may complain of "flashing lights" or transient visual obscurations (brief episodes of visual loss occurring in one or both eyes), often precipitated by changes in posture, such as standing up after bending over. Untreated chronic papilledema results in visual loss: central visual acuity is normal until late, and patients develop insidious progressive visual field constriction (▶ Fig. 9.18, ▶ Fig. 9.19, ▶ Fig. 9.20, ▶ Fig. 9.21, ▶ Fig. 9.22).

Formal visual field testing (Humphrey perimetry shown in ▶ Fig. 9.23) is often abnormal in papilledema. Blind spot enlargement and nasal defects are common initially (top, ▶ Fig. 9.23). They may progress, usually circumferentially, to involve the central 30 degrees of the visual field (middle). Severe devastating visual field loss (bottom) is often permanent if raised intracranial pressure is not promptly treated (note that even

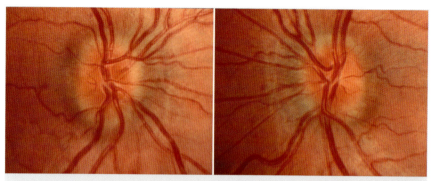

Fig. 9.18 Early papilledema. The disc borders are blurry and elevated. There is a peripapillary halo.

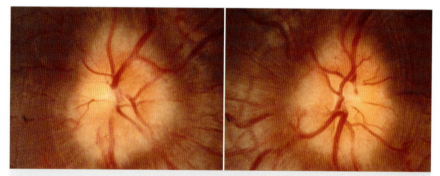

Fig. 9.19 Moderate papilledema. All borders are obscured, and the disc appears larger. The blood vessels are also obscured. There is a peripapillary halo.

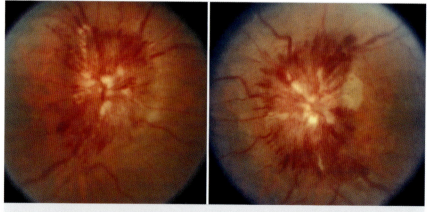

Fig. 9.20 Severe papilledema. The entire optic nerve head are elevated and obscured with numerous hemorrhages and exudates. The margins of the nerves and the vessels cannot be seen. The veins are dilated and tortuous.

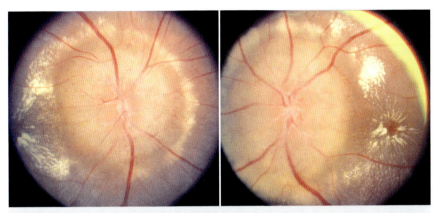

Fig. 9.21 Severe, chronic papilledema. The optic nerves protrude anteriorly with a dome-shaped appearance. There are exudates extending into the macula.

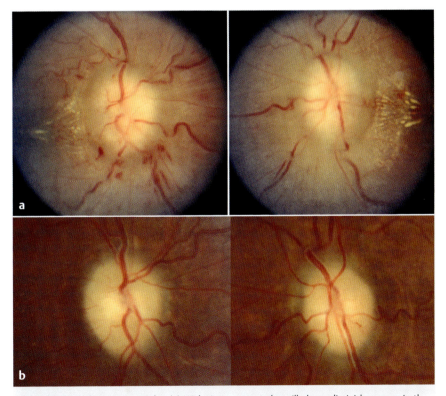

Fig. 9.22 Secondary optic atrophy. (**a**) With time, untreated papilledema diminishes, even in the setting of persistently elevated intracranial pressure. The discs become atrophic, and the retinal vessels become narrow and sheathed. (**b**) The nerves become flat and pale. Peripapillary changes persist from previous disc edema.

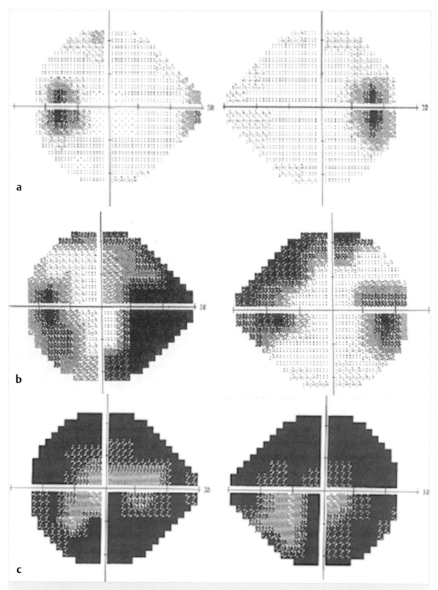

Fig. 9.23 Progression of visual field defects in papilledema (24–2 Humphrey visual fields). (**a**) Early changes with enlarged blind spots. (**b**) Constriction of visual fields, worse nasally. (**c**) Severe constriction.

with the severe visual field loss seen in the bottom example, visual acuity was still relatively preserved at 20/25 OD [right eye] and 20/40 OS [left eye]).

9.6 Idiopathic Intracranial Hypertension

Idiopathic intracranial hypertension (IIH), previously called pseudotumor cerebri, is defined as increased intracranial pressure with normal imaging and normal CSF contents. By definition, papilledema from a meningeal process or cerebral venous thrombosis should not be classified as IIH. Patients with IIH have symptoms and signs of raised intracranial pressure, such as headaches, nausea, pulsatile tinnitus, papilledema (and visual loss), and diplopia from unilateral or bilateral sixth nerve palsy. The management of the disease is based on the severity of headaches and the presence of visual loss, specifically visual field deficits.

9.6.1 Diagnosis of IIH

The criteria for the diagnosis of idiopathic intracranial hypertension are as follows:
- Signs and symptoms of raised intracranial pressure (including papilledema)
- No localizing neurologic signs, in an alert patient, other than abducens nerve paresis
- Normal neuroimaging studies (neuroimaging should include a good quality MRI scan ± magnetic resonance venography [MRV] or computed tomographic venography [CTV] to rule out cerebral venous thrombosis). Nonspecific signs of increased intracranial pressure are common and include empty sella, flattening of the globes, dilation of the optic nerve sheath, meningoceles, and stenosis of the intracranial transverse venous sinuses.
- Documented increased opening pressure (≥ 250 mm of water) but normal CSF composition
- Primary structural or systemic causes of elevated intracranial pressure excluded (e.g., chronic meningitis or cerebral venous thrombosis)

9.6.2 Cause of IIH

The cause of this disorder is unknown. It involves most often young, obese women and may be associated with other factors. The main factors associated with IIH are obesity or recent weight gain, sleep apnea syndrome, chronic anemia, and medications (vitamin A, isoretinoid, tetracycline, and cyclosporine).

9.6.3 Treatment of IIH

The goals of the management of IIH are to relieve headaches and diplopia and to preserve visual function (▶ Fig. 9.24). There is a high spontaneous remission rate.

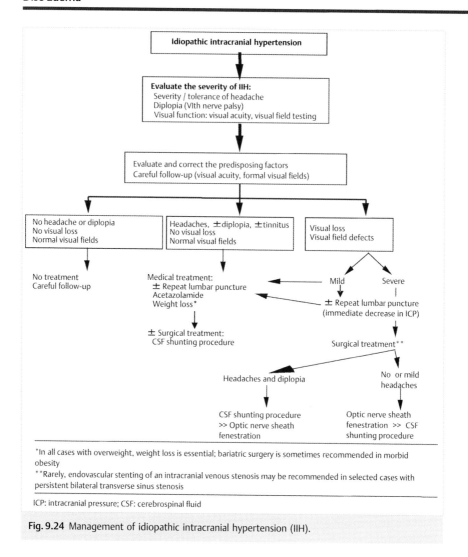

Fig. 9.24 Management of idiopathic intracranial hypertension (IIH).

The lumbar puncture performed as part of the workup is usually the first step of the treatment, as it immediately decreases the intracranial pressure (at least transiently). Headaches that do not improve (at least transiently) after lumbar puncture are unlikely to be entirely the result of raised intracranial pressure.

In rare cases, patients develop rapidly progressive visual loss that requires emergent surgical treatment. A brief course of intravenous steroids is sometimes helpful in this setting, but steroids should not be prescribed routinely or chronically in IIH (because of weight gain and rebound effect).

Surgical treatments in idiopathic intracranial hypertension include the following:
- CSF shunting procedures (performed by neurosurgeons) (▶ Fig. 9.25)
  - CSF drainage into the peritoneum most often
  - Lumboperitoneal shunt or ventriculoperitoneal shunt

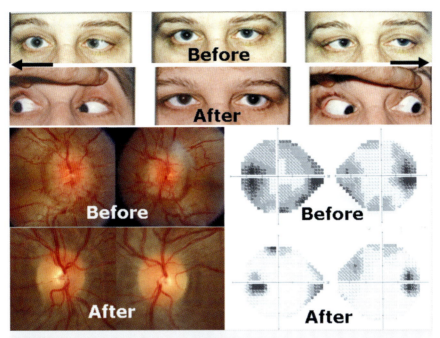

Fig. 9.25 Idiopathic intracranial hypertension. Improvement of symptoms and signs after a lumboperitoneal shunt procedure (top images: before shunt; bottom images: after shunt). There are bilateral sixth nerve palsies (bilateral abduction deficits), bilateral papilledema, and visual field defects.

- ○ Preferred when headaches are severe
- ○ Obstruction or disconnection requires a revision in about 50% of lumboperitoneal shunts.
- Optic nerve sheath fenestration (performed by ophthalmologists) (► Fig. 9.26)
  - ○ Decompression of the optic nerve by making a window into its dural sheath from a transconjunctival medial or lateral approach
  - ○ Done on the eye with the worst visual function first (often needs second eye surgery)
  - ○ Preferred when visual loss is predominant and headaches are mild
  - ○ The fenestration fails in up to one third of cases within 3 years.
- Endovascular venous stenting of a stenosed transverse sinus (performed by interventional neuroradiologists) (► Fig. 9.27)
  - ○ Most IIH patients have bilateral stenoses of the distal portion of the intracranial transverse venous sinus (► Fig. 9.27). Although these stenoses contribute to the intracranial hypertension (► Fig. 9.28), they are not necessarily the primary cause of increased intracranial pressure and they do not need to be treated in most patients.
  - ○ Rarely, endovascular stenting of a stenosed sinus can be proposed to decrease the intracranial venous hypertension and reduce the intracranial pressure.

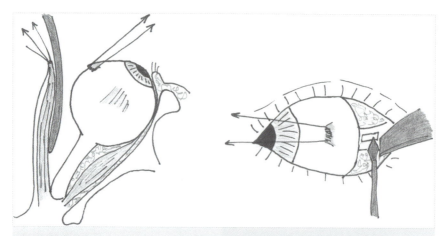

Fig. 9.26 Optic nerve sheath fenestration. The optic nerve sheath is exposed after a transconjunctival medial or lateral approach. A few slits or a window is made with a sharp blade into the sheath, allowing cerebrospinal fluid to escape (*arrows*).

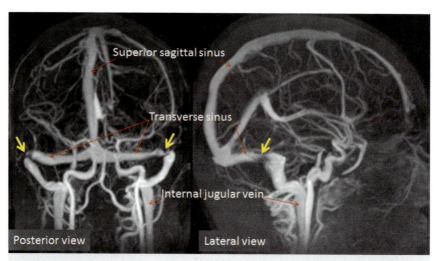

Fig. 9.27 Magnetic resonance venography with contrast showing the major intracranial venous sinuses (*red arrows*) and bilateral distal focal transverse venous stenoses (*yellow arrows*) in idiopathic intracranial hypertension. The left image shows the venous sinuses seen from behind, and the right image shows a lateral view of the venous sinuses.

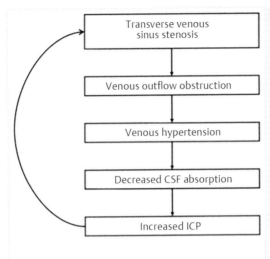

Fig. 9.28 Venous hypertension in idiopathic intracranial hypertension. The stenosed transverse venous sinuses impair venous return from the brain into the internal jugular vein, thereby increasing the intracranial venous pressure. The increase in venous pressure is responsible for impaired passive cerebrospinal fluid (CSF) resorption into the intracranial venous sinuses, contributing to intracranial hypertension. Increased intracranial pressure (ICP) results in collapse of the transverse venous sinuses, with resultant worsened transverse venous stenosis, with subsequent worsening of the intracranial venous hypertension.

10 Disorders of Higher Cortical Function

Unlike the anterior visual and geniculocalcarine pathways that deliver basic visual information from the eyes to the occipital cortex, association cortical visual areas (higher cortical areas) perform the more complex interpretation of visual information. Many of the syndromes of higher cortical dysfunction are secondary to a disconnection of the flow of visual information between the striate cortex and other cortical regions. When these areas are damaged, visual processing is abnormal despite often normal visual acuity and visual fields.

This chapter focuses on some of the main visual disorders of higher cortical function, particularly their clinical and radiologic findings and causes, commonly encountered in neuro-ophthalmology.

10.1 Classification

Disorders of higher cortical function are often grouped into two processing streams. The first stream, the inferior (ventral) or occipitotemporal pathway for object recognition, extends from below the calcarine fissure into the adjacent temporal lobe. It facilitates object recognition and color perception. Disorders here include achromatopsia, prosopagnosia, alexia, and topographagnosia.

The second stream, the superior (dorsal) or occipitoparietal pathway for object localization extends from the upper bank of the calcarine fissure into the adjacent parietal lobe. It processes visuospatial attributes, including location and motion. Disorders here include akinetopsia, Balint syndrome (simultagnosia, ocular apraxia, and optic ataxia), and hemineglect.

▶ Table 10.1 lists the clinical findings, recommended tests, associated clinical signs, and lesions associated with these higher cortical disorders.

10.2 Clinical and Radiologic Findings of Specific Disorders

10.2.1 Balint Syndrome

Balint syndrome results most frequently from bilateral parieto-occipital cortical or white matter injury, such as from watershed infarctions, progressive multifocal leukoencephalopathy, Alzheimer disease, and Creutzfeldt–Jakob disease. It associates (1) ocular apraxia (deficit in shifting gaze), (2) optic ataxia (defect in reaching under visual guidance), and (3) simultagnosia (inability to grasp the entire meaning of a picture despite an intact capacity to recognize the picture's individual constituent elements). Affected patients may be unable to identify a picture of a landscape, but they may be able to identify a small tree within the picture; alternatively, they may be able to read the individual 20/20 letters on the Snellen chart but may not be able to identify a whole word.

10.2.2 Gerstmann Syndrome

Gerstmann syndrome is caused by lesions in the dominant parietal lobe, and therefore, aphasia is often (but not always) present as well, which can make the diagnosis difficult or impossible.

Table 10.1 Clinical and radiologic findings of higher cortical visual disorders

Higher cortical disorder	Clinical finding	Test	Associated clinical signs	Brain lesion
Alexia without agraphia	Patient able to write but not read	Reading a text and writing	Right homonymous hemianopia Left occipital lobe and splenium of corpus callosum	
Hemiachromatopsia	Patient does not recognize colors in one hemifield	• Ishihara color plates • Farnsworth Lanthony	Ipsilateral homonymous superior quadrantanopia	Contralateral inferior occipitotemporal lobe
Prosopagnosia	Patient cannot recognize famous people or identify familiar faces	Identify famous people in magazine	• Alexia without agraphia • Visual agnosia • Bilateral superior altitudinal visual field defects	Bilateral inferior occipitotemporal lobes
Visual object agnosia	Patient is unable to identify objects by sight but can give a verbal description or recognize by another sensory modality	Name objects presented visually	• Alexia without agraphia • Prosopagnosia	Bilateral occipitotemporal lobes
Optic aphasia	Patient is unable to name visually presented objects or point to named objects (able to name and recognize what he or she hears or feels)	Name an object he or she sees	Right homonymous hemianopia	Left occipital lobe
Hemineglect (left)	Patient draws only the right half	Clock drawing	Inattention Left sensorimotor hemiparesis	Right inferior parietal lobe
Topographagnosia	Patient is unable to identify familiar landmarks and buildings	Gets lost in familiar surroundings	Prosopagnosia, Achromatopsia	Right inferior occipitotemporal lobes

Table 10.1 *(continued)*

Higher cortical disorder	Clinical finding	Test	Associated clinical signs	Brain lesion
Akinetopsia	Patient shows impairment of motion perception	Judge speed of approaching objects	Bilateral occipitotemporal cortex	
Simultagnosia	Patient identifies colors but cannot read numbers on the Ishihara color plates; identifies only part of the whole scene	Ishihara color plates Magazine pictures	Balint syndrome: Ocular apraxia Simultagnosia Optic ataxia	Bilateral parieto-occipital lobes
Ocular apraxia (psychic gaze paralysis, spasm of fixation)	Patient cannot look at an object that can be seen	Look at various objects on command	Part of Balint syndrome	
Optic ataxia (visuomotor ataxia)	Patient sees an object but cannot touch it	Touch various objects	Part of Balint syndrome	

Table 10.2 Differences between hemineglect and hemianopia

	Hemineglect	Hemianopia
Detecting stimuli:		
Awareness of defect	No	Yes
Modality	Often multimodal	Visual only
Extinction	Common	Unusual
Contralateral cueing	Improves neglect	No effect
Neglect tests:		
Line bisection bias	Ipsilesional	None or contralesional
Drawing (clock, etc.)	Lack of contralateral details	Normal
Exploring space:		
Contralateral saccade	Decreased	Increased
Object search test	Contralesional neglect	Contralateral emphasis
Side of hemispheric lesion	More often right (nondominant hemisphere)	Right or left

Gerstmann syndrome is a combination of right–left confusion, finger agnosia (loss in the ability to distinguish, name, or recognize the fingers), acalculia (acquired difficulty performing simple mathematical tasks), and agraphia (acquired inability to communicate through writing).

10.2.3 Hemineglect

Hemineglect usually occurs from lesions of the nondominant (right) hemisphere. Patients with hemineglect do not notice or respond to stimuli on the contralateral side. Hemineglect can affect not only vision but also other sensory and motor modalities. It is associated with damage to various components of a cerebral attentional network, which includes the inferior parietal lobe, the frontal cortex, and the thalamus.

▶ Table 10.2 lists the differences between hemineglect and hemianopia, although they can also coexist.

10.3 Causes of Disorders of Higher Cortical Functions

Cerebral disturbances of vision can be caused by any condition that affects the visual association cortices or subcortical white matter. They commonly result from bilateral cerebral lesions and are most often found in patients with cerebral hypoxia resulting in bilateral watershed infarctions or with bilateral infarctions in the territory of the posterior cerebral arteries, diffuse encephalopathy and encephalitis, and degenerative disorders producing dementia.

Computed tomography (CT) and magnetic resonance imaging (MRI) of the brain are sometimes normal or show nonspecific cerebral atrophy in most degenerative dementias. The diagnosis is often difficult and is delayed in patients in whom visual complaints predominate.

10.3.1 Posterior Cortical Atrophy

Posterior cortical atrophy is characterized by a progressive illness combining memory impairment, insight, and judgment impairment, alexia with or without agraphia, visual agnosia, and components of Balint syndrome, Gerstmann syndrome, and transcortical sensory aphasia (fluent aphasia with intact ability to repeat). Neuroimaging reveals cerebral atrophy, more severe posteriorly. Etiologies include Alzheimer disease and other dementias.

10.3.2 Alzheimer Disease

Alzheimer disease is a slowly progressive degenerative dementia that is often associated with visual disturbances (e.g., difficulty reading), which may predominate early in the course of the disease. Although these patients have numerous visual complaints (e.g., difficulty reading, difficulty seeing, and difficulty processing what they see), they have normal visual acuity and normal ocular examination, and frequently even normal visual fields, and the correct diagnosis is often delayed. Brain CT and MRI are often normal or show some posterior cerebral atrophy at the parieto-occipital junction. Functional imaging, such as positron emission tomography (PET) and single-photon emission computed tomography (SPECT), may help make the diagnosis.

10.3.3 Creutzfeldt–Jakob Disease

Creutzfeldt–Jakob disease is a rapidly progressive dementia that is usually lethal within a few months. Along with kuru, Gerstmann–Sträussler syndrome, and fatal familial insomnia, it comprises a group of dementing illnesses known as human transmissible spongiform encephalopathies. The Heidenhain variant of sporadic Creutzfeldt–Jakob disease manifests with early, prominent visual complaints (e.g., visual hallucinations, difficulty reading, homonymous hemianopia, and distortion of vision).

The diagnosis is based on the following:

- Normal conventional brain MRI with abnormal diffusion-weighted images
- Abnormal electroencephalogram (periodic activity)
- Positive testing for mutation 14–3–3 in the prion protein gene in the cerebrospinal fluid
- Abnormal brain biopsy

11 Abnormal Visual Perceptions: Hallucinations and Illusions

Abnormal visual perceptions are common in psychiatric disorders, ophthalmic disorders, and neurologic diseases, and can be due to numerous drugs and toxins.

In this chapter, the term *hallucination* refers to perception of a stimulus when, in reality, none is present, for example, when a patient with delirium tremens describes seeing bugs and snakes on the bedroom walls. The term *illusion* refers to misperception of a stimulus that is present in the external environment, for example, when an elderly individual interprets a chair in a poorly lit room as a person.

11.1 Psychiatric Disorders

Hallucinations are common in psychotic syndromes. They are most often complex and auditory. Isolated visual hallucinations are uncommon in psychiatric disorders.

> **Pearls**
>
> Primary psychiatric illnesses often cause visual illusions and hallucinations, which are usually associated with other perceptive abnormalities (usually auditory); they are not associated with altered mental status or focal neurologic signs.

11.2 Ophthalmic Disorders

11.2.1 Optical Causes

Optical causes of abnormal visual perceptions include alterations in the tear film (dry eyes and abnormalities in blinking), and irregularities in the cornea (keratoconus and corneal scarring) or the lens (cataract). Entoptic phenomena are visual experiences caused by ocular structures (e.g., floaters).

11.2.2 Retinal Disorders (Maculopathies)

Retinal disorders or maculopathies can produce visual hallucinations.

Metamorphopsias from macular disorders are best detected by the Amsler grid test. Macular edema produces micropsia (increased separation of retinal photoreceptors), and epiretinal membrane produces macropsia (when the photoreceptors are pushed together) (▶ Fig. 11.1).

Vitreoretinal traction is responsible for phosphenes (flashing lights). These are more apparent in a dark environment. Floaters (posterior vitreous detachment and vitreous debris) are most noticeable against a uniformly illuminated background. Outer retinal diseases, such as cancer-associated retinopathy, acute zonal occult outer retinopathy, and multiple evanescent white dot syndrome, may cause simple white flashing lights.

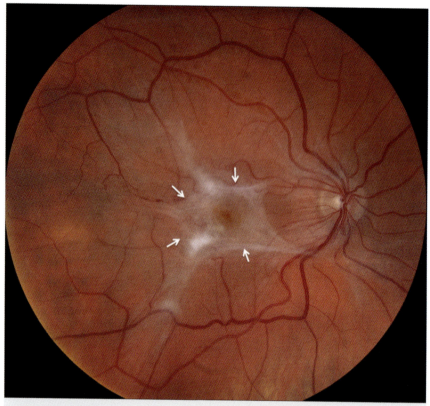

Fig. 11.1 Epiretinal membrane in the right eye responsible for decreased visual acuity and severe distortion of vision. Note the whitish membrane that pulls on the retina (*arrows*).

11.2.3 Optic Nerve Disease

Phosphenes are sometimes reported by patients with optic neuropathies. They are sometimes triggered by noise or moving the eye.

Pulfrich phenomenon, or the perception of an elliptical movement when observing a pendulum swinging in one plane, occurs in patients with unilateral or asymmetric optic neuropathies. It is a stereoillusion related to the difference in conduction delay between the two eyes.

11.2.4 Charles Bonnet Syndrome

Charles Bonnet syndrome is characterized by visual hallucinations associated with poor vision, such as in macular degeneration. Simple and complex visual hallucinations are present in up to 10% of patients with severe binocular visual loss, presumably because the normal visual cortex has been "released" from anterior visual pathway input. This syndrome is more common in the elderly.

The hallucinations are not stereotyped and involve vivid scenes of animals, flowers, and people. They may be episodic or continuous and are more common in the evening and when patients have their eyes open. Once patients are reassured, they often tolerate these hallucinations well, but treatment is usually unsuccessful.

11.3 Neurologic Disorders

A variety of encephalopathies or focal cerebral lesions can cause hallucinations and illusions. These symptoms are most often visual and tactile, whereas psychiatric hallucinations are most often auditory. They occur in awake or drowsy patients, who often are not aware that these are hallucinations and may become frightened.

11.3.1 Confusion and Dementia

Confusion and dementia can cause visual hallucinations and illusions.

Delirium tremens is associated with very frightening, well-formed visual hallucinations, including bugs, monsters, and snakes.

Lewy body dementia is commonly associated with visual hallucinations.

Other dementias, such as Alzheimer disease, Pick disease, human immunodeficiency virus (HIV) dementia, Huntington chorea, Creutzfeldt–Jakob disease, and multi-infarct dementia, may be associated with paranoid hallucinations and illusions.

Drugs used to treat Parkinson disease can also cause hallucinations.

11.3.2 Migraine

Numerous visual phenomena occur during the visual aura of migraine (▶ Table 11.1). These visual phenomena are often positive and therefore can be described as hallucinations.

Migrainous visual phenomena usually last between 10 and 30 minutes and progress over time (migrainous march) (see Chapter 6, ▶ Fig. 6.1). They may be associated with other neurologic symptoms, such as ipsilateral tingling and speech impairment, and are classically followed by migrainous headaches. Migraineurs are aware that the images they see are not real.

Table 11.1 Characteristics of visual phenomena in migraine with visual aura and occipital seizures

Characteristics	Migraine with visual aura	Occipital seizures
Visual phenomena	Positive and negative	Positive and negative
Color	Bright, scintillating, black and white	Colorful
Description	Simple, but with stereotyped progression from center to periphery; experienced in both eyes; often in a hemifield	Often simple (sparkles, pinwheel, bubbles, circles); experienced in both eyes; often in a hemifield
Duration	10 to 30 minutes (up to 1 hour)	A few seconds
Recurrence	Yes, often change sides, various patterns	Yes, often daily, stereotyped for each patient, same side
Associated symptoms	Migrainous headache after aura	Often isolated, or with other epileptic symptoms
Examination	Normal between attacks	May have visual field defect

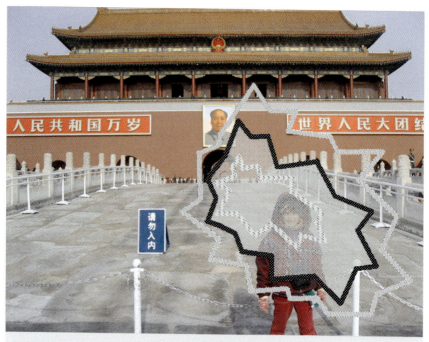

Fig. 11.2 Scintillating scotoma with zig-zag pattern highly suggestive of migraine.

Positive or negative visual phenomena are present in both eyes, either in the entire eye or in one hemifield. Phenomena include phosphenes, which are usually bright or white, and scintillating scotoma, described as progressively enlarging bright scotoma with sharp edges (▶ Fig. 11.2). Distortion of images with micropsia and macropsia (Alice in Wonderland syndrome) or tilting of objects can also occur.

11.3.3 Occipital Seizures

Occipital seizures can cause simple and colorful, positive or negative visual phenomena present in both eyes, including sparkles, pinwheels, bubbles, scotoma, and dots. Although they are often moving, they do not have the stereotyped progression observed in migraine. They are short in duration (usually lasting only a few seconds) and may be isolated. They are usually stereotyped for each patient.

Occipital seizures can occur with a variety of occipital lesions or as part of primary occipital seizures, which are more common in children.

11.3.4 Peduncular Hallucinosis

Peduncular hallucinosis is a rare neurologic syndrome characterized by vivid, usually well-formed, colorful hallucinations of people, animals, and complex scenes with motion. It is most often related to a midbrain infarction in the region of the peduncle, and is also likely a "release phenomenon" (▶ Fig. 11.3).

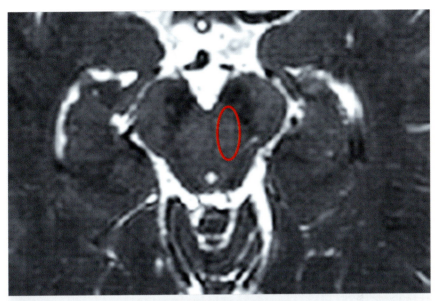

Fig. 11.3 Axial brain magnetic resonance imaging at the level of the midbrain, showing the cerebral location of lesions (*red circle*) classically producing peduncular hallucinosis.

Patients usually have sleep/wake disorders and are aware that these images are not real. The hallucination usually begins a few days after the lesion occurs and may persist for weeks to months.

11.3.5 Narcolepsy

Visual hallucinations are a common presenting complaint of narcolepsy. They are described as colorful images, which may involve people, animals, and panoramic scenes.

Patients often have a vague sense that someone else is in the room. They also realize that what they are experiencing is not a dream and that they are awake.

The classic tetrad of narcolepsy includes the following:

- Cataplexy (transient loss of muscle tone)
- Sleep paralysis (inability to move when the patient first wakes up)
- Sleep attacks (overwhelming sense of fatigue causing the patient to fall asleep for 10 to 30 minutes)
- Hypnogogic (entering sleep) and hypnopompic (awakening) hallucinations, lasting several minutes. The hallucinations can be visual, auditory, or tactile.

11.3.6 Palinopsia

Palinopsia is the continuation of visual sensations after cessation of visual stimuli or intermittent reappearance of images (visual perseveration or multiple afterimages) (▶ Fig. 11.4). The images are brief and recur periodically in a hemifield. Palinopsia also occurs as a release phenomenon involving lesions of the parietal and occipital lobes, most often in the nondominant hemisphere.

275

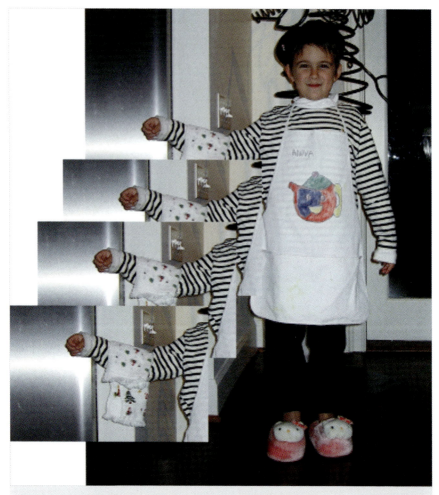

Fig. 11.4 Palinopsia with impression that the arm is duplicated many times in the left hemifield.

The following are the most common causes of palinopsia:
- Drugs: lysergic acid diethylamide (LSD), neuroleptics
- Migrainous visual aura
- Seizures: temporal, occipital
- Focal cerebral lesions: parietal and occipital lobe lesions, most often in the nondominant hemisphere
- Creutzfeldt–Jakob disease
- Encephalopathies: carbon monoxide poisoning, hepatic encephalopathy, hyperglycemia, and hypoglycemia

11.3.7 Polyopia (Cerebral Diplopia)

Polyopia, or cerebral diplopia, is a rare manifestation of occipital cortex lesions. The images are identical in the two eyes, and the number of images seen ranges from one and a half to hundreds. The diplopia or polyopia does not resolve by closing either eye and does not improve with pinhole glasses. There is often an associated homonymous hemianopia.

11.3.8 Dysmetropsia (Dysmegalopsia or Metamorphopsia)

Dysmetropsia (also known as dysmegalopsia or metamorphopsia) is a disorder of size perception, where objects can appear smaller (micropsia) or larger (macropsia). Causes include retinal disorders (most common; one eye only) and migraine (Alice in Wonderland syndrome; both eyes).

11.3.9 Visual Allesthesia

Visual allesthesia occurs when visual stimuli are transposed from one hemifield to another (▶ Fig. 11.5). It is usually brief, and most patients experience recurrent episodes. It is seen most often with parieto-occipital lesions or as part of the migrainous visual aura.

11.3.10 Sensation of Environment Tilt

The sensation of environment tilt phenomenon involves the acute tilt of the environment by 90 or 180 degrees (▶ Fig. 11.6). It is brief and spontaneously resolving.

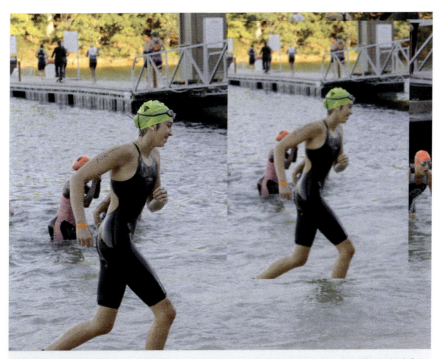

Fig. 11.5 Visual allesthesia with the impression that visual objects are transposed from the left visual field to the right. The transposed person is less distinct than the original and appears farther away. The phenomenon involves the background as well as the foreground.

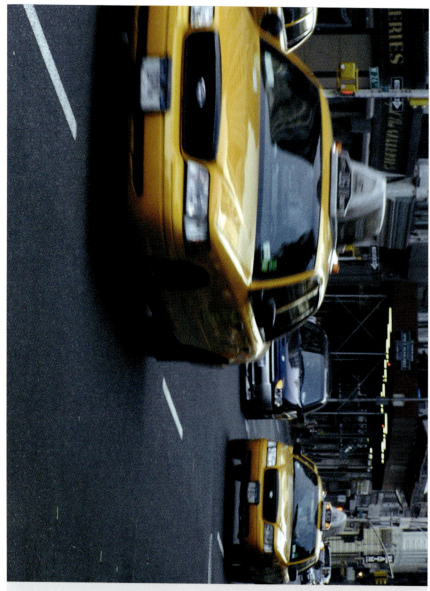

Fig. 11.6 Environmental tilt by 90 degrees in a migrainous patient.

The phenomenon is most often associated with the lateral medullary syndrome. It is also described in patients with occipital lesions or migraine with aura.

11.3.11 Riddoch Phenomenon

The Riddoch phenomenon involves perception of moving targets in a field otherwise blind to static stimuli due to an occipital lesion.

11.3.12 Blindsight and Residual Vision

It has been suggested that lesions of the geniculostriate pathway do not eliminate all visual function within the resulting blind region.

In blindsight, patients who state they are completely blind in one hemifield and are not aware of a visual stimulus in the blind hemifield, nevertheless guess at a level better than chance when asked about some property of the visual stimulus.

In residual vision, patients retain some awareness of the target within a dense visual field defect, suggesting a severe but relative hemianopia.

11.3.13 Oscillopsia

Oscillopsia is the illusion of movement of the environment, often due to any of the following:

- Abnormality of the vestibulo-ocular reflex caused by damage to the vestibular system
- Nystagmus
- Tullio phenomenon (noise-induced peripheral vestibular dysfunction)
- Superior oblique myokymia (one eye)
- Pulsating orbital mass (one eye)

11.3.14 Anton Syndrome

In Anton syndrome, patients with cerebral blindness (bilateral occipital lesions) are not aware of their visual loss and insist that they can see. It is a denial syndrome of unknown mechanism.

11.4 Drugs and Toxins

Numerous drugs and toxins produce visual hallucinations and illusions.

The following are some of the most common:

- Postoperative delirium: transient hallucinations after general anesthesia
- Hallucinogens:
  - Cocaine, LSD, marijuana, mescaline, opiates, phencyclidine hydrochloride (PCP), psilocybin and psilocin (hallucinogenic mushroom), and 3,4-methylenedioxy-N-methylamphetamine (MDMA; Ecstasy or Molly).
  - LSD is responsible for delayed impressions of déjà vu or flashbacks that may occur years after even a single LSD use.
- All anticholinergic agents (including atropine, scopolamine, and cyclopentolate)
- All antiparkinsonian agents (dopamine agonists, bromocriptine, anticholinergic agents, etc.)
- Antidepressants
- Antipsychotics
- Digoxin: toxic levels are associated with xanthopsia (illusion of abnormal colors—yellow and green are typical).
- Phosphodiestherase-5 inhibitors (erectile dysfunction medications): bluish vision
- Alcohol

Withdrawal of alcohol and benzodiazepines will also produce hallucinations.

12 The Pupil

Pupillary function is an important objective clinical sign in patients with visual loss and neurologic disease.

The mnemonic PERRLA (pupils equal, round, reactive to light, and accommodation) reminds us of the four questions we should ask in evaluating the pupils:
- Are the pupils equal in size?
- Are the pupils round or irregularly shaped?
- Do the pupils react to a light stimulus?
- If not, do they react to a near target?

The normal pupil varies in size, depending on the ambient illumination. Pupils are usually symmetrical in size, although physiologic anisocoria (the difference in size between the two pupils) of 0.4 mm or greater is seen in about 20% of individuals.

12.1 Examining the Pupils

Pupils should be tested in the dark with a bright light and with the patient fixating at distance (see Chapter 1, ▶ Fig. 1.16, ▶ Fig. 1.17, ▶ Fig. 1.18, ▶ Fig. 1.19, ▶ Fig. 1.20). When examining the pupils, you should record the following:
- Size (in millimeters)
- Presence of anisocoria
- Response to light (direct and consensual response)
- Presence of a relative afferent pupillary defect (RAPD)
- Dilation in the dark
- Constriction at near

When pupillary reactions are abnormal, slit lamp examination of the anterior segment and the iris may demonstrate abnormalities that may affect pupillary size and shape, such as synechiae, uveitis, iris tear, segmental contraction of the iris, iris tumor, and lens subluxation (▶ Fig. 12.1, ▶ Table 12.1).

> **Pearls**
>
> Shining a light in one eye of a normal subject causes both pupils to constrict equally. The pupillary response in the illuminated eye is called the *direct response*. The pupillary response in the eye that is not being illuminated is called the *consensual response*.

12.2 Clinical Anatomy and Physiology of the Pupils

Light directed into either eye normally produces bilateral pupillary constriction.

Each pupil receives both sympathetic (dilator muscle: active dilation) and parasympathetic (sphincter muscle: active constriction) innervation. The size of the pupils at any one moment is determined by the balance of the parasympathetic tone of the iris sphincter and the sympathetic tone of the iris dilator. This balance is in constant flux, so that pupil sizes change symmetrically from moment to moment.

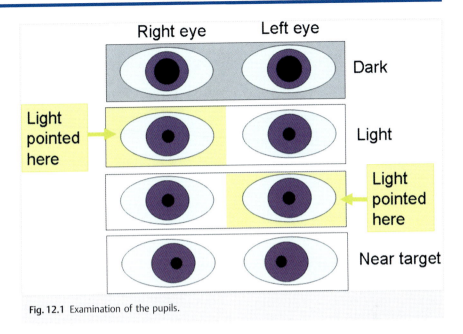

Fig. 12.1 Examination of the pupils.

Hippus is the normal rhythmic pupillary oscillation commonly seen when light stimulates either eye. Both pupils oscillate in synchrony, and the amplitude and frequency vary (▶ Table 12.2).

Changes in the pupil innervation will produce dilation or constriction of the pupil. Additionally, local problems such as lesions of the iris (tumor, iris synechiae on the lens, iris tears from trauma, and postsurgical pupil) may change the shape or alter the reactivity of the pupil.

Pupillary size results from the balance of actions of two opposing muscle groups of the iris: the dilator of the iris (responsible for dilation) and the sphincter pupillae (responsible for constriction). The size changes are reflex mechanisms in response to the amount of ambient light. These changes vary based on the patient's age, emotional state (adrenergic tone), state of arousal, and intraocular pressure.

▶ Fig. 12.2 shows the normal pupil and iris.

Table 12.1 Examination of the pupils (how to report the results)

	Right eye	Left eye
Dark	6 mm	6 mm
Light	3 mm	3 mm
Reaction to light	Brisk (3 +)	Brisk (3 +)
RAPD	No	No
Dilation in dark	Normal	Normal
Reaction at near	2 mm	2 mm

Abbreviation: RAPD, relative afferent pupillary defect.

Table 12.2 Pharmacologic effect of the sympathetic and parasympathetic systems on the pupil size

	Sympathetic (adrenergic) stimulation	Parasympathetic (cholinergic) blockage
Pupillary dilation	Stimulation of dilation: • Drugs: Phenylephrine, adrenaline, cocaine, amphetamines • Endogenous increase of adrenaline (pain, fear, pheochromocytoma, etc.)	Blockage of constriction: • Drugs: Tropicamide, cyclopentolate, homatropine, atropine • Lesion of the parasympathetic system: third nerve palsy; Adie pupil
	Sympathetic (adrenergic) blockage	Parasympathetic (cholinergic) stimulation
Pupillary constriction	Blockage of dilation: Lesion of the sympathetic system: Horner syndrome	Stimulation of constriction: Drugs: pilocarpine

12.2.1 Pupillary Light Reflex Pathway

Pupillary constriction to light is mediated via parasympathetic (cholinergic) nerve fibers that travel along the third cranial nerve. When light is shone into one eye, both pupils constrict symmetrically (direct and consensual response to light). Light information from retinal ganglion cells travels through the optic nerves, chiasm (where the nasal fibers decussate), and optic tracts to reach the pretectal nuclei of the dorsal midbrain (▶ Fig. 12.3).

Afferent pupillary fibers leave the optic tract before the lateral geniculate nucleus via the brachium of the superior colliculus to reach the pretectal nuclei (explaining why lesions of the geniculate nucleus, the optic radiations, or the visual cortex do not affect pupillary size or pupillary reactivity, and why lesions of the brachium of the superior colliculus can cause a relative afferent pupillary defect without visual loss).

Both pretectal nuclei receive input from both eyes, and each sends axons to both Edinger–Westphal nuclei (connections are bilateral but predominantly from the contralateral nucleus). Parasympathetic fibers for pupillary constriction leave the Edinger–Westphal nucleus and travel along the ipsilateral third cranial nerve to the ipsilateral ciliary ganglion within the orbit.

The postganglionic parasympathetic fibers innervate the ciliary muscle (for lens accommodation) and the pupillary sphincter muscle (for pupil constriction) in a proportion of 30:1. (This is important to understand the pathophysiology of the tonic [Adie] pupil.) Acetylcholine is released at the neuromuscular junction of the iris sphincter to result in pupillary constriction.

12.2.2 Relative Afferent Pupillary Defect

When light is directed into either eye, both pupils react equally. The brighter the light source, the greater the degree of bilateral pupillary constriction. Therefore, the amount of pupillary constriction from the same light source directed to either eye should be identical.

The RAPD, where stimulation of one eye causes both eyes to constrict less than stimulation of the other eye, is a very important objective sign of optic nerve disease. It can easily be detected at bedside, and it can also be quantified (see Chapter 1).

In unilateral optic nerve or retinal ganglion cell dysfunction, the light signal received by the brainstem efferent centers is relatively less when the same light source is

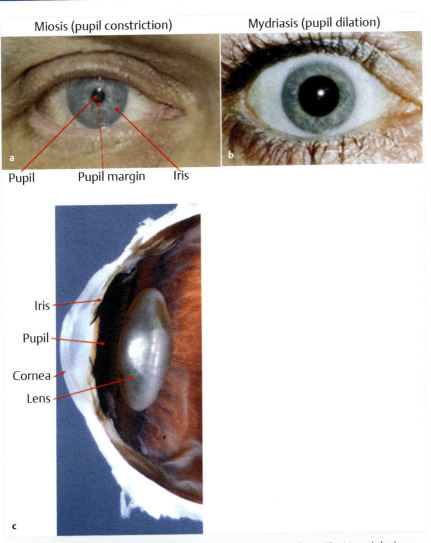

Miosis (pupil constriction) Mydriasis (pupil dilation)

Pupil Pupil margin Iris

Iris
Pupil
Cornea
Lens

Fig. 12.2 (a,b) The normal pupil and iris. **(c)** Sagittal cut of a normal eye. The iris and the lens separate the anterior chamber from the posterior chamber. The lens is immediately behind the iris, explaining why lens disorders or synechiae between the iris and lens (posterior synechiae) may change the pupil size and shape.

presented to the affected eye. Hence both pupils constrict less when the involved eye is stimulated and more when the normal eye is stimulated (▸ Fig. 12.4).

Pearls

A relative afferent pupillary defect will not cause anisocoria (inequality in size of the pupils).

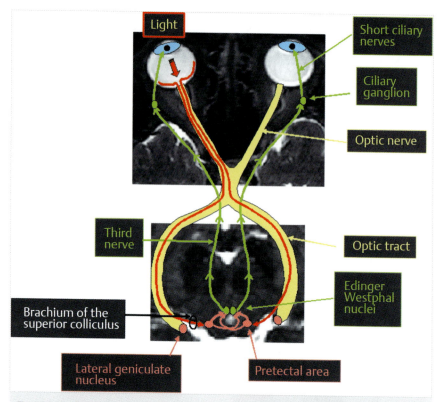

Fig. 12.3 Pupillary light reflex (parasympathetic pathway). The afferent pathway is shown in red, and the efferent pathway is shown in green.

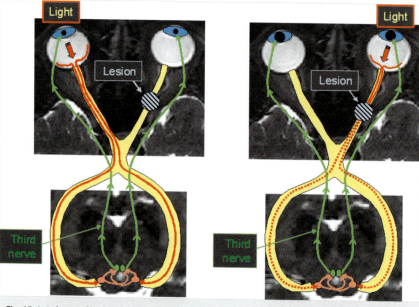

Fig. 12.4 Relative afferent pupillary defect (RAPD) in the left eye. A RAPD can be detected by comparing the light reaction between the two pupils.

A RAPD ipsilateral to visual loss indicates an optic neuropathy or severe retinal disease (in which case the retina looks abnormal on funduscopic examination). Ocular disease, such as corneal abnormalities, cataracts, and most retinal disorders, do not cause a RAPD.

A unilateral lesion in the pretectal nucleus or in the brachium of the superior colliculus will damage the pupillary fibers coming from the ipsilateral optic tract. This can produce a contralateral RAPD, just like in optic tract lesions, but without any visual loss or visual field defect.

By placing neutral-density filters over the normal eye, the examiner can neutralize the RAPD and quantitate its severity in log units (see Chapter 1). Filters usually range from 0.3 (small RAPD) to 1.8 (dense RAPD) log units.

The causes of RAPD include the following:

- Unilateral or asymmetric optic neuropathy (0.3 to 1.8 log units)
- Severe unilateral retinopathy (0.3– > 1.8 log units)
- Maculopathy with visual acuity worse than 20/200 (small RAPD of 0.3 log unit)
- Amblyopia (small RAPD of 0.3 log unit)
- Dense, unilateral cataract: may produce a small *contralateral* RAPD (the retina behind the dense cataract is dark adapted, and the light shines in all directions, causing excess retinal stimulation on the side of the dense cataract)
- Patching of one eye (or complete ptosis) may produce a transient contralateral RAPD (the patched eye has a dark-adapted retina and is hypersensitive to light; this can produce a contralateral RAPD of up to 1.5 log units for up to 30 minutes after the patch is removed).
- Optic tract lesions produce a contralateral RAPD (RAPD of 0.3–0.6 log unit), which is on the side of the homonymous hemianopia, the side opposite the lesion (see Chapter 3, ▶ Fig. 3.22).
- Lesions of the brachium of the superior colliculus or the pretectal nucleus produce a contralateral RAPD without visual loss or visual field defect.

> **Pearls**
>
> If a patient with a suspected optic neuropathy (regardless of the cause) has no RAPD, either the patient does not have an optic neuropathy, or the optic neuropathy is bilateral.

12.2.3 Pupillary Constriction with Accommodation

Pupillary constriction to a near stimulus is accomplished through the parasympathetic pathways. The near-reflex pathway bypasses the pretectal nuclei in the dorsal midbrain and descends directly to the area of the Edinger–Westphal nuclei from higher cortical centers.

The distinction between the light-reflex and near-reflex pathways forms the basis for some forms of pupillary light-near dissociation (i.e., pupils that do not react to light but react to near stimuli) in which the dorsal midbrain and pretectal nuclei are damaged, but the near-reflex pathways and the Edinger–Westphal nuclei are spared (▶ Fig. 12.5 and ▶ Fig. 12.6).

Because the afferent pathways serving the light reflex and the near reflex are anatomically distinct, patients with severe optic neuropathies will still have intact, brisk

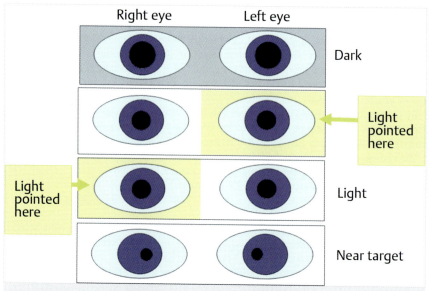

Fig. 12.5 Light-near dissociation. Because the afferent pathways serving the light reflex and the near reflex are anatomically distinct, patients with severe optic neuropathies will still have intact, brisk pupillary responses to near stimuli, while their pupils will not, or will only poorly, react to light (▶ Fig. 12.7).

pupillary responses to near stimuli, while their pupils will not, or will only poorly, react to light (▶ Fig. 12.7).

12.2.4 Pupillary Dilation

Pupillary dilation is mediated through sympathetic (adrenergic) pathways that originate in the hypothalamus (▶ Fig. 12.8).

The sympathetic pathway (oculosympathetic fibers) responsible for pupillary dilation is a three-neuron pathway:

- *First order neuron:* descends from the hypothalamus to the first synapse, which is located in the cervical spinal cord (levels C8–T2, also called the intermediolateral cell column or the ciliospinal center of Budge). In the midbrain, the sympathetic pathway is located close to the fourth nerve nucleus.
- *Second-order neuron:* travels from the sympathetic trunk, through the brachial plexus, and over the lung apex. It then ascends to the superior cervical ganglion (located near the angle of the mandible and the bifurcation of the common carotid artery).
- *Third-order neuron (distal to the superior cervical ganglion):* ascends within the adventitia of the internal carotid artery and through the cavernous sinus (where it is in close relation to the sixth cranial nerve) and joins the ophthalmic (V 1) division of the fifth cranial nerve to get into the orbit.

The oculosympathetic fibers innervate the iris dilator muscle, Müller muscles (small muscles in the upper eyelids responsible for a minor portion of upper lid elevation), and inferior tarsal muscle (equivalent of the Müller muscles in the lower eyelid).

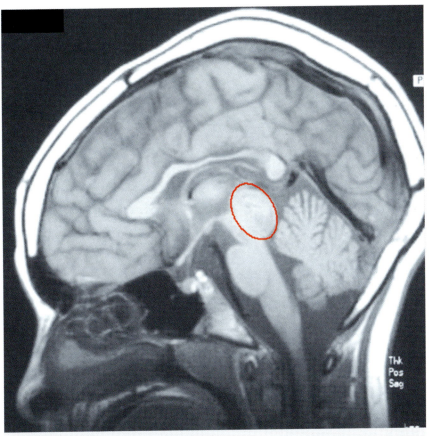

Fig. 12.6 Pretectal lesion producing light-near dissociation in a patient with a tectal mass (*red oval*) and dorsal midbrain syndrome.

The sympathetic fibers responsible for facial sweating and vasodilation branch off at the superior cervical ganglion from the remainder of the oculosympathetic pathway (explaining why patients with a third-order Horner syndrome usually do not have anhidrosis [loss of sweating]).

12.3 Pupillary Abnormalities in Coma

The metabolic causes of coma usually cause small reactive pupils (▶ Fig. 12.9). Many toxins and drugs also have effects on the size of the pupils. Finally, pharmacologic mydriasis can inadvertently occur in patients treated with aerosols after extubation.

12.4 Anisocoria

Patients with anisocoria, or inequality in the size of the pupils, usually present emergently and generate much anxiety in the emergency room. Indeed, anisocoria from a

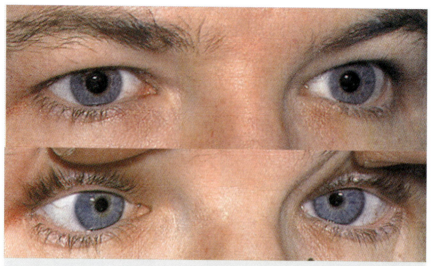

Fig. 12.7 Light-near dissociation from severe bilateral optic neuropathies. The pupils do not react to light (top) but constrict when focusing on a near target (bottom).

third nerve palsy may reveal an intracranial aneurysm, which may rupture and cause a life-threatening subarachnoid hemorrhage if not diagnosed promptly. The fear of an underlying life-threatening condition such as an intracranial aneurysm often leads physicians to obtain numerous tests. However, a simple and logical clinical approach that appreciates the mechanisms of anisocoria allows for prompt recognition of true emergencies and often avoids the need for invasive and costly testing in other cases.

12.4.1 Diagnosis

To determine the cause of anisocoria, the first step is to determine which pupil is abnormal—the large pupil or the small pupil—by carefully evaluating the pupillary reactions in the dark and in the light (▶ Fig. 12.10, ▶ Fig. 12.11, ▶ Fig. 12.12).

The next step is to look for associated symptoms and signs:
- A decreased palpebral fissure on the side of a small pupil suggests a Horner syndrome.
- Diplopia, ptosis, and impaired extraocular movements on the side of a large pupil point to a third nerve palsy.
- An isolated large pupil without ptosis or diplopia suggests Adie pupil or pharmacologic mydriasis.
- With mydriasis, patients often complain of decreased near vision (from impaired accommodation) and of sensitivity to light (photophobia).

12.4.2 Causes of Anisocoria

Physiologic Anisocoria

Physiologic anisocoria, a normal benign inequality of the pupils that may change from time to time, is seen in about 20% of the normal population (▶ Fig. 12.13).

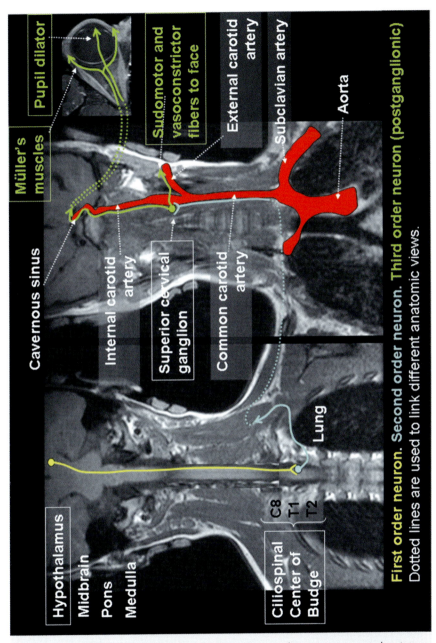

Fig. 12.8 Sympathetic pupillary pathways. The three-neuron pathways are represented on two different coronal views of the upper chest, neck, and head.

289

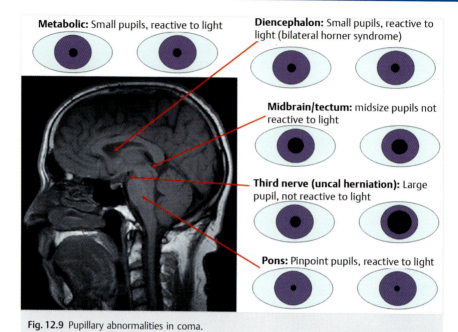

Metabolic: Small pupils, reactive to light

Diencephalon: Small pupils, reactive to light (bilateral horner syndrome)

Midbrain/tectum: midsize pupils not reactive to light

Third nerve (uncal herniation): Large pupil, not reactive to light

Pons: Pinpoint pupils, reactive to light

Fig. 12.9 Pupillary abnormalities in coma.

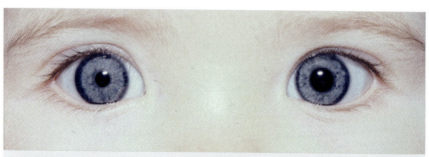

Fig. 12.10 Anisocoria. Is the left pupil larger than the right pupil, or is the right pupil smaller than the left pupil?

- Reviewing the patient's old photographs on a driver's license or ID (with magnifying glasses or the slit lamp) may help confirm the diagnosis, as physiologic anisocoria is usually persistent.
- The amount of anisocoria is usually equal in light and dark (may be slightly greater in the dark than in the light).
- The anisocoria is usually < 0.5 mm.
- Depending on the degree of ambient lighting, the anisocoria may seem to come and go.
- Occasionally, the anisocoria may switch sides.

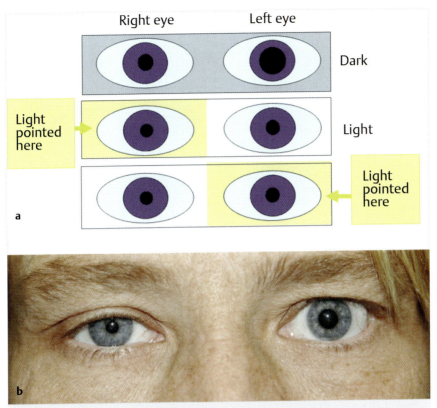

Right eye   Left eye

Dark

Light
pointed
here

Light

Light
pointed
here

a

b

Fig. 12.11 (a) The small (right eye) pupil is abnormal (it does not dilate well in the dark). The anisocoria is greater in the dark than in the light (indicating poor pupillary dilation on the abnormal side). This indicates an abnormality of the sympathetic system. (b) Right Horner syndrome. The right pupil does not dilate in the dark, and there is a decreased palpebral fissure on the right. Extraocular movements are full.

Ocular Causes of Anisocoria

The ocular examination of the anterior segment by an ophthalmologist using a slit lamp confirms the diagnosis (▶ Fig. 12.14, ▶ Fig. 12.15, ▶ Fig. 12.16, ▶ Fig. 12.17, ▶ Fig. 12.18, ▶ Fig. 12.19, ▶ Fig. 12.20, ▶ Fig. 12.21).

Structural defects of the iris can lead to anisocoria and abnormal pupillary shapes.

Congenital defects, such as aniridia, iris coloboma, congenital ectopic pupils, persistent pupillary membrane, polycoria, congenital heterochromia, iridocorneal endothelial (ICE) syndrome, and other developmental anomalies of the anterior segment, produce anisocoria, which usually presents in childhood.

Numerous acquired ocular conditions, such as intraocular inflammation (anterior uveitis), anterior segment ischemia, neovascularization of the iris, trauma, iris sphincter atrophy related to surgical or traumatic injury, mechanical distortion by an intraocular tumor, and angle closure glaucoma, also produce anisocoria. Associated visual loss, ocular redness, and ocular pain are usually present.

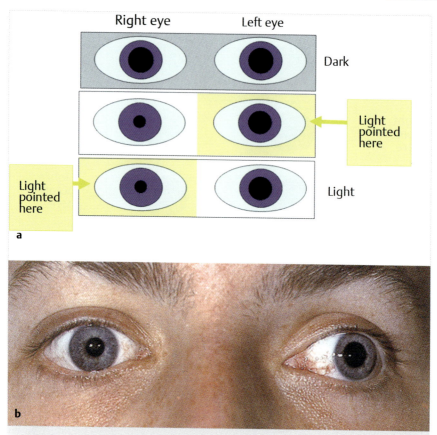

Fig. 12.12 (a) The large (left eye) pupil is abnormal (the large pupil does not constrict well in response to light). The anisocoria is greater in the light than in the dark (indicating poor pupillary constriction on the abnormal side). This indicates an abnormality of the parasympathetic system. (b) Left third nerve palsy. The left pupil does not constrict in response to light, and there is an adduction, elevation, and depression deficit of the left eye.

Miosis (the Small Pupil Is Abnormal)

Miosis, or excessive smallness or contraction of one pupil, is diagnosed when the small pupil does not dilate as well as the large pupil in dim light.

Miosis can be related to an ocular condition that keeps the small pupil from dilating (e.g., uveitis, previous ocular surgery, or pseudoexfoliation syndrome) or to pharmacologic constriction of the pupil (by drops, e.g., pilocarpine). Brimonidine tartrate (used topically to treat glaucoma) usually decreases the pupil size. This effect is not noticeable when patients place drops in both eyes, but it can induce anisocoria when used to treat unilateral glaucoma.

When the ocular and pharmacologic causes are excluded, pupillary miosis usually results from dysfunction of the ipsilateral sympathetic pathway, or Horner syndrome.

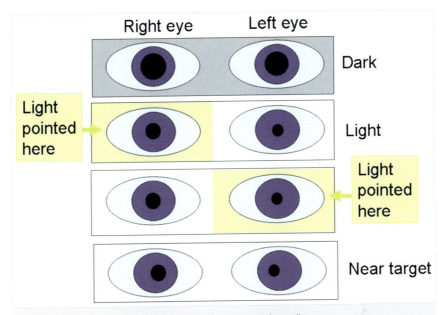

Fig. 12.13 Physiologic anisocoria (right pupil larger than left pupil).

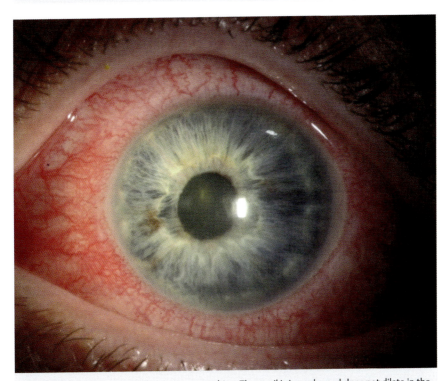

Fig. 12.14 Anterior uveitis with posterior synechiae. The pupil is irregular and does not dilate in the dark or with dilating drops. The intraocular inflammation produces adhesions between the iris and the lens (synechiae). Note the red eye.

293

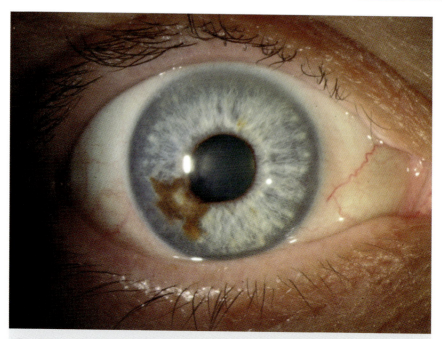

Fig. 12.15 Iris nevus. The pupil is irregular and does not dilate well in the dark.

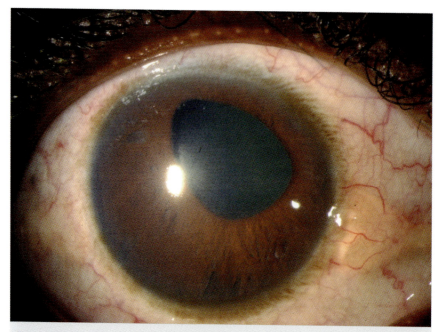

Fig. 12.16 Ectopic pupil from congenital dysgenesis of the anterior chamber. The pupil is dilated, irregular, and decentered.

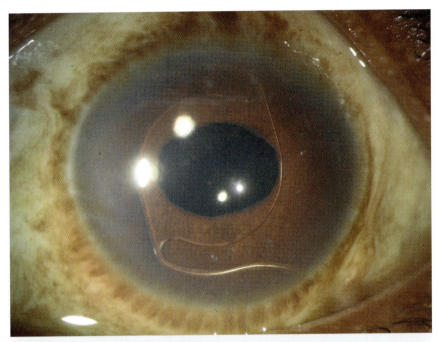

Fig. 12.17 Postsurgical pupil. The pupil is dilated and oval after complicated cataract surgery. The intraocular lens in the anterior chamber pulls on the iris.

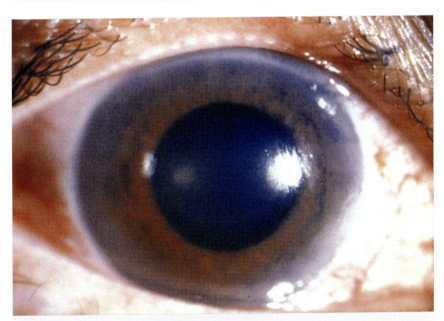

Fig. 12.18 Angle closure glaucoma. The pupil is dilated (nonreactive to light), with decreased vision and ocular pain; the eye is red, the intraocular pressure is elevated, and the cornea is edematous.

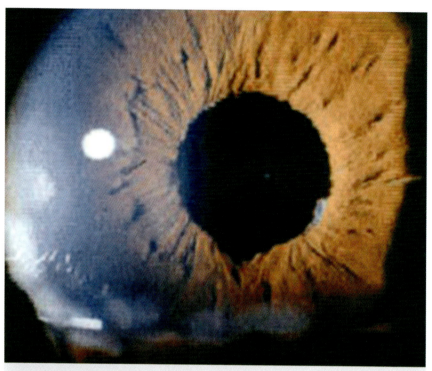

Fig. 12.19 Iris tears from trauma. The pupil is dilated, irregular, and poorly reactive to light because of iris tears.

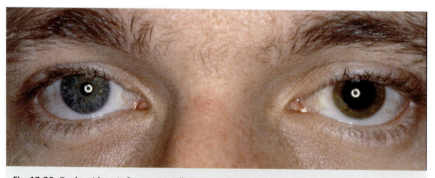

Fig. 12.20 Ocular siderosis from a metallic intraocular foreign body in the left eye. The left iris is hyperpigmented, and the left pupil is dilated and poorly reactive to light.

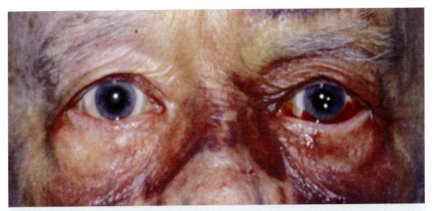

Fig. 12.21 Anisocoria after facial trauma. Both pupils are dilated, slightly irregular, and poorly reactive to light because of iris tears. There is a subconjunctival hemorrhage in the left eye.

Horner Syndrome (Oculosympathetic Paresis)

Features and Diagnosis

The signs of Horner syndrome include the following (▶ Fig. 12.22):

- Reduced palpebral fissure: mild ptosis involving both upper and lower lids due to paralysis of the Müller muscles innervated by the sympathetic pathway
- Pseudoenophthalmos because of the reduced palpebral fissure
- Unilateral miosis
- Dilation lag in the dark (slow dilation of the affected pupil)

Heterochromia in congenital Horner syndrome (lighter color on affected side) (▶ Fig. 12.23)

Associated neurologic symptoms and signs include the following:

- Anhidrosis of the ipsilateral face (loss of sweating) in preganglionic lesions (first- or second-order Horner syndrome)
- Brainstem and spinal cord symptoms and signs suggestive of a first-order Horner syndrome
- Arm pain, hand weakness, and history of neck surgery or neck trauma suggestive of a second-order Horner syndrome
- Ipsilateral facial pain suggestive of a third-order Horner syndrome

Pharmacologic testing confirms the diagnosis of Horner syndrome.

Cocaine drops are used but are difficult to obtain. Apraclonidine drops are now replacing cocaine for the diagnosis of Horner syndrome (apraclonidine is routinely used for glaucoma and is easy to obtain). The diagnosis of Horner syndrome with cocaine or apraclonidine can be performed in children, but apraclonidine should be avoided in young children less than 1 year of age (the punctum lacrima should be occluded with a finger while placing the drops to limit systemic effects in all children and in pregnant women).

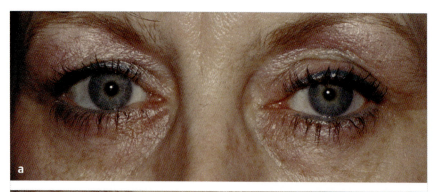

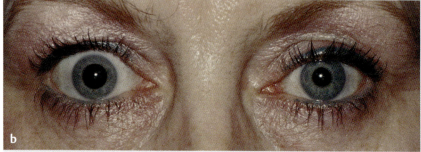

Fig. 12.22 Left Horner syndrome. (a) In the light. (b) In the dark (anisocoria is more obvious).

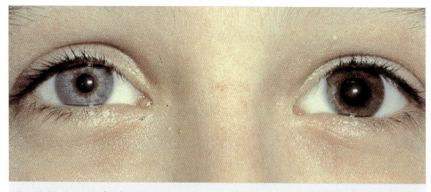

Fig. 12.23 Congenital right Horner syndrome with heterochromia (the affected side is lighter).

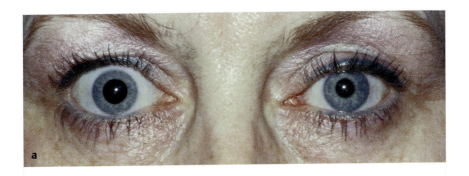

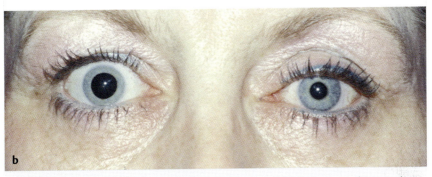

Fig. 12.24 Diagnosis of Horner syndrome with cocaine drops. (a) Left Horner syndrome in the dark. (b) Left Horner syndrome after cocaine (the Horner pupil does not dilate).

Testing with cocaine (▶ Fig. 12.24) involves the following:
1. Instill two drops of 4 or 10% cocaine in both eyes.
2. After 45 minutes to 1 hour,
   • the normal pupil dilates,
   • the Horner pupil dilates poorly, and
   • anisocoria increases.

Cocaine blocks the reuptake of norepinephrine at the sympathetic nerve synapse with the iris dilator. It causes pupillary dilation in eyes with intact sympathetic innervation and has no effect in eyes with impaired sympathetic innervation, regardless of the lesion location (little or no norepinephrine is being released into the synaptic cleft tonically).

To test with apraclonidine (Iopidine, Alcon, Fort Worth, TX; ▶ Fig. 12.25):
1. Instill two drops of 0.5 or 1.0% apraclonidine in both eyes.
2. After 30 to 45 minutes,
   • the normal pupil does not dilate,
   • the Horner pupil dilates,
   • anisocoria reverses, and
   • the palpebral fissure enlarges on the side of the Horner syndrome.

Apraclonidine is a direct alpha-receptor agonist (strong alpha-2 and weak alpha-1). It has no effect in eyes with intact sympathetic innervation and causes mild pupillary

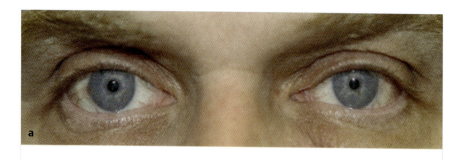

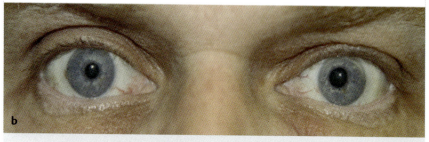

Fig. 12.25 Diagnosis of Horner syndrome with 0.5% apraclonidine drops. (**a**) Left Horner syndrome in the dark. (**b**) Left Horner syndrome after apraclonidine drops (the anisocoria is reversed, and the left upper eyelid is elevated).

dilation in eyes with sympathetic denervation, regardless of the lesion location (with denervation hypersensitivity, alpha-1 effect dilates the Horner pupil and elevates the ptotic lid). Apraclonidine reverses the Horner syndrome.

Localization

Horner syndrome is caused by a lesion anywhere along the sympathetic pathway that supplies the head, eye, and neck. Associated symptoms and signs usually allow localization of the lesion.

Pharmacologic testing helps localize the lesion along the sympathetic pathway (hydroxyamphetamine test) (▶ Fig. 12.26 and ▶ Fig. 12.27). Except for rare emergencies, pharmacologic localization of the lesion should ideally be performed before obtaining any neuroimaging in adults. It is usually not performed in young children in whom the test is poorly reliable.

Testing with hydroxyamphetamine involves the following:
1. Instill two drops of 1% hydroxyamphetamine in both eyes.
2. After 45 minutes,
   - the normal pupil dilates, and
   - the Horner pupil dilates poorly if the lesion is postganglionic (third order), or
   - the Horner pupil dilates if the lesion is preganglionic (first or second order).

Hydroxyamphetamine releases stored norepinephrine from the postganglionic adrenergic nerve endings. It causes pupillary dilation in eyes with intact sympathetic

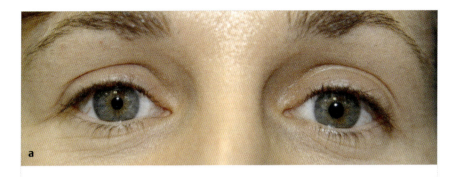

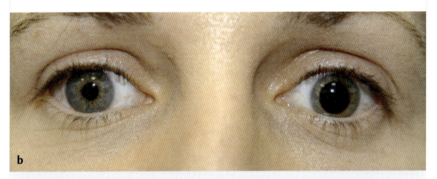

Fig. 12.26 Pharmacologic localization of third-order Horner syndrome using hydroxyamphetamine drops. (**a**) Right Horner syndrome in dim light. (**b**) Right Horner syndrome (third-order) after hydroxyamphetamine. The right pupil does not dilate as much as the left (the anisocoria is increased).

innervation or intact postganglionic fibers (▶ Fig. 12.27) and has no or partial effect in eyes with impaired sympathetic innervation from lesions involving the postganglionic fibers (no effect on third-order Horner syndrome).

Because cocaine may interfere with the uptake and efficacy of hydroxyamphetamine drops, it is recommended that at least 72 hours elapse between the two tests. This is why the diagnosis of Horner syndrome is most often made clinically and only the hydroxyamphetamine test is performed to localize the lesion prior to obtaining a directed workup.

Horner Syndrome in Adults

The evaluation of an adult with Horner syndrome is mostly based on lesion location.

The most classic cause of a first-order Horner syndrome is ipsilateral medullary infarction (Wallenberg syndrome); other causes are ipsilateral various thalamic, brainstem, and spinal cord lesions (▶ Fig. 12.28). Second-order Horner syndromes are most suggestive of neoplasm or trauma of the lower cervical spine, brachial plexus, or lung apex (▶ Fig. 12.29). Third-order Horner syndromes point to lesions of the internal carotid artery, such as dissection and cavernous sinus aneurysms (▶ Fig. 12.30). ▶ Table 12.3 summarizes the causes of Horner syndrome in adults.

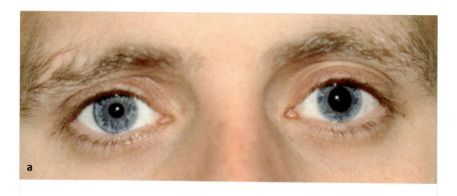

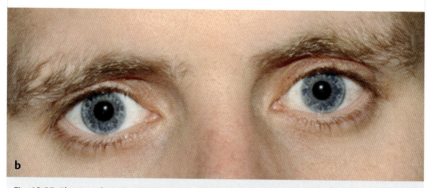

Fig. 12.27 Pharmacologic localization of second-order Horner syndrome using hydroxyamphetamine drops. (**a**) Right Horner syndrome after right brachial plexus injury. (**b**) After hydroxyamphetamine, both pupils dilate symmetrically, confirming a preganglionic lesion.

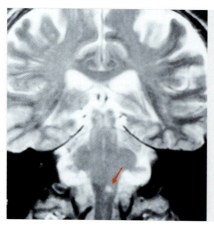

Fig. 12.28 Wallenberg syndrome (left lateral medullary infarction) (*arrow*) with first-order left Horner syndrome (T2-weighted coronal magnetic resonance imaging).

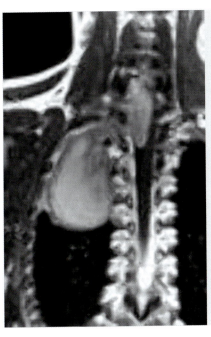

Fig. 12.29 Pancoast (Tobias) syndrome with second-order right Horner syndrome from a pulmonary apex mass (T1-weighted coronal magnetic resonance imaging with contrast).

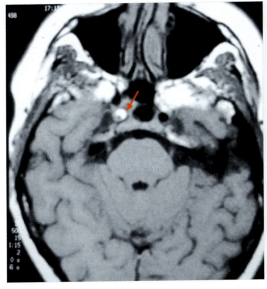

Fig. 12.30 Right internal carotid artery dissection (*arrow*) with right painful third-order Horner syndrome (T1-weighted axial magnetic resonance imaging).

Table 12.3 Most common causes of Horner syndrome in adults based on lesion location

Central (first order)	Preganglionic (second order)	Postganglionic (third order)
Hypothalamus • Stroke • Tumor Brainstem • Stroke (lateral medullary infarction) • Demyelination • Tumor Spinal cord (cervicothoracic) • Trauma • Syringomyelia • Tumor (intramedullary) • Demyelination • Myelitis • Arteriovenous malformation	Cervical spine disease Brachial plexus injury Pulmonary apical lesion • Apical lung tumor • Mediastinal tumors • Trauma • Cervical rib Iatrogenic (jugular or subclavian cannulation chest tube, thoracic surgery) Subclavian artery aneurysm Thyroid tumors	Superior cervical ganglion • Trauma • Jugular venous ectasia • Iatrogenic (surgical neck dissection) Internal carotid artery • Dissection • Aneurysm • Trauma • Arteritis • Tumor Skull base lesion • Nasopharyngeal carcinoma • Lymphoma Cavernous sinus lesion • Tumors • Pituitary tumor • Inflammation • Thrombosis • Carotid aneurysm Cluster headache

Pearls

The combination of an ipsilateral Horner syndrome (first-order) and contralateral superior oblique palsy (fourth nerve palsy) suggests a lesion of the trochlear nucleus or its fascicle in the brainstem.

The combination of an ipsilateral Horner syndrome (third-order) and an abducens paresis (sixth nerve palsy) suggests a lesion in the cavernous sinus (▶ Fig. 12.31 and ▶ Fig. 12.32).

An acute painful Horner syndrome should be presumed related to a dissection of the ipsilateral internal carotid artery unless proven otherwise. These patients are at risk of cerebral infarction and should be evaluated emergently.

In evaluating an adult with isolated Horner syndrome, ask about the duration of symptoms, the presence of pain, and other symptoms or signs. Next, determine the localization of the lesion to the first-order, second-order, or third-order neuron. Finally, conduct a physical examination (ocular, neurologic, neck, supraclavicular, and chest).

The tests ordered will vary depending on the lesion location, the presence of associated symptoms or signs, the urgency of the workup, and the radiologist's preference.

• For first- or second-order Horner syndrome, tests would include a chest X-ray, computed tomography (CT) or magnetic resonance imaging (MRI) of the chest (to view the pulmonary apex), and MRI with contrast of the head and neck. Magnetic resonance angiography (MRA) of the aortic arch or computed tomographic angiography (CTA) of the head and neck may be required.

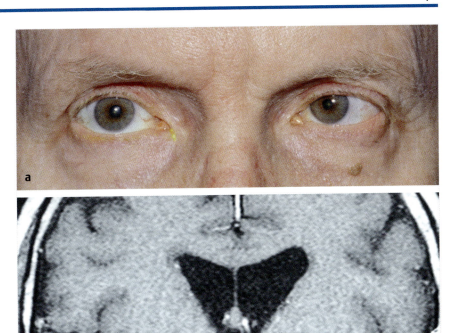

Fig. 12.31 (a) Left abduction deficit (sixth nerve palsy) with left Horner syndrome (miosis and reduced palpebral fissure). The association of a sixth nerve palsy and an ipsilateral Horner syndrome localizes the lesion to the cavernous sinus, where the sympathetic pathway is briefly in contact with the sixth nerve. (b) Coronal T1-weighted magnetic resonance imaging with contrast showing a large left cavernous sinus aneurysm (*red circle*).

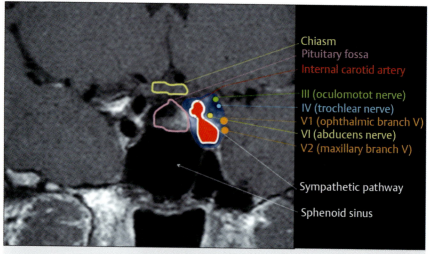

Fig. 12.32 Anatomy of the cavernous sinus showing the sympathetic pathway (*white*) around the internal carotid artery (*red*). The sixth nerve (*yellow*) is immediately next to the internal carotid artery.

- For third-order Horner syndrome, tests would include MRI with contrast of the head and MRA or CTA of the head and neck.
- If localization is unknown, image brain, neck, spinal cord, carotid arteries, and pulmonary apex (may require multiple imaging tests). The easiest test is a CT/CTA of the head, neck, and chest allows good examination of the brain and spine, of the soft tissues, and of large blood vessels in the head, neck, and chest as well as examination of the pulmonary apex.

Horner Syndrome in Infants and Children

The etiology of Horner syndrome in infants and children differs from that for the adult population. The classic causes include birth trauma, neuroblastoma, vascular anomalies of the large arteries, and chest surgery (▶ Table 12.4; ▶ Fig. 12.33 and ▶ Fig. 12.34).

Table 12.4 Most common causes of Horner syndrome in children

Congenital[a]	Acquired
Birth trauma related	Neuroblastoma
Cervical rib	Rhabdomyosarcoma
Congenital infections	Brainstem vascular malformations
Neuroblastoma	Brainstem tumors (glioma)
Congenital agenesis of the internal carotid artery	Demyelination (brainstem)
Idiopathic	Carotid artery dissection
	Neck trauma
	Postsurgical:
	Jugular cannulation
	Neck surgery
	Thoracic surgery
	Idiopathic

[a]Congenital causes occur within 4 weeks of birth.

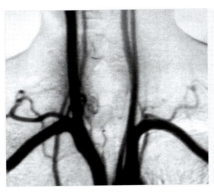

Fig. 12.33 Congenital agenesis of the left internal carotid artery (catheter angiogram).

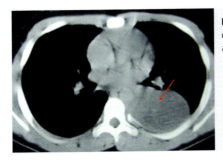

Fig. 12.34 Metastatic neuroblastoma (*red arrow*) on a computed tomographic scan of the chest in a child with a left Horner syndrome.

Pearls

An isolated Horner syndrome in a young child should prompt a workup for neuroblastoma.

In evaluating a young child with isolated Horner syndrome, first determine any history of birth trauma, then conduct a physical examination, checking for a supraclavicular or abdominal mass. To rule out a neuroblastoma, order an MRI scan of the head, neck, and chest with contrast; an MRI scan of the abdomen if there is high clinical suspicion; and tests for urinary catecholamines (vanillylmandelic acid [VMA] and homovanillic acid [HVA]). MRA scans of the neck and aortic arch are also often obtained.

MRI of the head, neck, and chest as well as MRA of the head and aortic arch can be performed in one test under sedation in a young child. MRI of the abdomen usually requires a separate test (and therefore another sedation) and is often not required in a child with isolated Horner and normal abdominal examination.

Treatment of Horner Syndrome

Most patients with Horner syndrome have no visual changes and tolerate a mild ptosis. Rarely, lid surgery is requested to correct a persistent ptosis. Topical apraclonidine temporarily (a few hours) corrects the ptosis associated with Horner syndrome and may be used intermittently for cosmetic reasons or when the ptosis reduces the superior visual field.

Mydriasis (the Large Pupil Is Abnormal)

When the larger pupil does not constrict as well as the small pupil in light, then the large pupil is abnormal (mydriasis). The clinical history and associated symptoms or signs, such as visual loss, diplopia, and ptosis, help in the diagnosis.

Investigations should be obtained only once the mechanism of mydriasis is understood. Indeed, the noncontrast head CT routinely ordered in the emergency room for a patient with mydriasis is useless and falsely reassuring.

Causes

Ocular Disorders

Ocular conditions that keep the large pupil from constricting (e.g., posterior synechia, angle closure glaucoma, previous ocular surgery, ocular trauma, pseudoexfoliation syndrome, and chronic mydriatic use) can produce mydriasis of various sizes; the pupil is not or is poorly reactive to light (see ▶ Fig. 12.14, ▶ Fig. 12.15, ▶ Fig. 12.16, ▶ Fig. 12.17, ▶ Fig. 12.18).

Traumatic Mydriasis

Pupillary dilation following ocular trauma often results from injury to the pupillary sphincter muscle. The pupil may be irregular and is typically large. Its reaction to light and accommodation varies, depending on the extent of the damage. Anisocoria is more evident in bright light as the pupil fails to constrict due to injury to the sphincter muscle. The pupillary abnormality is isolated without ptosis or diplopia (see ▶ Fig. 12.19).

Pharmacologic Mydriasis

Pharmacologic agents are a common cause of isolated unilateral or bilateral mydriasis. Drugs can produce mydriasis either by stimulation of the sympathetic innervation of the dilator pupillae or by inhibition of the parasympathetic innervation to the sphincter pupillae. Topical agents (e.g., ocular drops or toxins accidentally or purposely placed in the eye) usually cause a unilateral mydriasis, and systemic agents can cause bilateral mydriasis (▶ Table 12.5 and ▶ Table 12.6). Pharmacologic mydriasis can also occur when the patient touches a substance with effects on the autonomic system and then rubs an eye with the same fingers. Occasionally, patients using nebulized bronchodilators for asthma or bronchitis may notice anisocoria when the mask is not well adjusted and some mist reaches one eye. A number of solutions or drugs routinely used to treat dry eyes or allergic conjunctivitis may also induce pharmacologic mydriasis.

Table 12.5 Topical medications producing pharmacologic mydriasis

Parasympatholytic cycloplegic drugs	Sympathomimetic drugs
Atropine	Adrenaline
Homatropine	Phenylephrine (also used in topical allergy medications)
Cyclopentolate	Clonidine
Tropicamide	Apraclonidine

Table 12.6 Other agents producing pharmacologic mydriasis

Parasympatholytic cycloplegic agents	Sympathomimetic agents
Scopolamine patch (used for motion sickness) Contact with belladonna plant Exposure to chemicals, such as organophosphates (parasympatholytic agents used as pesticides) Use of bronchodilators (nebulizer)	Use of bronchodilators (nebulizer)

Pharmacologic mydriasis from topical agents, such as dilating drops, is usually large (pupil measures at least 7 or 8 mm) (▶ Fig. 12.35). The vision is decreased at near (cycloplegia with paralysis of accommodation), and the pupil does not react to light and does not constrict at near. The condition may last up to 10 days if atropine was placed in the eye.

Pharmacologic testing confirms the diagnosis of pharmacologic mydriasis:

1. Place two drops of dilute pilocarpine (0.1%) in both eyes to make sure this is not a tonic pupil (in which case, the dilated pupil will constrict because of denervation hypersensitivity, whereas the normal or pharmacologic pupil will not change).
2. If there is no response after 45 minutes, place two drops of pilocarpine 1 or 2% in each eye. The normal pupil will constrict. If the dilated pupil constricts only partially or not at all, the diagnosis of pharmacologic mydriasis is confirmed.

Dysfunction of the Ipsilateral Parasympathetic Pathway

Parasympathetic fibers for pupillary constriction travel along the third cranial nerve to the ipsilateral ciliary ganglion within the orbit. Therefore, third nerve palsies and tonic pupil (Adie pupil) from ciliary ganglion dysfunction may produce a mydriasis with a poorly or nonreactive pupil in response to light.

Tonic Pupil (Adie Pupil)

Tonic pupil is defined as isolated iris sphincter and ciliary muscle dysfunction resulting from damage to the ciliary ganglion or postganglionic short ciliary nerves (in the orbit), followed by aberrant reinnervation.

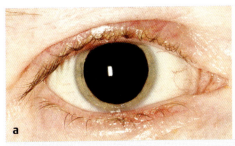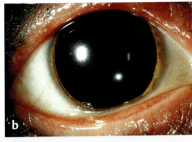

Fig. 12.35 (a) Pharmacologic mydriasis (topical dilating drops). (b) Large pharmacologic mydriasis (topical dilating drops).

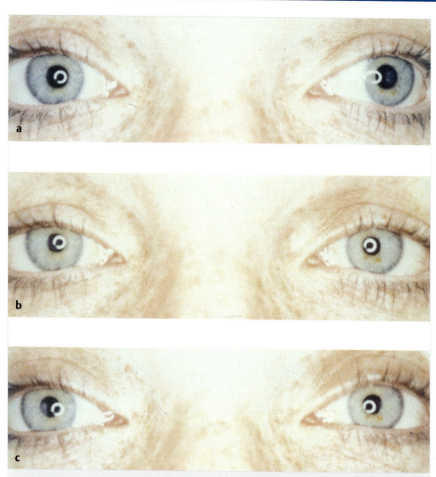

Fig. 12.36 Left tonic (Adie) pupil. **(a)** Pupils in the light (distance). The left pupil is larger and does not react to light. **(b)** When the patient is asked to look at a near target, both pupils constrict. **(c)** Forty-five minutes after dilute pilocarpine (0.10%) is placed in both eyes, the tonic pupil (left) constricts. Dilute pilocarpine has no effect on the normal pupil.

Clinical symptoms and signs of tonic pupil (► Fig. 12.36, ► Fig. 12.37, ► Fig. 12.38) include the following:

- Large pupil that does not react or reacts poorly to light
- Better constriction when looking at a near target (because the ratio of fibers that serve accommodation compared with pupilloconstriction is about 30:1, there is an overwhelming amount of regenerating accommodative fibers that respond to a near stimulus but may aberrantly regenerate to the pupil sphincter muscle; this explains the light-near dissociation classically found in a tonic pupil)
- Slow tonic redilation of the pupil from near to distance because of sphincter muscle denervation supersensitivity
- Patients often complain of blurry vision at near (accommodation paralysis) and sensitivity to light (from the large pupil).

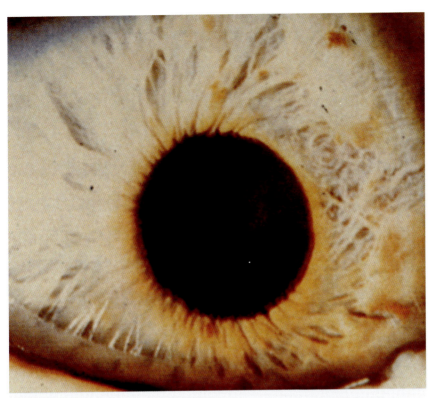

Fig. 12.37 The tonic pupil is irregular with segmental contraction (from 6 to 12 o'clock) in response to bright light.

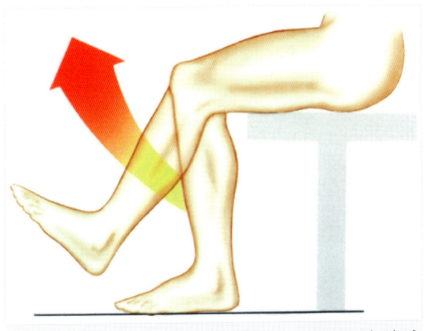

Fig. 12.38 In Adie syndrome, deep tendon reflexes are absent. (From Rohkamm R. Color Atlas of Neurology. New York, NY: Thieme; 2004:41. Reprinted with permission.)

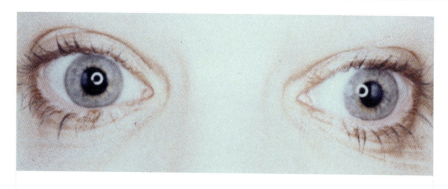

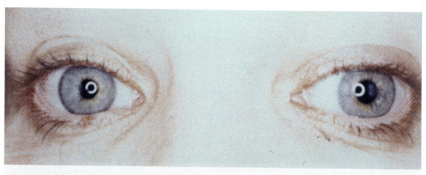

Fig. 12.39 Pharmacologic confirmation of the tonic pupil. (a) Right tonic pupil in the dark. The right pupil is larger and is not reactive to light. (b) Constriction of the right tonic pupil after dilute pilocarpine (0.1%).

Pharmacologic testing confirms the diagnosis of Adie pupil. Dilute pilocarpine can be used to make a pharmacologic diagnosis of tonic pupil (▶ Fig. 12.39). Supersensitivity of denervation makes the tonic pupil sensitive to dilute pilocarpine. Within 5 to 7 days of denervation, cholinergic supersensitivity of the end-organ begins. It is demonstrated by placing two drops of dilute pilocarpine (0.1%) in both eyes. If the iris sphincter has cholinergic supersensitivity, the larger pupil (tonic pupil) becomes smaller than the normal pupil 30 to 45 minutes after instillation of the dilute pilocarpine (the dilute pilocarpine has no effect in the normal eye). Dilute pilocarpine can be made by mixing 0.1 mL of 1% pilocarpine with 0.9 mL of sterile saline in a 1 mL tuberculin syringe.

Causes of tonic pupil include a variety of local processes affecting the ciliary ganglion in the orbit, such as trauma, tumor, ischemia (giant cell arteritis), and infection (viral, e.g., herpes zoster virus or herpes simplex virus, or syphilis). It may happen after laser panretinal photocoagulation and as part of a more widespread autonomic process (diabetes, amyloidosis, and Sjögren syndrome). Adie syndrome is idiopathic in women ages 20 to 40. This syndrome is often characterized by absent lower extremity deep tendon reflexes. It is unilateral in most cases but may become bilateral over years in about 20% of patients.

The evaluation of the patient with a tonic pupil is based mostly on other symptoms or signs, history of trauma or infection, and the patient's age, and may include blood count, erythrocyte sedimentation rate, C-reactive protein, fasting glucose, hemoglobin

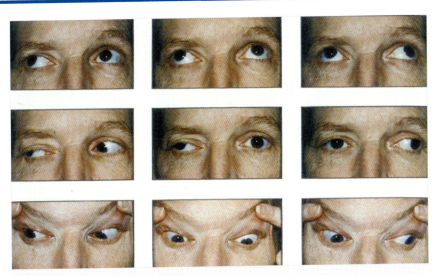

Fig. 12.40 Right third nerve palsy with mydriasis.

A1C, syphilis and human immunodeficiency virus (HIV) testing, and orbital imaging. Most often, however, confirmation of an Adie pupil with pharmacologic testing, especially in women ages 20 to 60, is satisfactory, and no workup is performed.

Over time, tonic pupils tend to become smaller ("little old Adies"). Patients may need reading glasses to correct the accommodation paralysis. Some patients wear tinted glasses because of photophobia. Although dilute pilocarpine corrects the mydriasis and may be used occasionally for cosmetic purposes, its chronic use is not recommended.

Third Nerve Palsy

Mydriasis from isolated third nerve palsy is essentially always associated with an extraocular movement deficit (responsible for diplopia) and/or ptosis (see Chapter 13).

The signs and symptoms of third nerve palsy are ptosis, mydriasis, and abnormal extraocular movements, with impaired adduction, depression, and elevation. Some patients have incomplete third nerve palsy, but there is always some ptosis and diplopia from mild extraocular muscle deficits (▶ Fig. 12.40).

A completely isolated mydriasis is extremely unlikely to be related to a third nerve palsy and should be evaluated clinically and with pharmacologic testing to rule out an Adie pupil or pharmacologic mydriasis prior to obtaining any further workup.

Not all third nerve palsies have pupil involvement. Pupil involvement is common in nuclear, fascicular, and subarachnoid third nerve palsies. Because the pupillary fibers are located superficially, they are vulnerable to compressive processes such as aneurysmal mass effect, various tumors such as pituitary apoplexy, and uncal herniation (▶ Fig. 12.41 and ▶ Fig. 12.42).

The evaluation of the patient with a third nerve palsy depends on associated symptoms and signs, the pattern of oculomotor nerve involvement, and the age of the patient. The approach to the patient with a third nerve palsy is detailed in Chapter 13.

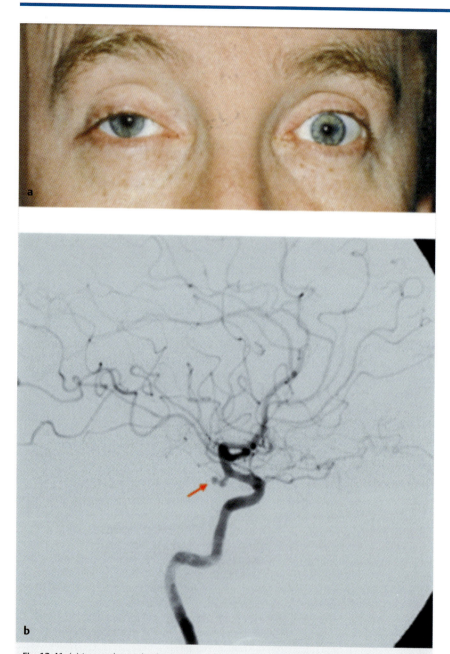

Fig. 12.41 (a) Incomplete right third nerve palsy with mild ptosis, mild mydriasis, and limitation of adduction, depression, and elevation of the right eye. (b) Cerebral angiogram showing a posterior communicating artery aneurysm compressing the right third nerve (*arrow*).

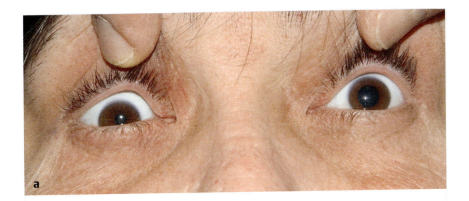

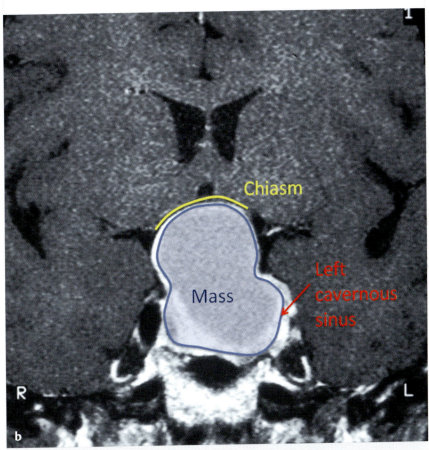

Fig. 12.42 (a) Complete left third nerve palsy with ptosis, mydriasis, and limitation of adduction, depression, and elevation of the left eye. (b) Coronal T1-weighted magnetic resonance imaging with contrast showing a large pituitary tumor invading the left cavernous sinus.

The approach to the patient with anisocoria is detailed in ▶ Fig. 12.43.

12.5 Other Pupillary Abnormalities

12.5.1 Tadpole Pupil

Tadpole pupil is an irregular pupil that resembles a tadpole (▶ Fig. 12.44). It is a benign phenomenon that is spontaneously reversible. The pupil undergoes sectoral dilation lasting for a few minutes before returning to normal (segmental spasm of the iris dilator muscle). Tadpole pupil may occur multiple times for several days or a week and then disappear.

12.5.2 Midbrain Correctopia

Midbrain correctopia refers to eccentric or oval pupils occasionally seen in patients with rostral midbrain lesions.

12.5.3 Argyll Robertson Pupils

Argyll Robertson pupils are small (< 2 mm), irregular pupils (almost always bilateral). They are characterized by no reaction to light, normal near response (light-near dissociation), often iris atrophy and iris transillumination defects, and poor dilation with drops. The condition is classically described in patients with tertiary syphilis, is common in diabetes, and may happen in encephalitis.

12.5.4 Light-Near Dissociation

Light-near dissociation refers to pupils that do not react to light but react to near stimuli (▶ Table 12.7).

12.5.5 Paradoxical Pupillary Reactions

Paradoxical pupillary constriction in dim illumination after exposure to light can be observed in children with severe congenital retinopathies, such as congenital stationary night blindness and congenital achromatopsia.

12.5.6 Benign Episodic Pupillary Mydriasis

Also known as springing pupil, benign episodic pupillary mydriasis usually occurs in young, healthy individuals. It lasts from a few minutes to a few hours and is sometimes associated with migraine-like headaches. The condition resolves spontaneously and is not associated with any underlying disorder.

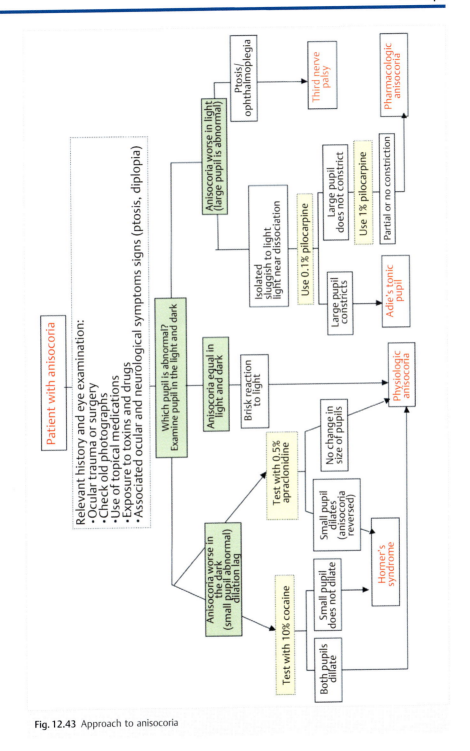

Fig. 12.43 Approach to anisocoria

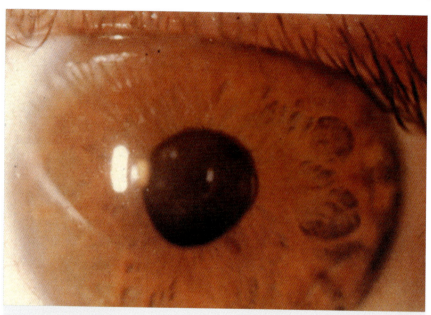

Fig. 12.44 Tadpole pupil.

Table 12.7 Causes of light-near dissociation

Cause	Lesion location	Mechanism of light-near dissociation
Severe loss of vision	Anterior visual pathway (retina, optic nerves, chiasm)	Damage to retina or optic nerve
Laser panretinal photocoagulation, retinal cryotherapy	Short posterior ciliary nerves	Aberrant reinnervation of the iris sphincter by accommodative fibers
Tonic (Adie) pupil	Ciliary ganglion	Aberrant reinnervation of the iris sphincter by accommodative fibers
Argyll Robertson pupils (loss of pretectal light input to the Edinger–Westphal nucleus)	Tectum of the midbrain	Any lesion of the tectum of the midbrain (syphilis is the most classic cause, but not the most common)
Aberrant regeneration of the third nerve	Course of the third nerve	Aberrant reinnervation of the iris sphincter by fibers meant for the extraocular muscles or for the ciliary body (accommodation)
Peripheral neuropathy	Short posterior ciliary nerves	Axonal loss

12.5.7 Bilateral Mydriasis

Bilateral large pupils that do not react to light are observed during generalized tonic clonic seizures, although in rare cases unilateral ictal mydriasis or miosis may occur. In coma patients, this condition is often associated with brain death. Bilateral large pupils in an awake patient are usually physiologic (more obvious in dim light, or produced by increased adrenergic state in young patients who are anxious or in pain) or pharmacologic (such as after cocaine use). Bilateral and symmetrical tonic pupils are rare.

12.5.8 Spasm of the Near Triad (Spasm of Convergence)

Spasm of the near triad (also known as spasm of convergence) is a disorder in which intermittent overaction of all three components of the near triad—miosis, accommodation, and convergence—occur. This disorder can mimic a unilateral or bilateral abduction deficit. The pupils constrict when the patient "attempts" to abduct each eye, confirming the voluntary convergence (▶ Fig. 12.45). Because the near triad is under voluntary control, this disorder is usually functional (nonorganic) and not related to an underlying lesion.

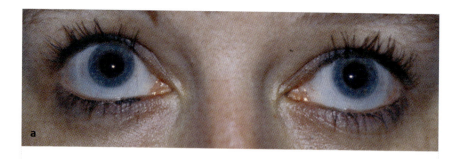

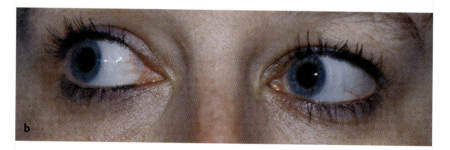

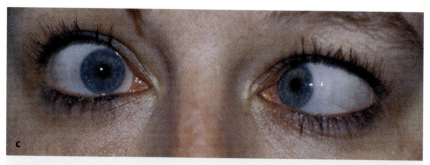

Fig. 12.45 Spasm of the near triad. (**a**) The patient looks straight at distance, and both pupils are normal. (**b**) The patient looks to the right, and the pupil size is unchanged. (**c**) The patient claims to be unable to abduct the left eye and complains of binocular horizontal diplopia. Note the bilateral miosis, confirming that the patient is using her near triad.

13 Diplopia

The goal of all normal eye movements is to place and maintain an object of visual interest on each fovea simultaneously to allow visualization of a single, stable object. Any deviation from normal eye movement will degrade vision and will often give the perception of double vision (diplopia). Diplopia is a common complaint and often reveals an underlying neurologic disorder.

The first step in evaluating a patient who is complaining of diplopia is to determine whether the diplopia is *monocular* (persists when the patient closes one eye) or *binocular* (resolves when the patient closes either eye).

13.1 Monocular Diplopia

Monocular diplopia is *not* related to a neurologic disorder and usually results from an optical problem (e.g., abnormal diffraction of light within the eye). It is almost always secondary to an ocular disease (e.g., cataract) or a refractive problem (e.g., astigmatism or issues with glasses).

It is typically alleviated when the patient looks through a pinhole (opaque panel perforated with one or multiple holes of 1 to 1.5 mm diameter). The holes restrict incoming light rays to a narrow path that bypasses refractive irregularities and presents a single, focused image to the retina. If monocular diplopia is due to an optical problem, the pinhole will usually make the secondary images disappear (▶ Fig. 13.1).

Any uncorrected refractive error or media opacity may be responsible for monocular diplopia. Not all refractive errors can be fully corrected with glasses. In cases of monocular diplopia, correction with contact lenses should be tried.

Lens opacities in the visual axis are a common cause of monocular diplopia, which resolves after cataract surgery (▶ Fig. 13.2).

Other causes of monocular diplopia include corneal surface irregularity (e.g., irregular astigmatism from pterygium or keratoconus, corneal edema, corneal scar, problem with contact lens, dry eye syndrome), post–cataract surgery (e.g., eccentric implant, tilted implant, multifocal implant, posterior capsular opacification), and retinal surface irregularity (e.g., macular edema, epiretinal membrane).

Damage to the visual association areas may very rarely produce duplicative images. In this case, the monocular diplopia or polyopia is present in *both* eyes (the patient sees

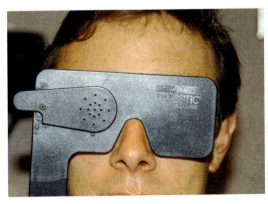

Fig. 13.1 Pinhole. The patient reads letters through small holes. Improvement of visual acuity suggests a refractive error or a media opacity. Monocular diplopia secondary to optical aberrations resolves or improves when looking through a pinhole.

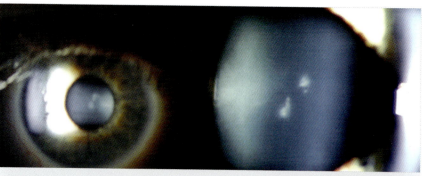

Fig. 13.2 Lens opacities responsible for monocular diplopia. The lens opacities (better seen on the enlarged photo on the right) are in the visual axis and are responsible for abnormal diffraction of incoming light.

double with either eye covered) and is *identical* in both eyes. Cerebral monocular diplopia is often monocular polyopia (i.e., more than two images).

Monocular diplopia or polyopia from cerebral lesions, however, is rarely an isolated finding; homonymous visual field defects are usually present, and other higher-order visual deficits such as alexia, prosopagnosia, and visual agnosia may be noted (see Chapters 10 and 11).

13.2 Binocular Diplopia

When the diplopia is binocular, it results from ocular misalignment secondary to dysfunction of the extraocular muscles, neuromuscular junction, ocular motor cranial nerves, or the internuclear and supranuclear pathways of eye movement control (▶ Fig. 13.3).

13.3 Understanding Eye Movements

Movements of the eyes are produced by the six extraocular muscles that are innervated by cranial nerves III (oculomotor nerve), IV (trochlear nerve), and VI (abducens nerve). To change visual fixation or to maintain fixation on an object that is moving relative to the observer, the eyes have to move with exquisite precision, and both eyes must move together. This requires a high degree of coordination of both the individual muscles to each eye and the muscle groups in each orbit. To achieve this, the nuclei of cranial nerves III, IV, and VI are controlled as a group by higher centers in the brainstem and the cerebrum.

Eye movements can be classified as follows, based on their role in vision:
1. Those that hold images steady on the retina
   - *Fixation:* holds the image of a stationary object on the fovea when the head is immobile
   - *Vestibular (vestibulo-ocular reflex [VOR]):* holds the image steady on the retina during brief head movements (tested using the oculocephalic reflex)
   - *Optokinetic:* holds the image steady on the retina during sustained head movements

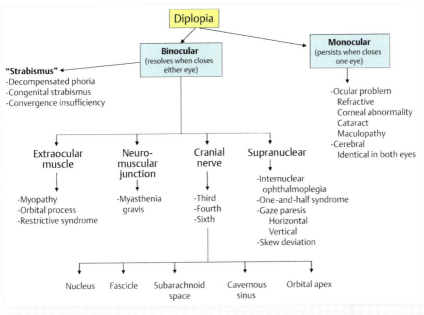

Fig. 13.3 Diagnosis of diplopia.

2. Those that direct the fovea to an object of interest
   - *Saccades:* bring the image of an object of interest rapidly onto the fovea
   - *Smooth pursuit:* holds the image of a small moving target on the fovea
   - *Vergence:* moves the eyes in opposite directions (convergence or divergence) so that images of a single object are held simultaneously on both fovea

Six muscles are responsible for eye movements:
- Medial rectus muscle: performs adduction
- Lateral rectus muscle: performs abduction
- Superior and inferior rectus muscles: elevate and depress the eye, respectively, performing these functions best when the eye is abducted.
- Superior and inferior oblique muscles: work using a sling/pulley mechanism, with insertions of the muscles being located toward the posterior portion of the globe. The oblique muscles serve as rotators of the eye about the vertical and horizontal axis as the eye is viewed (clockwise or counterclockwise torsion), but also serve to elevate or depress the eye in adduction.
   - *Superior oblique muscle:* primarily intorts the eye (rotates the superior aspect of the globe toward the nasal bridge about the vertical axis, clockwise in the case of the right eye as viewed by the examiner); this muscle also depresses the eye in adduction.
   - *Inferior oblique muscle:* extorts the eye but also serves as an elevator in adduction.

In the primary position of gaze, the superior and inferior oblique and superior and inferior rectus muscles all perform a combination of vertical and torsional actions.

323

Table 13.1 Action of the extraocular muscles

Extraocular muscle	Primary action	Secondary action	Tertiary action
Lateral rectus	Abduction	None	None
Medial rectus	Adduction	None	None
Superior rectus	Elevation	Incyclotorsion	Adduction
Inferior rectus	Depression	Excyclotorsion	Adduction
Superior oblique	Incyclotorsion	Depression	Abduction
Inferior oblique	Excyclotorsion	Elevation	Abduction

13.3.1 Laws of Ocular Motor Control

An *agonist muscle* moves the eye toward the desired direction. An *antagonist muscle* moves the eye away from the desired direction. According to Sherrington's law of reciprocal innervation, whenever an agonist muscle receives an excitatory signal to contract, an equivalent inhibitory signal is sent to the antagonist muscle of the same eye (e.g., in left gaze the right medial rectus is excited while the right lateral rectus is inhibited). *Yoke muscle pairs* are pairs of muscles (one from each eye) that move both eyes toward the same direction (e.g., the left lateral rectus and the right medial rectus contract simultaneously in leftward gaze). According to Hering's law of equal innervation, during conjugate eye movements, the muscles in the yoke muscle pair receive equal innervation so that the eyes move together.

13.3.2 Actions of the Extraocular Muscles

The primary action of an extraocular muscle is its major effect on the eye while the eye is looking straight ahead (in primary position). The secondary and tertiary actions of an extraocular muscle are additional effects on the eye while it is in primary position (▶ Table 13.1, ▶ Fig. 13.4).

During the clinical examination, the primary position refers to the position when the eyes look straight ahead. The patient is then asked to look right, left, up, and down and then to look up and right, down and right, up and left, and down and left (▶ Fig. 13.5).

The superior and inferior oblique muscles also rotate the eye, out for the inferior oblique (extorsion) and in for the superior oblique (intorsion) (▶ Fig. 13.6, ▶ Fig. 13.7, ▶ Fig. 13.8).

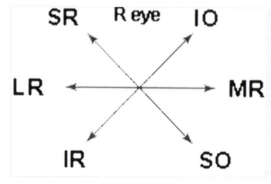

Fig. 13.4 Action of the six extraoculomotor muscles (right eye, examiner's view). LR, lateral rectus, innervated by the abducens nerve (cranial nerve [CN] VI). SO, superior oblique, innervated by the trochlear nerve (CN IV); SR, superior rectus; IO, inferior oblique; MR, medial rectus; IR, inferior rectus. All are innervated by the oculomotor nerve (CN III), which also innervates the levator palpebrae and the pupil.

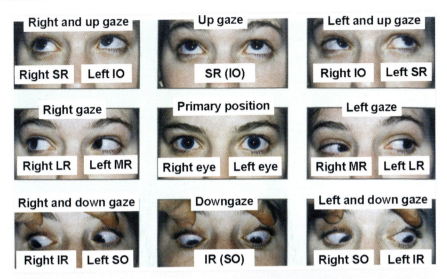

Fig. 13.5 Full extraocular movements in a normal subject (examiner's view). The eye movements must be examined in the nine cardinal positions of gaze. IO, inferior oblique; IR, inferior rectus; LR, lateral rectus; MR, medial rectus; SO, superior oblique; SR, superior rectus.

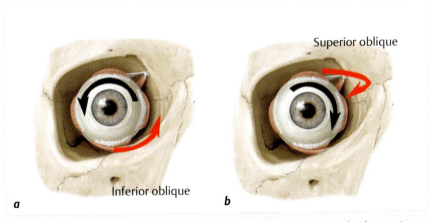

Fig. 13.6 Cyclotorsion effect of the oblique muscles (on the right eye) as seen by the examiner. (a) The right inferior oblique extorts the right eye. (b) The left superior oblique intorts the right eye. The red arrow shows the action of the muscle, the black arrow demonstrates the resultant movement of the eye. (Adapted from From Schuenke M, Schulte E, Schumacher U, Ross LM, Lamperti ED, Voll M. THIEME Atlas of Anatomy, Head and Neuroanatomy. Stuttgart, Germany: Thieme; 2007. Illustration by Karl Wesker.)

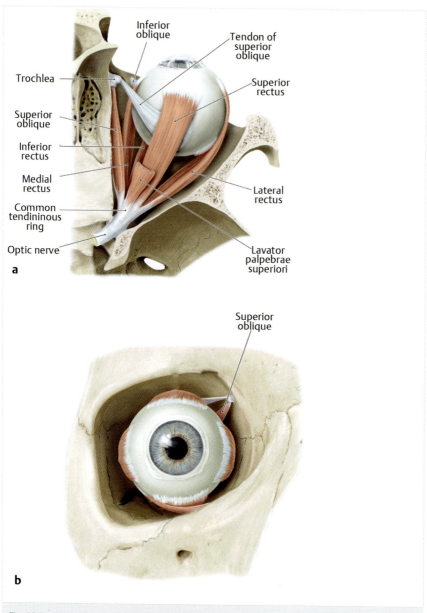

Fig. 13.7 Extraocular muscles in the orbit (right eye seen from above (**a**) and from the front (**b**)). (From Schuenke M, Schulte E, Schumacher U, Ross LM, Lamperti ED, Voll M. THIEME Atlas of Anatomy, Head and Neuroanatomy. Stuttgart, Germany: Thieme; 2007. Illustration by Karl Wesker.)

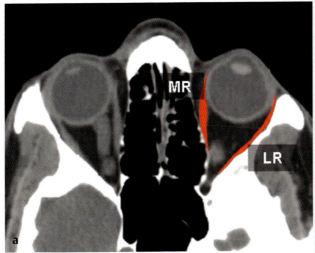

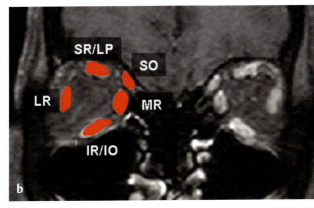

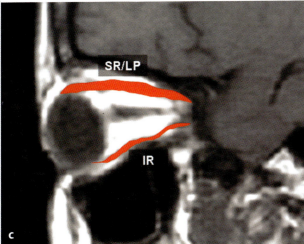

Fig. 13.8 (a) Extraocular muscles on an axial computed tomographic scan of the orbits. The medial and lateral recti (in red) are seen on this cut. (b) Extraocular muscles on a coronal magnetic resonance imaging (MRI) scan of the orbits (medial rectus, inferior rectus, and inferior oblique complex; lateral rectus; superior rectus; and superior oblique are in red). The levator palpebra cannot be distinguished from the superior rectus. (c) Sagittal MRI of the orbits showing the superior and inferior recti. IO, inferior oblique; IR, inferior rectus; LP, levator palpebra; LR, lateral rectus; MR, medial rectus; SO, superior oblique; SR, superior rectus.

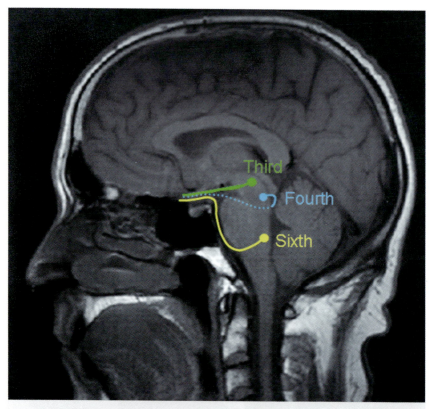

Fig. 13.9 Sagittal cut of the brain showing the origin of the ocular motor cranial nerves.

13.3.3 Cranial Nerves

The three ocular motor cranial nerves (III, IV, and VI) innervate the six extraocular muscles of each eye, the major eyelid elevator, and the parasympathetics (for pupillary constriction and lens accommodation) (▶ Fig. 13.9).

The third cranial nerve (oculomotor nerve) innervates the medial rectus, inferior rectus, superior rectus, inferior oblique, and levator palpebrae muscles, and it provides the parasympathetic pathway (pupillary constriction and accommodation).

The fourth cranial nerve (trochlear nerve) innervates the superior oblique muscle.

The sixth cranial nerve (abducens nerve) innervates the lateral rectus muscle.

All cranial nerves originate in the brainstem, where their nuclei are located. Each nerve has a short course within the brainstem (fascicle) prior to emerging and traveling in the subarachnoid space. Then all ocular motor cranial nerves enter the cavernous sinus and the superior orbital fissure to reach their corresponding extraocular muscles in the orbit. It is essential to understand the anatomical course of each cranial nerve to evaluate a patient with a cranial nerve palsy. By looking at accompanying signs, it is generally possible to accurately localize the lesion (▶ Fig. 13.10).

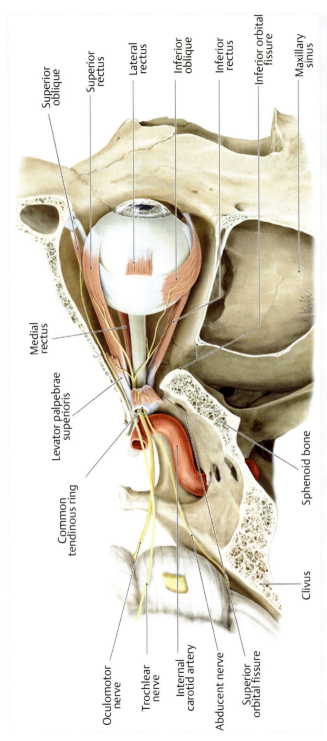

Fig. 13.10 Course of the third, fourth, sixth, and fifth cranial nerves (sagittal view). (From Schuenke M, Schulte E, Schumacher U, Ross LM, Lamperti ED, Voll M. THIEME Atlas of Anatomy, Head and Neuroanatomy. Stuttgart, Germany: Thieme; 2007. Illustration by Karl Wesker.)

13.3.4 Internuclear and Supranuclear Pathways

The initiation of conjugate eye movements is controlled by pathways and centers above the third, fourth, and sixth nerve nuclei (supranuclear pathways) and by interconnections among these nuclei (internuclear pathways). Inputs from the vestibular system (vestibulo-ocular pathways) also play an important role in the maintenance of eye position with head movement.

13.4 Examination of Eye Movements

Commonly Confused Ocular Motility Terms

Strabismus
This term is commonly used to describe ocular misalignment. It is a nonspecific term that does not indicate the underlying mechanism. It is, however, often used by ophthalmologists to describe congenital ocular deviation (i.e., congenital strabismus) rather than acquired ocular deviations. Neurologists do not use this term.

Comitance/Incomitance
Ocular misalignment (or strabismus) may be comitant or incomitant.
- With *comitant (or concomitant) strabismus*, the magnitude of ocular deviation is the same in all directions of gaze and does not depend on the eye used for fixation.
- With *incomitant (or noncomitant) strabismus*, the deviation varies in different directions of gaze. Most incomitant strabismus is caused by a paralytic or a mechanical restrictive process. The deviation is the largest when the eyes turn in the direction of the paralytic muscle. The deviation in incomitant strabismus also varies with the eye used for fixation. When the normal eye is fixating, the amount of misalignment is called the *primary deviation*. When the paretic eye is fixating, the amount of misalignment is called the *secondary deviation*. The secondary deviation is larger than the primary deviation in incomitant strabismus because an increase in innervation is needed for a paretic eye to fixate a target. By Hering's law, the contralateral yoke muscle also receives more innervation, resulting in a larger deviation.

Causes of incomitant misalignment are as follows:
- Extraocular muscle disease
- Myasthenia gravis
- Third, fourth, or sixth nerve palsy
- Internuclear ophthalmoplegia
- One-and-a-half syndrome

Causes of comitant misalignment are as follows:
- Early childhood strabismus
- Loss of fusion (severely decreased vision in one eye)
- Acquired vergence disturbance (convergence, divergence)
- Long-standing sixth nerve palsy (spread of comitance)
- Skew deviation

Phoria/Tropia

A phoria (heterophoria) is an ocular deviation that occurs only when binocular fixation is disturbed, such as when one eye is covered. When viewing an object with both eyes, a subject with a phoria is capable of aligning the eyes to achieve fusion (single binocular vision). The descriptive prefixes (*eso-, exo-, hyper-*) are used to describe the heterophoria.

A tropia (heterotropia) is present even when both eyes are viewing and may result in diplopia. Similarly, the descriptive prefixes (*eso-, exo-, hyper-*) are used to describe the heterotropia.

Although phorias are very common in the general population, a phoria or a tropia has the same localization value in a patient with new-onset binocular diplopia.

Right and Left Designations of Phorias and Tropias

When a horizontal strabismus is incomitant and one eye is obviously deviated, then it makes sense to say "right esotropia" or "right exotropia." In comitant horizontal strabismus, both eyes contribute equally to the problem, and the side is not designated. However, for vertical deviation, a side must be designated. Generally, the term *hypertropia* is preferred to *hypotropia,* and the patient is said to have a "right hypertropia" or a "left hypertropia" depending on which eye is higher. But "right hypertropia" or "left hypotropia" say the same thing: the right eye is higher than the left eye. These terms are describing the position of each eye only as it relates to the other and do not indicate the side of the pathological process. For example, a patient with a left third nerve palsy and an elevation deficit of the left eye may be described as having a "right hypertropia."

Ocular Motor Nerves/Oculomotor Nerve

Ocular motor nerves refers to all three cranial nerves involved in ocular movements.

The oculomotor nerve is cranial nerve III alone.

13.4.1 Assessing Ocular Motility

The objective of the motility examination is to evaluate the integrity of the supranuclear and internuclear pathways, ocular motor nuclei, and ocular motor nerves and their muscles. Ductions (monocular eye movements) and versions (conjugate eye movements of both eyes) should be checked in the nine cardinal positions of gaze ("look up, look down, look right, look left") (▶ Fig. 13.11).

The examiner should assess the eye movement by recording it as a percentage of normal.

For example, an abduction deficit in an isolated right sixth nerve palsy would be recorded as follows (▶ Fig. 13.12):
- Incomplete abduction of the right eye (20% of normal)
- Normal elevation, adduction, and depression of the right eye
- Full left eye movements
- Absence of ptosis
- Normal pupils

Another way to record eye movements is to use a scale from − 4 to 0 (with − 4 being complete paresis) and 0 being full eye movement (discussed later in chapter, ▶ Fig. 13.25c). With this scale, the incomplete abduction deficit shown in ▶ Fig. 13.12 would be described as a − 3 abduction of the right eye.

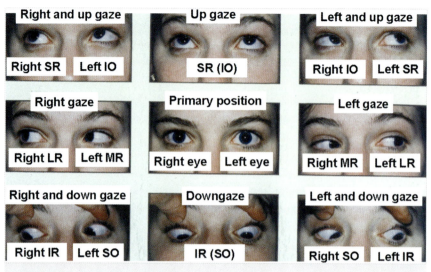

Fig. 13.11 Full extraocular movements in a normal subject. IO, inferior oblique; IR, inferior rectus; LR, lateral rectus; MR, medial rectus; SO, superior oblique; SR, superior rectus.

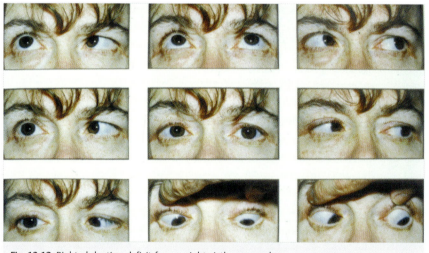

Fig. 13.12 Right abduction deficit from a right sixth nerve palsy.

Paresis or Restriction

When movements of one or both eyes are limited, it is important to determine whether the limitation is due to a *paresis* of the muscle or a *restriction* of the muscle. For example, an abduction deficit from a sixth nerve palsy results from a paresis of the lateral rectus muscle. On the other hand, an abduction deficit from an enlarged medial rectus in thyroid eye disease results from restriction of the

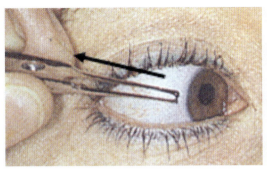

Fig. 13.13 The right eye is deviated toward the nose. The examiner pulls on the conjunctiva with forceps while asking the patient to look to the right to verify that the right eye movements are not restricted.

medial rectus. Additionally, an elevation deficit of one eye after an orbital floor fracture is most often due to a restriction of the inferior rectus that is bruised or trapped within the fracture.

In cooperative patients, the forced duction test allows differentiation between paresis and restriction (▶ Fig. 13.13) and is performed as follows:

- Instill two drops of topical anesthetic in the eye.
- Attempt to move the eye by pushing on the deviated globe with a cotton tipped swab or by pulling on the conjunctiva with forceps, while asking the patient to look in that direction.
- Inability of the examiner to move the eye suggests restriction.

Bell Phenomenon

With eye closure, there is a normal upward rotation of the eye. This is called the Bell phenomenon. It keeps the cornea from being exposed during sleep.

This normal reflex is easily visible in patients with peripheral facial nerve paralysis who attempt to shut their eyes (▶ Fig. 13.14).

In normal patients, it can be checked by having the patient try to close the eyes while the examiner holds the lids open.

In a patient with limited up gaze, a normal Bell phenomenon indicates a supranuclear defect with intact nuclear and infranuclear function (e.g., the Bell reflex is preserved despite up gaze paresis in Parinaud (dorsal midbrain) syndrome but is absent in a complete third nerve palsy or myopathy).

Saccades

Saccades, or fast eye movements, are tested by having the patient refixate between two targets. This can be easily performed by having the patient look at the examiner's nose and then at an eccentrically placed finger: "look at my nose, look at my finger" (▶ Fig. 13.15).

Pursuit

To test the pursuit system, the patient is asked to keep his or her head still and to follow a target (the examiner's finger) ("follow my finger").

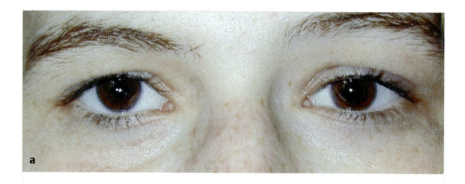

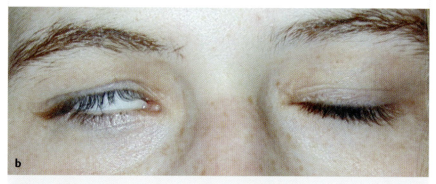

Fig. 13.14 Right peripheral facial nerve palsy. (a) The right palpebral fissure is larger than the left (lagophthalmos). (b) With attempted eye closure, the Bell phenomenon is seen in the right eye.

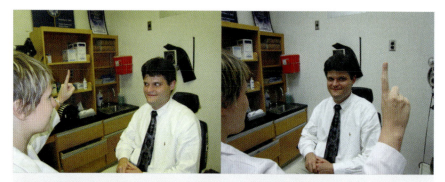

Fig. 13.15 Testing saccades by asking the patient to look from one finger to the other.

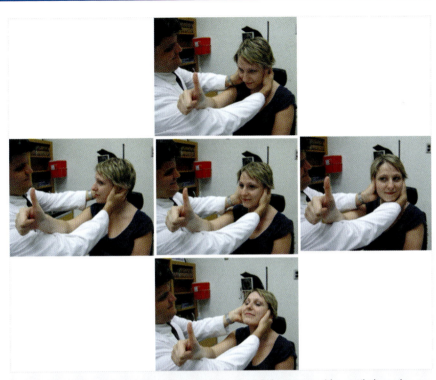

Fig. 13.16 Testing oculocephalic responses. The oculocephalic response (the vestibulo-ocular reflex) can be evaluated by having the patient fixate on a stationary target (the examiner's nose or the patient's own thumb), while the examiner gently rotates the head (horizontal), then extends and flexes the neck (vertical).

Oculocephalic Responses

Oculocephalic responses are used to test the vestibulo-ocular reflex and need to be tested in all patients with horizontal or vertical gaze paresis. Normally, the eyes should deviate conjugately in the direction opposite the head turn (▶ Fig. 13.16). Oculocephalic responses should not be tested in trauma patients who may have spinal lesions. Abnormal eye movements that are overcome by oculocephalic maneuvers are likely supranuclear (or nonorganic).

Vergences

Vergences are binocular eye movements in which the two eyes move in opposite directions (the eyes need to converge to see a single image at near, and need to diverge to see a single image at distance).

Convergence can be evaluated by having the patient look at his or her thumb or other accommodative target as it is brought toward the nose. Both eyes should adduct and there will be pupillary constriction and accommodation of the lens (the "near triad") (▶ Fig. 13.17). Convergence insufficiency is a common cause of binocular horizontal diplopia when the patient is reading. Patients develop an exotropia at near (to be discussed).

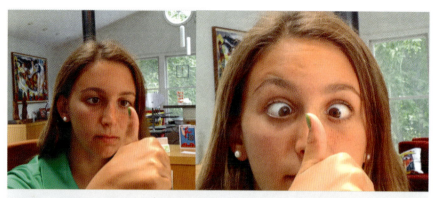

Fig. 13.17 Testing convergence.

13.4.2 Assessing Ocular Misalignment

When a patient complains of binocular diplopia, there must be ocular misalignment. If you conclude that the "extraocular movements are full," it usually means that you were not able to visualize small extraocular motor deficits. This is when the cover–uncover test, the cross-cover test, the red glass test, or the Maddox rod test becomes very helpful.

The Cover–Uncover Test

This test is based on evoking a fixational eye movement. In nearly all cases of ocular misalignment, one eye fixates the target while the other deviates. If the fixating eye is covered, the deviating eye will move to fixate the target. This test requires good vision and an attentive patient.

Procedure

The patient is instructed to fixate on a distant target while the right eye is covered. The left eye is observed to determine if it makes a fixational saccade toward the straight-ahead (primary) position. The direction of movement must be noted. Following removal of the cover from the right eye and after a delay of a few seconds, the left eye is covered and the right eye is watched for a fixational movement (▶ Fig. 13.18).

This cover–uncover maneuver should be repeated on each eye until the observations are consistent. If a fixational eye movement repeatedly occurs in the same direction, a "manifest misalignment" or a "tropia" can be diagnosed as follows:

- An outward movement denotes a convergent misalignment, or *esotropia*.
- An inward movement denotes a divergent misalignment, or *exotropia*.
- A downward movement denotes a *hypertropia*.
- An upward movement denotes a *hypotropia*.

The type of misalignment in primary position, right, left, up, and down gaze should be noted (see ▶ Fig. 13.18).

The Cross-Cover Test

This test is used to determine if there is latent misalignment not revealed by the cover–uncover test. It is based on eliciting a fixational eye movement, like the cover–uncover

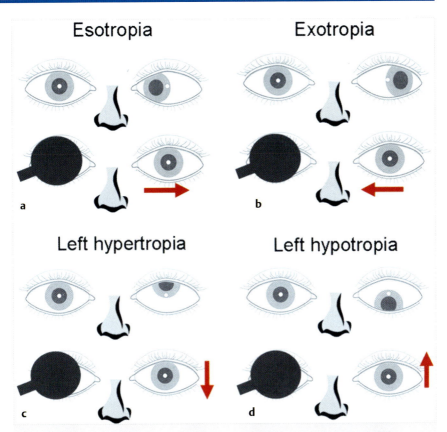

Fig. 13.18 Cover–uncover test. (**a**) Esotropia (the eyes are deviated in). (**b**) Exotropia (the eyes are deviated out). (**c**) Left hypertropia (the left eye is higher than the right eye). (**d**) Left hypotropia (the left eye is lower than the right eye). The red arrows show the movement of the uncovered eye during the cover-uncover test.

test. However, it interferes with binocular vision to bring out any latent misalignments that might be suppressed by a force called binocular fusion. This force is normally exerted to avoid double vision when both eyes are viewing a target.

Procedure

After covering the right eye as before, and after a 1 second pause, the cover is quickly moved across the nasal bridge to cover the left eye. Pausing 1 second, the cover is shifted back to cover the right eye, then the left eye, and so on, alternately covering the two eyes. One observes whether the eye being uncovered is shifting its position, the observations being recorded as with the cover–uncover maneuver. If a consistent fixational eye movement that was not present with the cover–uncover test is elicited, a latent misalignment, or phoria, is identified. Phorias, particularly exophorias, are so common in normal individuals that they may be considered physiological unless the degree of misalignment is incomitant (i.e., varies from one gaze position to another). When the cross-cover test does not elicit any eye movement, the patient is said to be orthophoric (▶ Fig. 13.19).

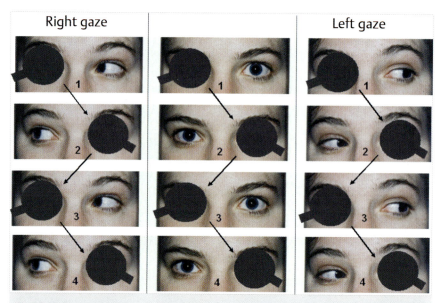

Fig. 13.19 Cross-cover test–orthophoric in horizontal gaze. The occluder is shifted from one eye to the other as demonstrated in successive frames 1 through 4. The patient is tested while looking straight first (middle column), then when looking to the right (left column), then when looking to the left (right column).

The test is repeated in all directions of gaze to make sure that the patient is orthophoric in right, left, up, and down gazes (▶ Fig. 13.20).

In the patient with a complaint of horizontal diplopia, the cross-cover test may show an abduction deficit (▶ Fig. 13.21).

In the patient with a complaint of new vertical diplopia, the *three-step test* is critical in looking for a fourth nerve palsy (▶ Fig. 13.22).

- *Step 1:* Because there is a right hyperdeviation in straight-ahead gaze, there must be a deficit in the depressor muscles of the right eye (inferior rectus, superior oblique) or the elevator muscles of the left eye (superior rectus, inferior oblique).
- *Step 2:* If the hyperdeviation is greater on left gaze than on right gaze, a vertical muscle active in left gaze is weak—either the right superior oblique or the left superior rectus.
- *Step 3:* Tilting the head to either side evokes an otolith-mediated ocular righting response ("ocular tilt reaction") designed to keep the eyes close to the plane of the horizon. In the right head tilt position, the right eye needs to intort (superior oblique, superior rectus), and the left eye needs to extort (inferior oblique, inferior rectus). If the right eye's superior oblique is weak, then the only available "intorter" in that position is the intact right superior rectus. Because the primary action of the superior rectus is elevation, the depressor force of the weak superior oblique will be overwhelmed by the elevator force of the intact superior rectus, and the right globe will move upward. As for the left eye, its intact inferior oblique upward pull is neutralized by its intact inferior rectus downward pull, so the globe does not move vertically. Left head tilt evokes an ocular counter-rolling motion that uses four intact muscles, so that neither eye moves vertically.

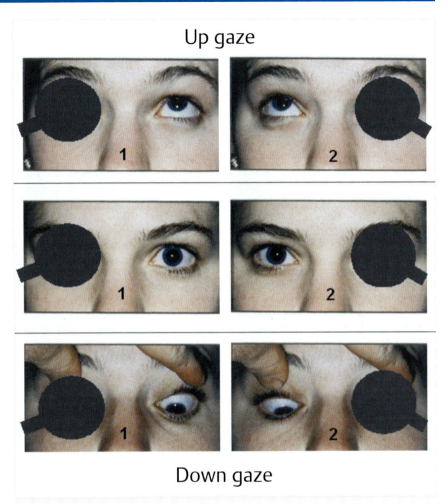

Up gaze

Down gaze

Fig. 13.20 Cross-cover test–orthophoric in vertical gaze. The occluder is shifted from one eye to the other (i.e., frame 1 to frame 2). The patient is tested first while looking straight ahead (middle row), then while looking up (top row), then while looking down (bottom row).

Quantification of the Ocular Deviation

The ocular misalignment can be quantified by determining the power of the prism necessary to neutralize the ocular deviation (▶ Fig. 13.23). The prism is placed over one eye, with the apex of the prism (point) pointed in the direction in which the eye is deviated: base out for an esotropia, base in for an exotropia, and base down on the right eye for a right hypertropia (▶ Fig. 13.24; "*the apex of the prism points toward the deviation*").

Each eye is then alternatively covered as the amount of prism (measured in prism-diopters) is slowly increased. When the eyes no longer move on alternate-cover testing, the deviation has been neutralized and the amount of prism required can be read on

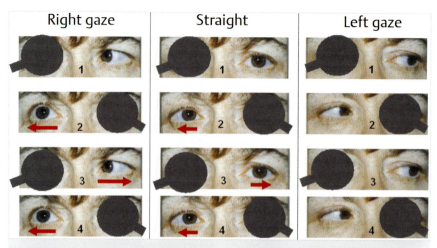

Right gaze	Straight	Left gaze

Fig. 13.21 Cross-cover test–right abduction deficit. The patient is tested while looking straight first (middle column), then when looking to the right (left column), then when looking to the left (right column). In straight-ahead gaze, covering the left eye elicits an outward deviation of the right eye (*arrow*), indicating an esotropia. The deviation is worse in right gaze and absent in left gaze, suggesting a right abduction deficit. The red arrows show the movement of the uncovered eye during the cross-cover test.

the prism or the prism bar. This measurement can be done in all cardinal positions and at near, as well as with head tilt.

Pearls

Measurement of the ocular deviation in prism-diopters reliably quantifies the ocular deviation. It is very useful for follow-up and to verify stability prior to considering eye muscle surgery for diplopia.

The same technique of prism quantification can be used during the red glass test or the Maddox rod test. With horizontal and vertical deviations, the same prism techniques can be used, and prisms of different orientations can be combined at the same time.

Communicating the Results of the Examination

The eye movements can be described in several ways (▶ Fig. 13.25 and ▶ Fig. 13.26).

The Red Glass Test

The red glass test relies on the patient's ability to report the location of two different-colored lights. By convention the red filter is placed in front of the right eye (▶ Fig. 13.27). This maneuver is then repeated for all the relevant positions of gaze (▶ Fig. 13.28). The patient is requested to stare straight ahead at a bright light. If the eyes are aligned, the patient will report one red-tinged light; however, if they are out of alignment, the patient describes one white and one red light. The extent of separation of images horizontally and vertically is determined.

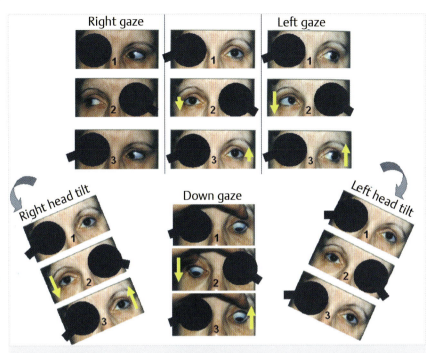

Fig. 13.22 Cross-cover test–right superior oblique paresis (fourth nerve palsy). The patient is tested while looking straight first (middle column), then when looking to the right (left column), then when looking to the left (right column). Down gaze and head tilt are subsequently tested. The three-step test measures ocular alignment in (1) straight-ahead gaze [step 1]; (2) right and left gaze [step 2]; (3) straight-ahead gaze with the head tilted right and then tilted left [step 3]. When the head is erect, the patient has a small right hyperdeviation (hypertropia) in straight-ahead gaze; the patient has normal alignment in right gaze, but a large right hyperdeviation in left gaze. In right head tilt, the patient has a very large right hyperdeviation; in left head tilt, the patient's eyes are aligned. The patient also has a large right hypertropia in down gaze. The yellow arrows show the movement of the uncovered eye during the cross-cover test.

With an esotropia or esophoria, the red image (as seen by the right eye) will appear to the patient as displaced to the right of the white image (▶ Fig. 13.29).

With an exotropia or exophoria, the red image (as seen by the right eye) will appear to the patient as displaced to the left. One way to remember this rule of horizontal misalignment is that there is an X in exotropia. This means that the red image viewed by the right eye crosses over to the left of the white light in an exotropia (▶ Fig. 13.30).

With a right hypertropia (▶ Fig. 13.31), the red image will appear displaced below the white image; with a left hypertropia, the red image will appear displaced above the white image. One way to remember the rule for vertical deviations is that there is an R in sunrise. The red image sits below the white light (the sun) in a right hypertropia.

The red glass test is more sensitive to small amounts of misalignment than the cover test, but it requires an attentive and verbally adept patient. Some patients have difficulty estimating spacing intervals, especially when the eyes are misaligned in two planes; the red glass test using the Maddox rod improves reliability under these circumstances.

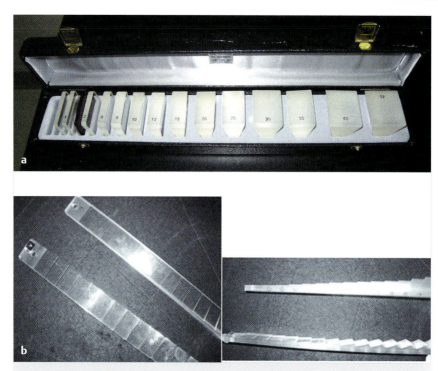

Fig. 13.23 Types of prisms used to quantify the ocular deviation. (a) Single prisms. (b) Prism bars.

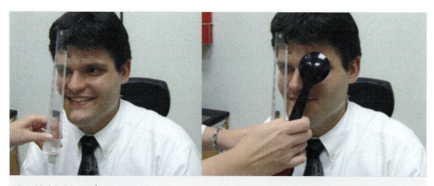

Fig. 13.24 Prism–alternate cover test.

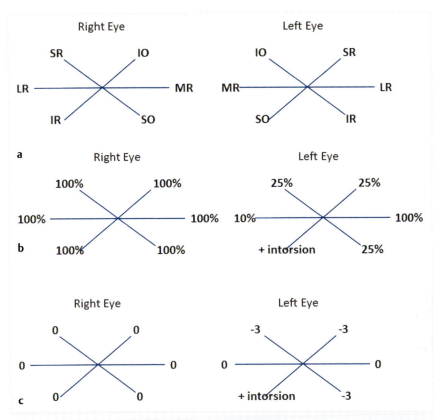

Fig. 13.25 (a) Diagram for transcription of eye movements. (b) Example of limitation of eye movements in the left eye using the percentage method. Only abduction and intorsion are normal in the left eye. There is only 25% of normal elevation and depression of the left eye, and only 10% of normal adduction. (c) Using the 0 to – 4 scale, abduction of the left eye would be 0, and elevation, depression, and adduction would be – 3. These measurements suggest a left third nerve palsy. IO, inferior oblique; IR, inferior rectus; LR, lateral rectus; MR, medial rectus; SO, superior oblique; SR, superior rectus.

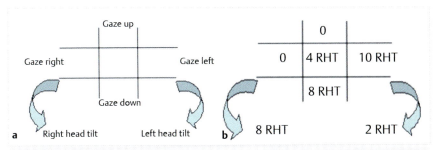

Fig. 13.26 (a) Diagram for transcription of eye movements (with cross-cover test). (b) Example of a right hypertropia (RHT) measuring 4 prism diopters in primary position, increasing to 8 prism diopters in down gaze, resolving in right gaze and up gaze, and increasing to 10 prism diopters in left gaze. With right tilt, there is an 8 prism diopter right hypertropia, and with left head tilt, it improved to 2 prism diopters. These measurements indicate a right fourth nerve palsy.

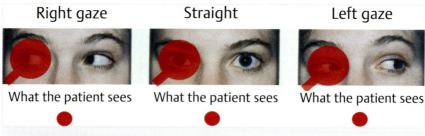

Fig. 13.27 Red glass test—orthophoric in horizontal gaze.

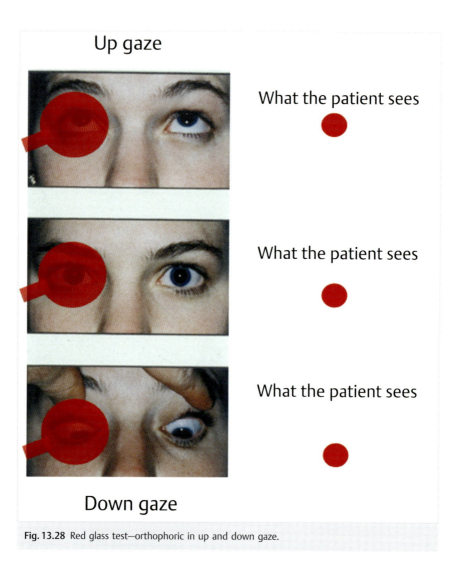

Fig. 13.28 Red glass test—orthophoric in up and down gaze.

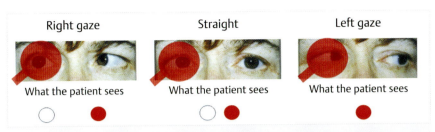

Fig. 13.29 Red glass test—right abduction deficit. With the red glass placed over the right eye, the patient reports that, in straight-ahead gaze, the red light appears to the right and the white light to the left, indicating an esotropia. In right gaze, the separation increases, indicating a greater esotropia in right gaze. In left gaze, the patient sees only a single red-tinged light.

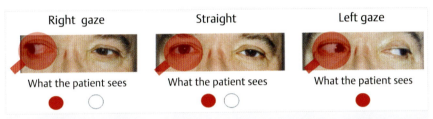

Fig. 13.30 Red glass test—left adduction deficit. With the red glass placed over the right eye, the patient reports that, in straight-ahead gaze, the red light appears to the left and the white light to the right, indicating an exotropia. In right gaze, the separation increases, indicating a greater exotropia in right gaze (this patient has a partial left third nerve palsy with an adduction deficit of the left eye). In left gaze, the patient sees only a single red-tinged light.

The Maddox Rod Test

The Maddox rod itself consists of a stack of transparent red plastic cylinders. When placed between a light source and the eye, it produces an image of a straight red line oriented at 90 degrees to the axis of the cylinders (▶ Fig. 13.32).

Thus, when the Maddox rod is held before the eye with cylinders oriented vertically, the viewer sees a point light source as a horizontal red line. When the Maddox rod cylinders are oriented horizontally, the red line is seen as vertical. This optical phenomenon allows the examiner to assess misalignment first in the horizontal plane, then in the vertical plane.

13.4.3 Testing for Horizontal and Vertical Deviation

The Maddox rod is used in the same way as the red glass, except that the patient is tested in all relevant gaze positions twice—first with the cylinders oriented horizontally and then with the cylinders oriented vertically (▶ Fig. 13.33 and ▶ Fig. 13.34).

For horizontal deviations, the Maddox rod is placed in front of the right eye with the cylinders oriented horizontally. When there is no horizontal ocular deviation (orthophoric), the patient sees the light through the red line. When the line is seen to the right of the light (uncrossed diplopia), there is an esotropia (▶ Fig. 13.35). When the line is seen to the left of the light (crossed diplopia), there is an exotropia (▶ Fig. 13.36).

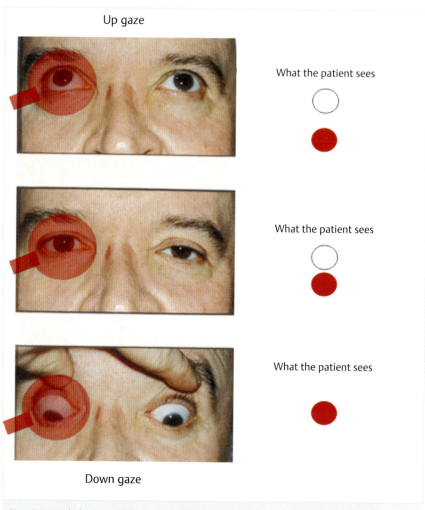

Up gaze

What the patient sees

What the patient sees

What the patient sees

Down gaze

Fig. 13.31 Red-glass test—right hypertropia. There is a subtle elevation deficit of the left eye (partial left third nerve palsy), and the patient complains of binocular vertical diplopia in primary position and when looking up. With the red glass placed over the right eye, the patient reports that, in straight-ahead gaze, the red light appears below the white light, indicating that the right eye is higher than the left eye (right hypertropia). In up gaze, the separation increases, indicating a greater deviation. In down gaze, the patient sees only a single red-tinged light, indicating no vertical deviation.

For vertical deviations, the Maddox rod is placed in front of the right eye, with the cylinders oriented vertically; the patient looks at the examiner's light. The patient sees a white light and a horizontal red line. When there is no vertical ocular deviation (orthophoric), the patient sees the light through the red line (see ▶ Fig. 13.34). When the light is seen above the line, there is a right hypertropia (▶ Fig. 13.37). When the light is seen below the line, there is a right hypotropia (or left hypertropia).

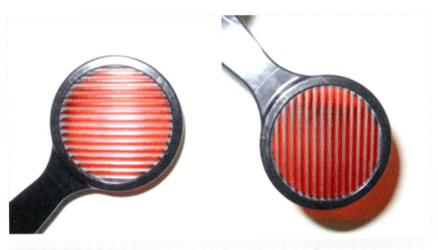

Fig. 13.32 Maddox rod with cylinders oriented horizontally and vertically.

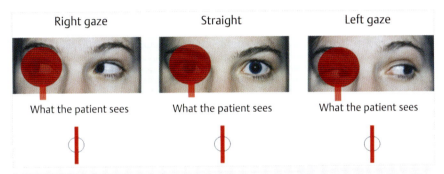

Fig. 13.33 Maddox rod test—no horizontal deviation. The Maddox rod is placed in front of the right eye, with the cylinders oriented horizontally. The patient looks at the examiner's light. The patient sees a white light and a vertical red line. When there is no horizontal ocular deviation (orthophoric), the patient sees the light through the red line.

Testing for Cyclotorsion

The double Maddox rod test helps demonstrate and quantify cyclotorsion: Maddox rod lenses are placed over each eye in a trial frame (by convention, red in front of right eye and white in front of left eye), with the cylinders oriented vertically (each at the 90 degree mark). As the patient is viewing a hand-held light at distance, two separate horizontal lines will be seen, one with each eye (right eye: red line; left eye: white line). The patient is asked to align the two lines so that they are parallel to each other and the floor by rotating the dials of the trial frame (▸ Fig. 13.38 and ▸ Fig. 13.39).

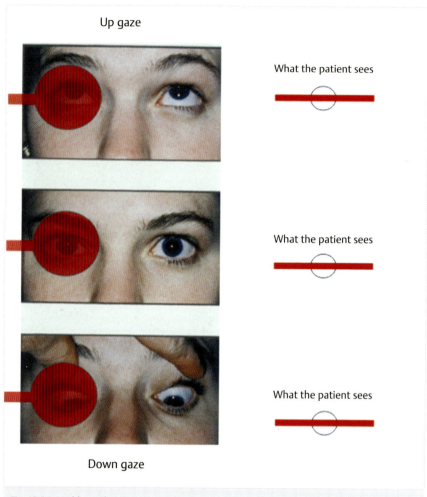

Up gaze

What the patient sees

What the patient sees

What the patient sees

Down gaze

Fig. 13.34 Maddox rod test—no vertical deviation. The Maddox rod is placed in front of the right eye, with the cylinders oriented vertically. The patient sees a white light and a horizontal red line when looking at the examiner's light.

13.4.4 Testing Uncooperative Patients or Young Children

- Observe spontaneous eye movements and eye position to determine whether the ocular alignment is normal.
- Use the Hirschberg test (corneal reflection test).
- Try the uncover–cover test with a noisy target such as a toy.

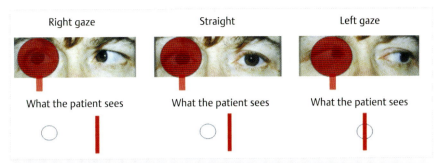

Fig. 13.35 Maddox rod test—right abduction deficit (esodeviation). When the Maddox rod with cylinders oriented horizontally is placed in front of the right eye as the patient gazes straight ahead, a vertical red line appears 1 inch to the right of the white light. In right gaze, the vertical red line appears 3 inches to the right, and in left gaze, the vertical red line intersects the white light.

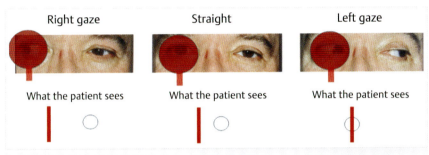

Fig. 13.36 Maddox rod test—left adduction deficit (exodeviation). A vertical red line appears 1 inch to the left of the white light when the Maddox rod with cylinders oriented horizontally is placed in front of the patient's right eye in a straight-ahead gaze. In right gaze, the vertical red line appears 3 inches to the left, and in left gaze, the vertical red line intersects the white light.

The Hirschberg and Krimsky Tests

In uncooperative patients or in children, ocular deviations can be assessed using corneal reflexes. When a fixation light is held 33 cm from a patient, the corneal light reflex should be centered in each pupil and should be symmetric. When the light reflex is deviated from the center of the pupil, there is a tropia (▶ Fig. 13.40).

Hirschberg test: the deviation of the corneal light reflex from the center of the pupil can be estimated in millimeters (see green arrow in ▶ Fig. 13.41):

1 mm decentration = 7 degrees of ocular deviation = 14 prism-diopters

The deviation of the light reflex is measured as follows:
- Edge of pupil: 15 degrees = 30 prism-diopters
- Middle iris: 30 degrees = 60 prism-diopters
- Edge of iris: 45 degrees = 90 prism-diopters

Krimsky test: using the Hirschberg test, prisms of increasing power can be placed in front of the *fixating eye* until both corneal reflexes are centered. The prism with

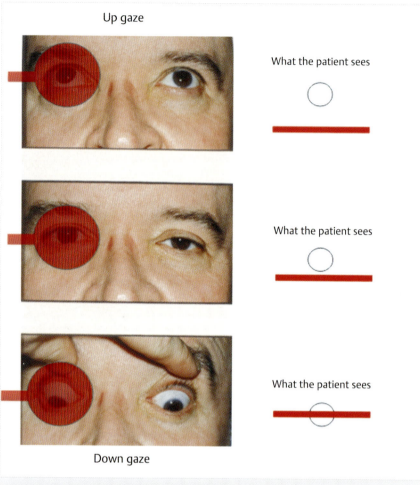

Fig. 13.37 Maddox rod test—right hypertropia. In the case of a subtle elevation deficit of the left eye (partial left third nerve palsy), with the Maddox rod placed over the right eye, the patient reports that, in straight-ahead gaze, the red line appears below the white light, indicating that the right eye is higher than the left eye (right hypertropia). In up gaze, the separation increases, indicating a greater deviation. In down gaze, the patient sees the red line intersect the white light, indicating no vertical deviation.

sufficient power to achieve centration of the light reflex indicates the magnitude of the deviation (▶ Fig. 13.42).

- Esotropia: orient the prism base out
- Exotropia: orient the prism base in
- Hypertropia: orient the prism base up (over the fixating eye); most often patients fixate with the normal eye (the hypertropic eye is deviated upward); hence the need to place the prism base up over the normal fixating eye.
- Hypotropia: orient the prism base down (over the fixating eye); most often patients fixate with the normal eye (the hypotropic eye is deviated downward); hence the need to place the prism base down over the normal fixating eye.

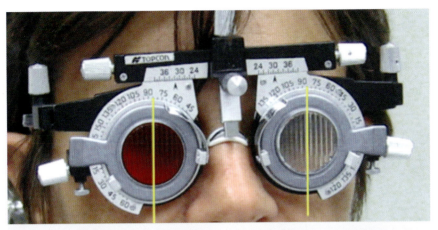

Fig. 13.38 Double Maddox rod testing in a patient with no deviation (the yellow lines show the orientation of the Maddox rods).

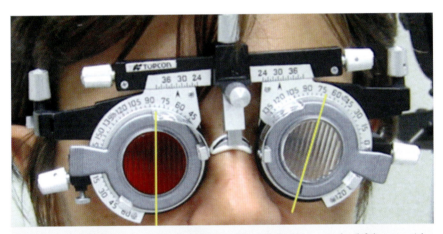

Fig. 13.39 Double Maddox rod testing in a patient with a left fourth nerve palsy (left hypertropia). The patient shows excyclotorsion of the left eye while the right eye is not torted (the yellow lines show the orientation of the Maddox rods).

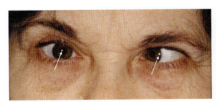

Fig. 13.40 Demonstration of an esotropia by the Hirschberg test. Note the corneal light reflex in each eye (*arrows*).

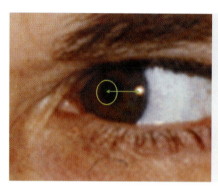

Fig. 13.41 Deviation of the corneal light reflex from the center of the pupil (*green circle*) in esotropia (*green arrow*).

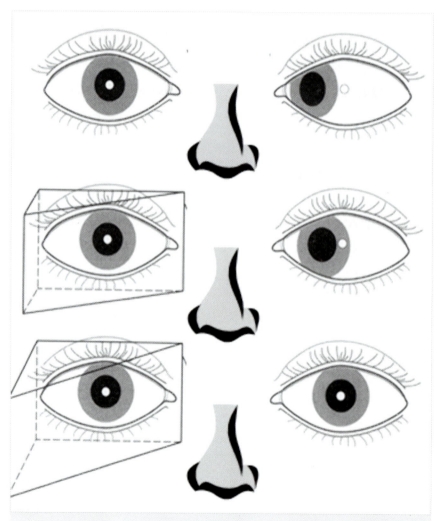

Fig. 13.42 Measurement of the esotropia by Krimsky test (prisms base out are placed in front of the fixating eye; the tip of the prism points toward the ocular deviation).

13.4.5 Testing Comatose Patients

Eye movements are assessed using reflex maneuvers. In the oculocephalic reflex, the eyes should deviate conjugately in the direction *opposite* the head turn. Dysconjugate horizontal eye movements suggest a sixth nerve palsy, internuclear ophthalmoplegia, or third nerve palsy. Oculocephalic eye movements are typically preserved in cerebral hemisphere injury. Oculocephalic maneuvers should not be performed in patients with cervical injury.

If the patient does not have any oculocephalic eye movements (or if testing them is contraindicated), caloric testing can help evaluate eye movements.

After examination of the external auditory canal to exclude a rupture of the tympanic membrane or cerumen impaction, 30 to 60 mL of ice-cold water is irrigated into the patient's ear with the head angled 30 degrees above the horizontal (to align the horizontal semicircular canals perpendicular to the floor). The eyes deviate slowly toward the irrigated ear in patients with intact brainstem function, followed by a fast corrective phase in the opposite direction to reset the eyes, and then the cycle repeats. Warm water stimulation produces a contralateral slow phase and ipsilateral fast phase.

The direction of the caloric response is named after the *fast* phase:
(remember: COWS for cold—opposite, warm—same)

Pearls

The goals of the evaluation of the diplopic patient are as follows:
1. Recognize the ocular misalignment.
2. Characterize the misalignment.
   - Determine the type of deviation: esotropia, exotropia, hypertropia.
   - Quantify the misalignment (prisms).
   - Ascertain whether it is comitant (same amount of deviation in all directions of gaze) or incomitant (varies from one direction of gaze to another).
   - Determine whether it maps to a cranial nerve or suggests a muscle or neuromuscular junction lesion.
3. Describe the pupils, visual acuity, and fundus.
4. Look for orbital signs.
5. Look for associated neurological signs.

These findings allow you to do the following:
- Localize anatomically the lesion responsible for the diplopia.
- Make hypotheses regarding the mechanism of the lesion.
- Obtain further testing to confirm your clinical impression.

13.5 The Diagnosis of Binocular Diplopia

It is important to determine by clinical examination whether the lesion responsible for diplopia involves the extraocular muscles, the neuromuscular junction, a cranial nerve, or the internuclear or supranuclear pathways.

13.5.1 The Lesion Is in the Extraocular Muscles

Disorders of the extraocular muscles (and neuromuscular junction) can produce a wide range of abnormal eye movements. Their clinical manifestations are not limited by the scope of a single cranial nerve or supranuclear process. These disorders are frequently bilateral, involve the levator palpebrae and the orbicularis oculi, and never involve the pupil. They can result in total bilateral ophthalmoplegia and are sometimes associated with systemic manifestations. Numerous disorders can involve the extraocular muscles directly (myopathy) or can involve the orbit and impair the free movements of the muscles in the orbit.

Diseases of the extraocular muscles can produce motility disturbances in two ways: weakness (paresis) or restriction.

- The disease process can affect the muscle's ability to contract and cause weakness, or paresis.
- The muscle's movements may be restricted by local disease (such as inflammation, fibrosis, trauma, tumor). In this case, the eye is pulled in the direction of the abnormal muscle (▶ Fig. 13.43).

A forced duction test allows differentiation between paresis (the paretic eye moves easily when pushed or pulled) and restriction (the restricted eye does not move). This test can be painful and may be difficult to interpret (see ▶ Fig. 13.13).

Differential Diagnosis of Enlarged Extraocular Muscles

Enlarged ocular muscles may result most commonly from the following:
- Thyroid eye disease
- Inflammatory disorders
  - Idiopathic orbital inflammation with myositis (inflammatory orbital pseudotumor)
  - Immunoglobulin G4 (IgG4) related disease
  - Wegener granulomatosis
  - Sarcoidosis
  - Crohn disease and inflammatory bowel syndrome
  - Connective tissue diseases
- Tumors
  - Lymphoma
  - Metastatic tumors
  - Rhabdomyosarcoma
- Infections
  - Trichinosis
- Orbital venous congestion
  - Carotid cavernous fistula
  - Carotid cavernous thrombosis
- Infiltration
  - Amyloidosis

Thyroid Eye Disease

Thyroid eye disease (Graves disease) is an autoimmune disorder characterized by enlargement of the extraocular muscles and an increase in orbital fat volume.

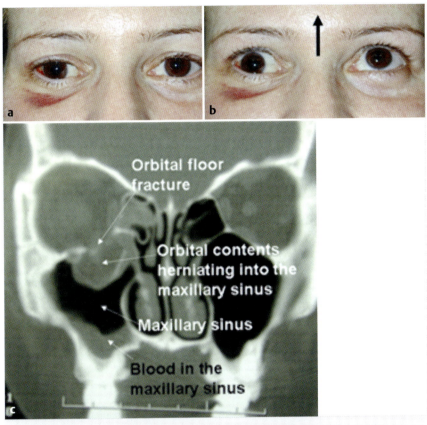

Fig. 13.43 (a) Trauma to the right eye with mild ecchymosis. The right eye does not elevate with attempted up gaze (b). (c) Coronal computed tomographic scan of the orbits without contrast showing a fracture of the right orbital floor. There is herniation of the orbital contents (including inferior rectus and inferior oblique muscles), resulting in restriction of elevation of the right eye.

Clinical Presentation

Thyroid eye disease is usually easily suspected clinically when patients present with the following:

- Unilateral or bilateral proptosis
- Lid retraction with lid lag in down gaze
- Ptosis (rare and should indicate possible associated myasthenia gravis)

- Orbital congestion with periorbital edema, puffiness of the eyelids, chemosis (these signs are worse in the morning)
- Diplopia with restricted eye movements (restricted elevation of the eye and esotropia are most common because of the classic involvement of the inferior and medial recti) (▶ Fig. 13.44 and ▶ Fig. 13.45)
- Visual loss, which can occur from the following:
  - Ocular surface disorder (dry eyes are common)
  - Exposure keratopathy (in the setting of severe proptosis)
  - Compressive optic neuropathy by the enlarged extraocular muscles
  - Glaucoma (increased intraocular pressure is common in thyroid eye disease)

Thyroid dysfunction in patients with thyroid eye disease is variable: 90% of patients are hyperthyroid and up to 6% of patients are euthyroid. There is no correlation between the thyroid hormone levels and the orbital disease. However, some treatments administered to treat hyperthyroidism (such as radioactive iodine) often worsen the orbital manifestations of Graves disease.

> **Pearls**
>
> The inferior rectus muscle is commonly involved in thyroid eye disease, causing restricted up gaze. The medial rectus muscle is the second most commonly involved muscle (causing an esotropia), followed by the superior and lateral rectus muscles.

Diagnosis

- Diagnosis relies mostly on clinical presentation and imaging: diagnosis of thyroid eye disease is sometimes based only on the findings of enlarged extraocular muscles on a computed tomographic (CT) scan or magnetic resonance imaging (MRI) of the orbits.
- Thyroid function tests are often normal.
- Autoantibodies (antithyroglobulin and antiperoxidase antibodies) are sometimes present and indicate an autoimmune disorder.

Treatment

- Treat thyroid abnormalities.
- Lubricate the cornea; temporary tarsorrhaphy may be required if there is corneal exposure.
- Treat elevated intraocular pressure.
- Elevate the head of bed at night to decrease orbital congestion.
- Use ocular occlusion and prisms for diplopia.
- Administer steroids (usually oral prednisone, except in cases of compressive optic neuropathy, in which case high-dose intravenous steroids may be preferred).
- If surgery is necessary, do orbital decompression first, followed by strabismus surgery and lid repair.
- Radiation therapy of the orbits is sometimes helpful.
- Encourage patients to discontinue cigarette smoking, which is associated with a worse prognosis for thyroid eye disease.

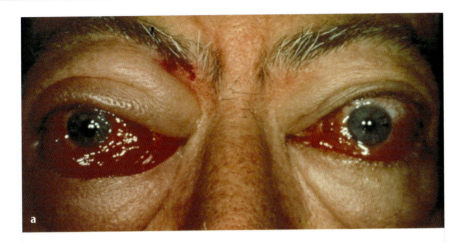

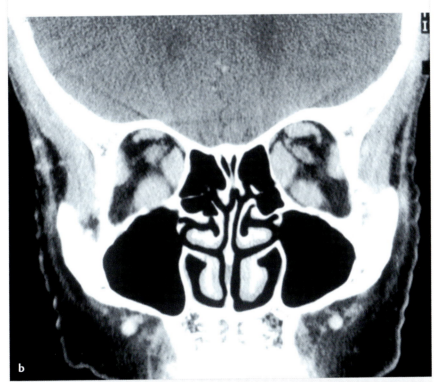

Fig. 13.44 Restricted eye movement from thyroid eye disease. **(a)** The eyes in primary position. There is severe proptosis with lid retraction, chemosis, and corneal exposure. The eye movements are diffusely restricted. **(b)** Coronal computed tomographic scan of the orbits with contrast showing enlargement of all extraocular muscles.

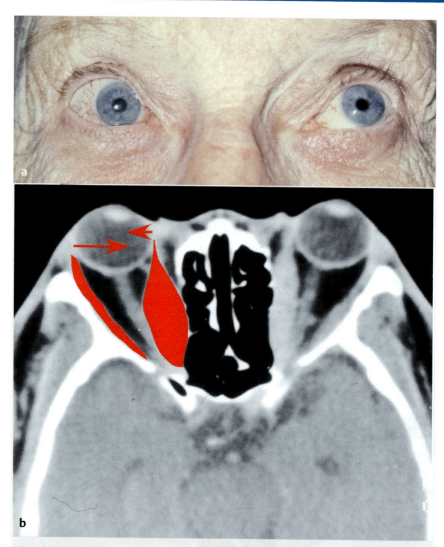

Fig. 13.45 Restricted eye movement from thyroid eye disease. (a) Position of the eyes in up gaze. The right eye does not elevate. There is mild conjunctival hyperemia and lid retraction. The proptosis is mild. (b) Axial computed tomographic scan of the orbits with contrast showing enlargement of the medial recti and normal lateral recti in both eyes. There is a right abduction deficit (*small red arrow*) related to restriction of the enlarged medial rectus muscle. The adduction of the right eye (*long red arrow*) is normal.

Table 13.2 Comparison of thyroid eye disease and inflammatory orbital pseudotumor

Thyroid eye disease	Inflammatory orbital pseudotumor
Common	Rare
Usually bilateral	More often unilateral
Chronic disease	Acute or subacute onset
No pain or mild discomfort	Pain often severe
Inferior rectus and medial rectus are most often affected	Any extraocular muscle is affected
Lid retraction	Ptosis
Response to steroids often moderate	Response to steroids often dramatic

Pearls

Thyroid eye disease is the most common cause of unilateral and bilateral proptosis. Thyroid eye disease and idiopathic orbital inflammation (orbital pseudotumor) can usually be differentiated based on clinical and radiologic characteristics (▶ Table 13.2, ▶ Fig. 13.46 and ▶ Fig. 13.47).

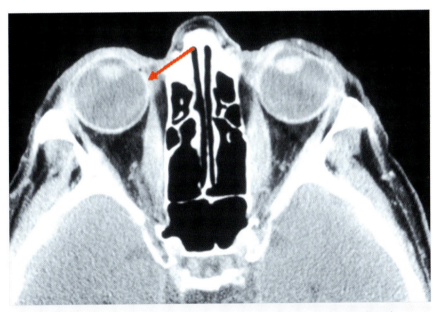

Fig. 13.46 Axial computed tomographic scan of the orbits with contrast showing thyroid eye disease. Enlargement and enhancement of both medial recti sparing the tendon itself (*arrow*). The orbital fat is not enhancing.

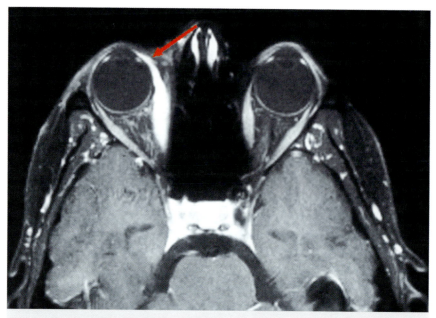

Fig. 13.47 Axial T1-weighted magnetic resonance imaging of the orbits with fat suppression and contrast showing orbital inflammatory pseudotumor. Enlargement and enhancement of the right medial rectus extending to the tendon itself (*arrow*). The orbital fat is also enhancing on the right.

Myositis

Inflammation of extraocular muscles can occur in the setting of any orbital inflammatory syndrome (such as nonspecific inflammation from orbital pseudotumor or Wegener granulomatosis) or any orbital infection (orbital cellulitis).

Clinical Presentation

Orbital myositis classically represents with a painful orbital symptoms, which includes the following:
- Pain over the eye or periorbital region
- Orbital syndrome
  - Periorbital swelling
  - Proptosis
  - Redness of the eye, chemosis
  - Possible visual loss from optic neuropathy
- Diplopia with limitation of eye movements
- Ptosis or lid retraction (if major proptosis)
- Imaging of the orbit (MRI of the orbits with fat suppression and contrast or CT of the orbits with contrast) confirms the diagnosis by showing enlargement and enhancement of the extraocular muscles and their tendons, as well as enhancement of other orbital structures (fat, sclera, optic nerve sheath).

Infectious Myositis

Trichinosis is a parasitic infection (undercooked meat is the vector) with a predilection for muscles. It is an acute systemic myositis involving the extraocular muscles associated with bilateral periorbital edema, diarrhea, eosinophilia, and fever.

Infectious orbital cellulitis and orbital or periosteal abscesses can result in ophthalmoplegia and diplopia. Infectious sinusitis involving the facial sinuses adjacent to the infected orbit is common, particularly in children (▶ Fig. 13.48).

Treatment with broad spectrum antibiotics and surgical drainage usually results in dramatic improvement.

Noninfectious Inflammatory Myositis, or Idiopathic Orbital Inflammation (Pseudotumor)

In most cases, inflammatory orbital myositis is due to "idiopathic inflammation" of the orbital contents, also called orbital pseudotumor (▶ Fig. 13.49). There is no infection and no underlying systemic disorder.

Diagnosis

The diagnosis is suspected clinically in an otherwise healthy patient presenting with unilateral or bilateral acute or subacute orbital syndrome associated with pain. Diplopia is very common, and visual loss can occur as a result of adjacent inflammation of the optic nerve or of the sclera.
- Infectious orbital cellulitis is ruled out by the following:
  - Absence of fever
  - Absence of associated sinusitis or abscess on imaging
  - Normal white blood cell count
- General examination and blood tests rule out an underlying systemic disorder such as IgG4 related disease, Wegener granulomatosis, sarcoidosis, Crohn disease, connective tissue diseases.

Clinical Presentation

All orbital structures can be involved in idiopathic orbital inflammation (orbital pseudotumor), explaining the various clinical presentations of this syndrome:
- Extraocular muscles
  - Myositis, which produces ophthalmoplegia
- Orbital fat
  - Proptosis
- Optic nerve sheath
  - Perineuritis and disc edema
- Optic nerve
  - Optic neuritis and visual loss (optic neuropathy)
- Sclera
  - Posterior scleritis and visual loss
- Lacrimal gland
  - Dacryoadenitis with eyelid swelling

Pain is usually severe, although sclerosing forms of orbital pseudotumor may have a more chronic indolent course.

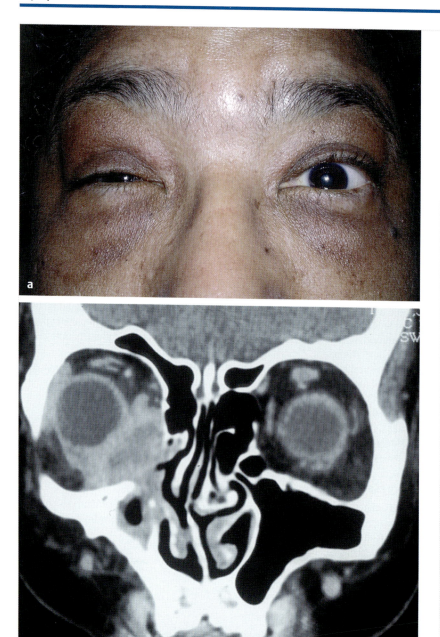

Fig. 13.48 (a) Right orbital cellulitis with ptosis, ophthalmoplegia, pain, and periorbital edema and redness. (b) Coronal computed tomographic scan of the orbits with contrast showing an inferior orbital abscess with bone erosion and adjacent sinusitis.

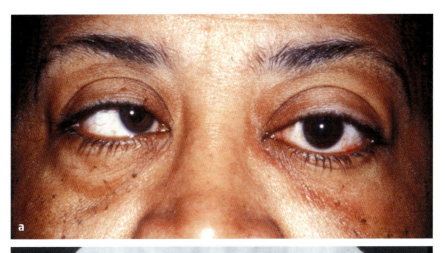

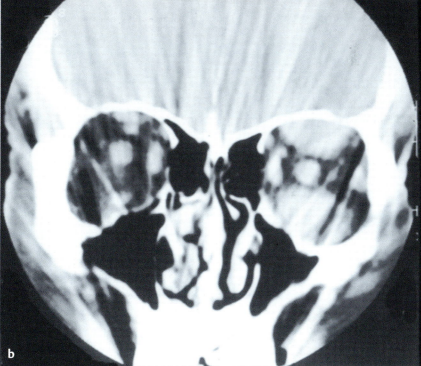

Fig. 13.49 (a) Left idiopathic orbital inflammation with myositis. Eye movements with attempted left gaze showing left proptosis, ptosis, periorbital swelling, and conjunctival hyperemia. The left eye does not abduct (restriction of all eye movements). (b) Coronal computed tomography of the orbits without contrast demonstrating very large extraocular muscles in the left orbit, consistent with myositis.

The inflammation may also extend into the cavernous sinus, resulting in multiple cranial nerve palsies. A similar disorder can involve the intracranial meninges and is called pachymeningitis.

Treatment

Orbital pseudotumor usually responds dramatically to steroid treatment. Symptoms and signs improve within a few hours after receiving steroids. When there is visual loss, intravenous steroids are usually preferred to oral prednisone.

Steroids need to be tapered very slowly, and steroid dependence (rebound during taper or after discontinuation) is common. For this reason, steroid-sparing agents or radiation of the orbit is sometimes recommended. Lubrication of the cornea and management of intraocular pressure are important during the acute phase.

Myositis of the Superior Oblique Muscle or Its Tendon

This produces an acquired Brown syndrome. The eye does not elevate in adduction (there is a downshoot of the eye in adduction).

Sometimes, Brown syndrome is intermittent (the superior oblique tendon is intermittently blocked in the pulley), and the patient hears a "snap" when the tendon releases and the eye fully elevates.

Orbital Tumors

Lymphoid tumors (e.g., lymphoma or leukemia) and metastases can involve extraocular muscles in the orbit and can present as a subacute or acute orbital syndrome associated with pain. An orbital biopsy should be considered in all patients with presumed "myositis" and a known history of cancer.

Metastases of breast cancer are commonly associated with enophthalmos rather than proptosis, presumably because of associated orbital fat atrophy and fibrosis (▶ Fig. 13.50).

> **Pearls**
>
> An orbital biopsy should be considered in all patients with presumed "myositis" and a known history of cancer and in patients with atypical orbital pseudotumor (e.g., no or mild pain, recurrence).

By compromising free movements of extraocular muscles in the orbits, orbital tumors can cause various degrees of ophthalmoplegia (▶ Fig. 13.51).

Trauma

Orbital trauma can restrict free movements of the globe in the orbit and often results in diplopia. Sudden orbital compression (e.g., tennis ball hitting the eye) can produce a blowout fracture of the orbital floor, entrapping the inferior rectus and other orbital tissue in the fracture. Elevation of the eye is restricted by the entrapped muscle, and depression of the eye is also generally poor because the muscle cannot constrict normally (▶ Fig. 13.43).

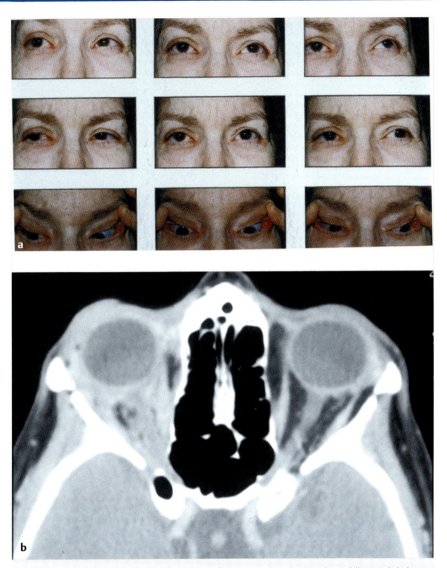

Fig. 13.50 (a) Painful diffuse ophthalmoplegia of the right eye, which is also mildly enophthalmic. This patient has a history of breast cancer. (b) Axial computed tomographic scan of the orbits with contrast showing enhancement of the entire right orbit. An orbital biopsy confirmed a metastasis from breast cancer.

Orbital fracture can also result in contusion of the extraocular muscle; hemorrhage in the extraocular muscle, with subsequent fibrosis; or orbital hemorrhage. Acute (and also sometimes delayed) enophthalmos and inferior orbital nerve damage (responsible for hypoesthesia and numbness of the inferior orbital rim and of the ipsilateral cheek) commonly accompany orbital floor fractures. A medial blowout fracture is also possible

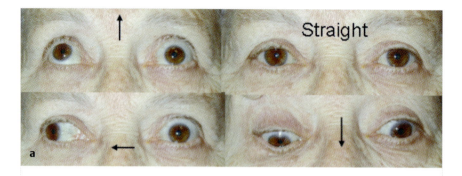

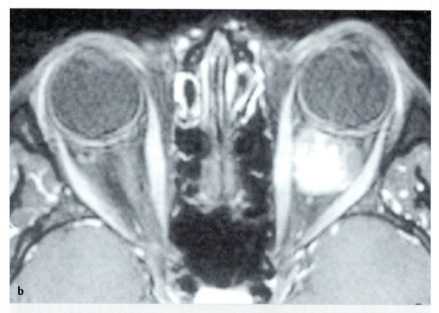

Fig. 13.51 (a) Restriction of the eye movements in the left eye. There is very subtle left proptosis, and visual function is normal. (b) Axial T1-weighted magnetic resonance imaging of the orbits with contrast and with fat suppression showing a mass in the left orbit.

and results in entrapment of the medial rectus with an abduction deficit that may mimic a sixth nerve palsy (▶ Fig. 13.52).

Other mechanisms of diplopia after head trauma include trauma to a cranial nerve (fourth nerve palsy most common, followed by sixth and third nerve palsies), carotid-cavernous fistula, brainstem lesion, subarachnoid hemorrhage with cranial nerve palsies, and raised intracranial pressure with sixth nerve palsy.

Giant Cell Arteritis and Orbital Ischemia

Chronic orbital ischemia (e.g., patient with common or internal carotid occlusion with poor collateral circulation, or patient with systemic vasculitis such as giant cell arteritis)

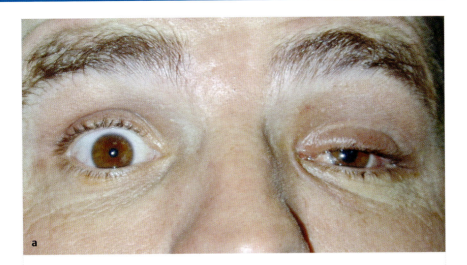

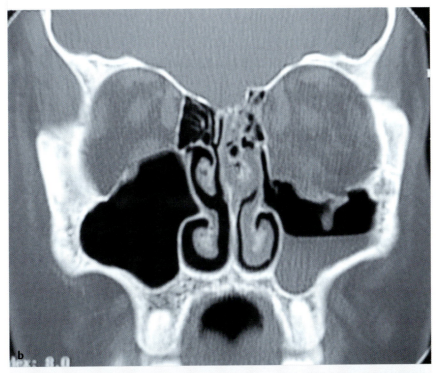

Fig. 13.52 (a) Left enophthalmos with mild periorbital ecchymosis and ptosis after trauma to the left orbit. (b) Coronal computed tomographic scan of the orbits without contrast showing a left orbital fracture (medial wall and floor). There is blood in the maxillary and ethmoid sinuses.

can result in ischemia of an extraocular muscle, thereby producing diplopia, usually with pain. The diplopia is often transient and can be horizontal or vertical. At least 10% of patients with permanent visual loss from giant cell arteritis report having episodes of transient diplopia within the weeks preceding loss of vision (see Chapter 20).

> **Pearls**
>
> Giant cell arteritis needs to be ruled out in all elderly patients with transient or permanent diplopia.

Bony Deformation of the Orbit

Bony deformations change the shape of the orbit and also change the orientation of the orbital walls. In addition to compressing intraorbital structures, these changes modify the way the extraocular muscles move in the orbit and often produce diplopia.

Fibrous Dysplasia

Fibrous dysplasia is a benign bone condition in which normal bone is replaced by immature bone and osteoid in a cellular fibrous matrix. This results in expansion of the bone, further resulting in pain; deformation of the face, orbit, and cranium; and compression of adjacent structures (▶ Fig. 13.53). Diplopia is common secondary to displacement of the globe and of the ocular muscles, as well as cranial nerve palsies. Associated visual loss happens when there is compression of the optic nerve (usually at the level of the optic canal).

Surgical debulking is often performed to improve the craniofacial deformity and to relieve cranial nerve compression. Surgical decompression of the orbital apex and optic canal is performed when there is a progressive optic neuropathy.

Agenesis of the Sphenoid Wing

Agenesis of the sphenoid wing occurs classically in the setting of neurofibromatosis type 1. It results in herniation of the intracranial contents into the orbit (▶ Fig. 13.54).
Clinically, patients present with the following:
- Pulsatile proptosis (pulsations of the cerebrospinal fluid push directly on the eye)
- Variable diplopia
- Various degrees of visual loss when the optic nerve is compressed

If the visual function is normal, there is usually no treatment necessary.

Silent Sinus Syndrome

Patients who have chronic maxillary sinusitis develop atrophy of the maxillary sinus with resultant lowering of the ipsilateral orbital floor (which constitutes the superior wall of the maxillary sinus). This may result in displacement of the orbital contents and ipsilateral hypoglobus, often with an elevation deficit of the eye. These patients may have binocular vertical diplopia, worse in up gaze (▶ Fig. 13.55 and ▶ Fig. 13.56).

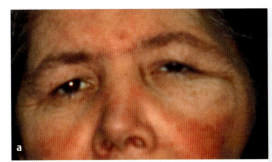

Fig. 13.53 (a) Fibrous dysplasia with abnormal external appearance. Note the deformation of the left side of the face with elevation and distortion of the left orbit. (b) Axial computed tomographic scan of the brain (bone window) showing fibrous dysplasia involving the frontal bone and the cheeks.

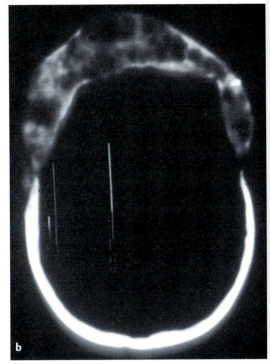

Progressive Myopathies Commonly Affecting the Extraocular Muscles

The syndrome of chronic progressive external ophthalmoplegia (CPEO) is characterized by progressive limitation of eye movements and ptosis (often over many years). The pupils are always normal. Commonly, patients do not complain of diplopia because their eyes remain relatively straight in primary position. The most common first complaint of diplopia occurs with reading because of convergence insufficiency.

Several disorders can present with CPEO, and often there are other neurologic signs such as diffuse facial and limb myopathy. In general, imaging is normal, and the extraocular muscles are not enlarged. Myopathies affecting the extraocular muscles are often associated with systemic myopathy and cardiomyopathy. Therefore, all patients

369

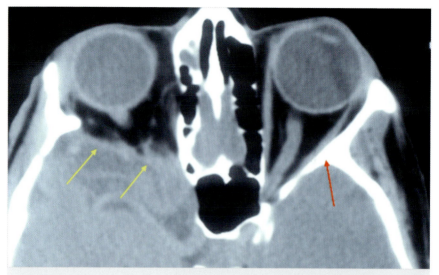

Fig. 13.54 Axial computed tomographic scan showing agenesis of the sphenoid wing (*yellow arrows*) on the right. The red arrow shows the normal sphenoid wing on the left.

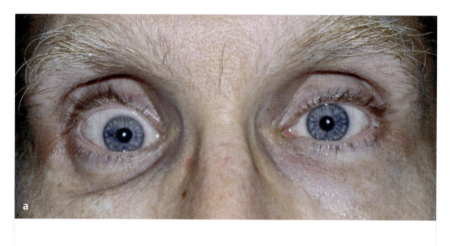

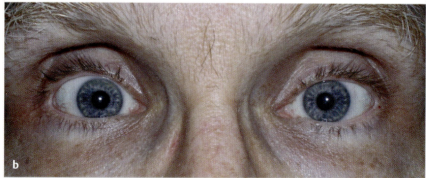

Fig. 13.55 (a) Right silent sinus syndrome with right hypoglobus. The right eye is deviated downward and there is an elevation deficit of the right eye. (b) Same patient after surgical repair. The right hypoglobus is resolved.

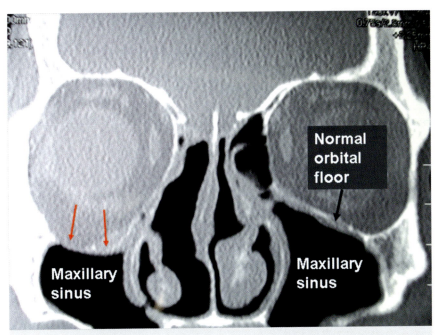

Fig. 13.56 Coronal computed tomographic scan of the orbits and facial sinuses showing deformation and expansion of the right orbit with low orbital floor (*red arrows*) consistent with right silent sinus syndrome.

with ocular myopathy need to have an electrocardiogram. Finding a cardiac conduction block may be life-saving. Myasthenia gravis needs to be ruled out.

Mitochondrial Myopathies

In mitochondrial disease, CPEO can occur any time from infancy to old age, and the onset is typically insidious. Ophthalmoplegia and ptosis may be isolated or associated with other neurologic or systemic abnormalities (▶ Fig. 13.57, ▶ Fig. 13.58, ▶ Fig. 13.59).

- *Common neurologic findings:* facial, bulbar, and limb myopathies, deafness, ataxia, spasticity, peripheral neuropathy, gastrointestinal myopathy and neuropathy, vestibular dysfunction, dementia, episodic encephalopathy or coma, and calcification of the basal ganglia
- *Associated ocular features:* optic atrophy, pigmentary retinopathy, corneal opacities, corneal edema, and cataracts
- *Systemic manifestations:* involve the cardiac, endocrine, skin, or skeletal systems and include cardiac conduction abnormalities, short stature, diabetes mellitus, delayed sexual maturation, hypogonadism, hypomagnesemia, hypoparathyroidism, hypothyroidism, and respiratory insufficiency.

The Kearns–Sayre syndrome is a subset of CPEO in which neurologic and systemic abnormalities figure most prominently.

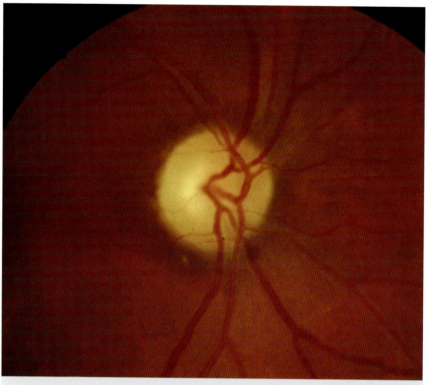

Fig. 13.57 Optic atrophy in a patient with chronic progressive external ophthalmoplegia.

Clinical diagnostic criteria include the following:
- Onset prior to age 20
- CPEO
- Retinal pigmentary degeneration
- At least one of the following:
  - Cardiac conduction abnormalities
  - Elevated cerebrospinal fluid protein (> 100 mg/dL)
  - Cerebellar dysfunction

The other neurologic and systemic abnormalities associated with mitochondrial myopathies (as already described) occur commonly in patients with Kearns–Sayre syndrome.

Muscle biopsy shows ragged red fibers (demonstrated on modified trichrome stain); they can be seen in limb and extraocular muscles in nearly all cases of Kearns–Sayre syndrome and in some patients with isolated CPEO.

Mitochondrial DNA analysis of skeletal muscle tissue of some CPEO patients reveals rearrangements of segments of mitochondrial DNA in the form of deletions and duplications.

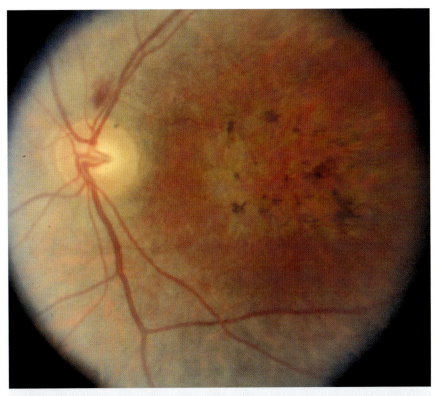

Fig. 13.58 Pigmentary retinopathy in a patient with chronic progressive external ophthalmoplegia.

Other Mitochondrial Diseases That Can Have Ophthalmoplegia

Myopathy involving the extraocular muscles is common in most mitochondrial diseases.
- MELAS syndrome (*m*itochondrial *e*ncephalopathy, *l*actic *a*cidosis, and *s*troke-like episodes)
- MNGIE syndrome (*m*itochondrial *n*eurogastrointestinal *e*ncephalomyopathy)
- SANDO syndrome (*s*ensory *a*taxic *n*europathy, *d*ysarthria, and *o*phthalmoplegia)
- Leigh syndrome (subacute necrotizing encephalomyelopathy)

Myotonic Dystrophy (▶ Fig. 13.60)

- Most common adult-onset muscular dystrophy
- Autosomal dominant (trinucleotide repeat on chromosome 19)
- Anticipation common (age of onset is younger in successive generations)
- Bilateral ptosis with progressive ophthalmoplegia
- Characteristic cataract ("Christmas tree")
- Progressive weakness of distal muscles with myotonia (involuntary delayed relaxation following contraction, such as the inability to let go after a sustained grip)
- Typical facies with frontal balding, facial weakness, long face, temporal wasting
- Cardiac conduction defects

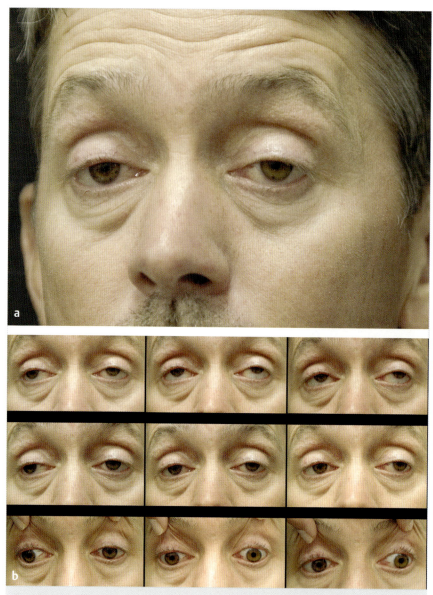

Fig. 13.59 (a) Bilateral ptosis encroaching on the visual axis. (b) Diffuse limitation of eye movements in chronic progressive external ophthalmoplegia. The patient is straight in primary position, and he does not have diplopia. He moves his head to look laterally. The pupils are normal.

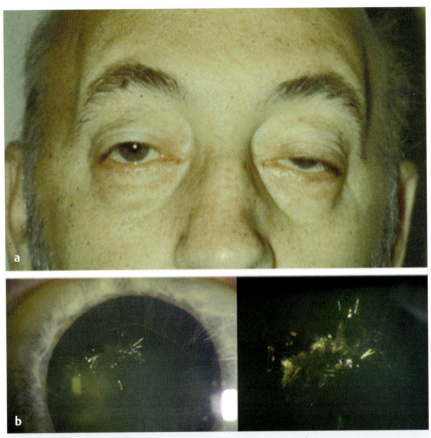

Fig. 13.60 (a) Bilateral ptosis and typical facies of myotonic dystrophy. (b) Lens opacities typical of myotonic dystrophy. Colorful spokes resembling a Christmas tree ("Christmas tree cataract").

Oculopharyngeal Dystrophy

- Autosomal dominant (trinucleotide repeat on chromosome 14)
- More common in French Canadians
- Presents late in life
- Bilateral ptosis with progressive ophthalmoplegia
- Dysphagia

Congenital and Developmental Disorders Affecting the Extraocular Muscles

Numerous congenital abnormalities affecting the extraocular muscles may result in eye movement abnormalities in young children.

Agenesis of the Extraocular Muscles

Congenital Agenesis of the extraocular muscles is rare; most cases involve only one muscle.

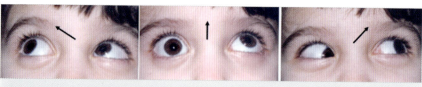

Fig. 13.61 Congenital right Brown syndrome. Attempted up gaze showing elevation deficit of the right eye.

Anomalies of Extraocular Muscle Origin and Insertion

The following disorders are responsible for various abnormalities of eye movement in young children.

Brown Syndrome

Patients with Brown syndrome have an elevation deficit of the affected eye secondary to restriction of the superior oblique tendon. The eye does not elevate when the eye is in adduction (there is a downshoot of the eye in adduction). Brown syndrome may be congenital or acquired.

Congenital Brown syndrome (▶ Fig. 13.61)
- Arises from congenitally short or inelastic tendon of the superior oblique muscle resulting in mechanical restriction of elevation of the eye when adducted
- Is commonly associated with normal binocular vision without amblyopia

Acquired Brown syndrome
- Can occur as a result of orbital trauma, an orbital inflammatory or infectious process, or after orbital injections
- Is often associated with pain at the level of the trochlea (superior medial corner of the orbit)
- Can result from rheumatoid arthritis

Congenital Adherence of Extraocular Muscles

- Adhesion between the sheaths of the lateral rectus and inferior oblique muscles, causing deficient abduction of the eye (usually bilateral)
- Adhesion between the sheaths of the superior rectus and superior oblique muscles, causing deficient elevation of the eye

Congenital Myopathies

Congenital myopathies make up a group of congenital systemic myopathies also affecting the extraocular muscles and causing ptosis and bilateral ophthalmoplegia.
- Myotubular myopathy (centronuclear myopathy)
- Nemaline myopathy
- Central core myopathy
- Multicore myopathy

Congenital Fibrosis of the Extraocular Muscles (CFEOM)

- Rare cause of ocular motility restriction, usually familial
- Presents in childhood

- Any individual extraocular muscle, or combination of muscles, may be replaced by fibrotic tissue, resulting in variable degrees of ophthalmoplegia and ptosis. The syndrome of CFEOM is associated with anomalies of the cranial nerves and their nuclei and is part of the *congenital* cranial dysinnervation disorders, similar to Duane syndrome, Möbius syndrome, and congenital facial palsy.
- Amblyopia is common.

13.5.2 The Lesion Is at the Neuromuscular Junction

Ocular Myasthenia and Myasthenia Gravis

Myasthenia gravis is essentially the only disease to clinically affect extraocular neuromuscular junction transmission. It presents with isolated ptosis or diplopia in 50% of cases.

- Autoimmune disorder
- Autoantibodies directed against the postsynaptic acetylcholine receptors block or destroy the receptors. This decreased number of functional acetylcholine receptors results in deficient synaptic transmission at the level of the junction between the motor nerve endings and the muscle.
- Because the amount of acetylcholine present in the synapse fluctuates, there is fatigability, which is the hallmark of myasthenia gravis: on repeated or sustained contraction, fewer receptors are available for activation and the strength of the muscle diminishes.

Clinical Presentation of Ocular Myasthenia

- Unilateral or bilateral fluctuating ptosis (▶ Fig. 13.62) that may worsen in bright sunlight, perhaps because of an increased stimulus to blink
- Fluctuating binocular diplopia
- Symptoms and signs typically worsen after exercise or when patients are tired.
- Ptosis and extraocular movement fluctuate even during the examination.
- The symptoms and signs improve with rest (sleep test).
- The ptosis often improves when ice is applied on the ptotic eyelid (ice test).
- Ptosis is very common but may be absent (▶ Fig. 13.63).
- Myasthenia can mimic any abnormal eye movement.
- The ophthalmoparesis can involve all the extraocular muscles or can be limited to one muscle or one group of muscles, thereby mimicking a pupil-sparing third nerve palsy, a sixth nerve palsy, or even an internuclear ophthalmoplegia. The neuro-muscular junctions innervated by the third nerve are particularly susceptible to involvement by myasthenia.
- Diffuse, bilateral ophthalmoplegia with sparing of the pupil is highly suspicious for ocular myasthenia (▶ Fig. 13.64).
- The orbicularis muscles (used to close the eyes very tightly) are often also weak: it is then easy to force the eyes open.
- The pupils are always normal.
- Findings fluctuate from one examination to another and during the examination. After some rest, the ptosis and diplopia often resolve.
- Ocular myasthenia may be isolated or may precede (sometimes by a few months or years) or accompany systemic myasthenia.

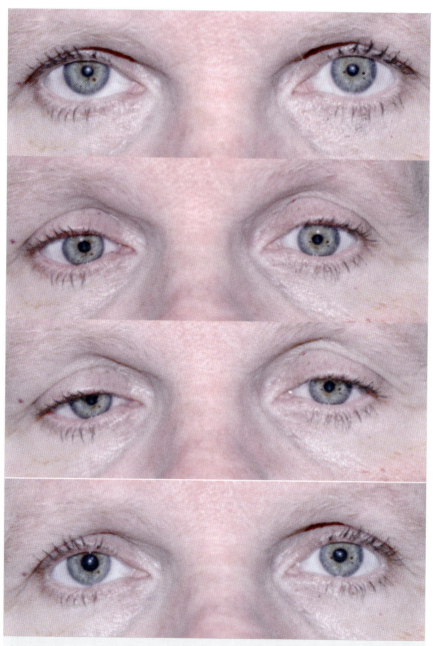

Fig. 13.62 Ocular myasthenia with fluctuating ptosis and esotropia during the examination. Top: at the beginning of the examination. Middle two photos: after sustained up gaze, there is ptosis and diplopia from esotropia. Bottom: after rest, the ptosis and esotropia are improved.

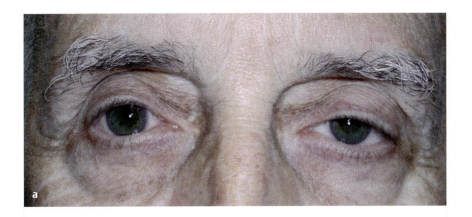

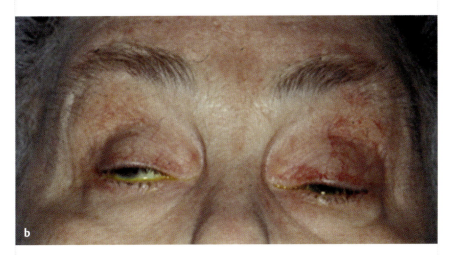

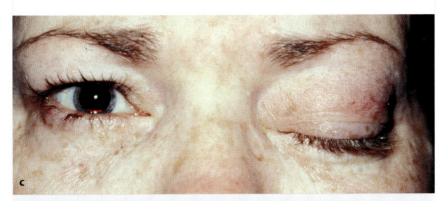

Fig. 13.63 All degrees of unilateral or bilateral ptosis can occur in ocular myasthenia.
(a) Mild bilateral asymmetric ptosis. (b) Severe bilateral ptosis. (c) Complete unilateral ptosis.

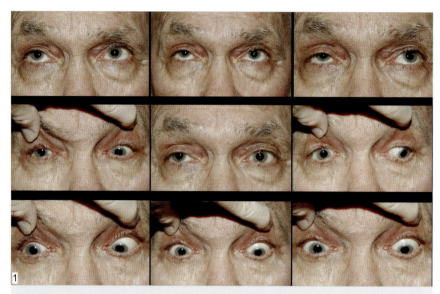

Fig. 13.64 Bilateral ophthalmoplegia from myasthenia gravis.

- In systemic myasthenia, there can be proximal diffuse weakness of the extremities, change in voice (hoarseness or nasal quality), swallowing difficulties, and respiratory compromise. Systemic myasthenia is a medical emergency, particularly when respiration and swallowing are affected.

Pearls

Between 50 and 60% of patients presenting with purely ocular myasthenia will progress to develop generalized disease, and the vast majority of those who do will do so within 1 to 2 years. Generalized myasthenia gravis can be an emergency because patients may develop respiratory distress and swallowing difficulties.

Pearls

In myasthenia gravis, the pupils are always normal and there is no pain.

Causes of Myasthenia Gravis

- Autoimmune disorder in most cases
- Rarely a paraneoplastic disorder
- There is an association in some patients between myasthenia and thymus enlargement or thymoma.
- Myasthenic syndrome may be induced by medications affecting neuromuscular transmission (curares, penicillamine). Autoimmune myasthenia gravis is often worsened by medications (curares, aminoglycosides, penicillamine, β-blockers, benzodiazepines).

Evaluation of the Patient with Suspected Ocular Myasthenia

The diagnosis of myasthenia is suspected clinically. A definite diagnosis is made when the clinical signs are reversed by the administration of a drug increasing the concentration of acetylcholine in the synapse (acetylcholinesterase inhibitor), when serum acetylcholine receptor antibodies are detected, or when there is electromyographic demonstration of muscle fatigability.

Examination and History

Examine the eyelids and eye movements.
- Are the signs fluctuating?
- Do the signs worsen with repetitive movements and sustained up gaze?
- Are the orbicularis muscles weak?
- Are the pupils normal?

Check for systemic involvement.
- Is there any proximal weakness?
  - Ask the patient to get up from a chair without using the hands 10 times in a row.
  - Ask the patient to raise both arms repetitively.
- Is the patient's voice normal?
- Does the patient have any difficulty swallowing (coughs while eating or drinking)?
- Is the patient short of breath?
  - Ask the patient to count to 60 without breathing.

Determine the cause.
- List the patient's medications.
- Any history of cancer?
- Any other autoimmune disease (such as thyroid disease)?

Confirm the diagnosis.
- Sleep test
- Ice test
- Administration of edrophonium (Tensilon test)
- Blood test for acetylcholine receptor antibodies (positive in up to 50% of patients with ocular myasthenia and in about 80 to 90% of patients with generalized myasthenia)
- Electromyography (single fiber electromyography is most accurate)
- Other tests
  - CT of the chest with contrast looking for a thymoma
  - Thyroid function tests
  - Autoantibody panel looking for other autoimmune diseases

Edrophonium (Tensilon) Test

Edrophonium is a short-acting acetylcholinesterase inhibitor that increases the concentration of acetylcholine at the synapse and, therefore, temporarily reverses signs of myasthenia gravis. It is given intravenously and its effects last 2 to 3 minutes. Side effects include sweating, fasciculations, diarrhea, abdominal cramps, palpitations, or bradycardia. Although it is generally well tolerated, hypotension, vagal reactions, and even respiratory or cardiac arrest are possible; it should be avoided in patients with known respiratory or cardiac diseases and in the elderly.

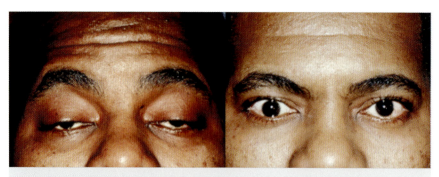

Fig. 13.65 Dramatic improvement of bilateral ptosis 1 minute after injection of 4 mg of edrophonium, confirming the diagnosis of ocular myasthenia.

1. Identify an examination parameter to observe for improvement after edrophonium administration (ideally, ptosis).
2. Establish venous access.
3. Monitor blood pressure and heart rate.
4. Prepare edrophonium (10 mg in 1 mL syringe), 1 mg atropine, saline flush (10 mL), blood pressure and heart rate monitoring equipment.
5. Inject 2 mg edrophonium test dose, flush intravenously (IV), observe for improvement or side effects for 1 minute. If definite improvement results, stop the test. You have a positive result.
6. Repeat step 4 every 1 to 2 minutes with 2 mg edrophonium until improvement of the chosen parameter is obtained, side effects occur, or 10 mg of edrophonium is administered.
7. Alternatively, give a 5 mg edrophonium bolus after uneventful test dose and observe for improvement or side effects (▶ Fig. 13.65).

Treatment of Myasthenia Gravis

The treatment of myasthenia gravis is mostly based on the clinical presentation and includes the following:

- Patients with generalized myasthenia should be evaluated emergently by a neurologist.
- Patients are instructed to go to the emergency room if they develop respiratory distress or swallowing difficulties.
- Medications associated with triggering or worsening of myasthenic symptoms and signs need to be discontinued (give the patient a list of forbidden medications).
- Treatment with pyridostigmine, a long-acting acetylcholinesterase inhibitor, is sometimes only partially effective for ophthalmoplegia.
- Corticosteroids (prednisone) are sometimes indicated if there is failure of pyridostigmine.
- Immunosuppressants are sometimes indicated for rebounds despite prednisone and as steroid-sparing agents.
- Thymectomy is indicated in all cases with a thymoma and in patients with severe generalized myasthenia.
- Symptomatic treatment of ptosis and diplopia: prisms and surgical procedures (on residual ptosis or strabismus) are sometimes necessary and should be performed in stable patients not responding to medical therapy. Ptosis crutches (mounted on glasses to keep the eyelids open) may be helpful.

Thyroid Eye Disease in Association with Myasthenia

Thyroid eye disease is the autoimmune disorder most commonly associated with ocular myasthenia. Each disease occurs more frequently in patients with the other disease than in the general population, attesting to the autoimmune origin of both disorders. Differentiating thyroid eye disease from myasthenia gravis can be challenging because both disorders present with painless bilateral ophthalmoplegia sparing the pupils.

Remember that thyroid eye disease produces proptosis, periorbital swelling, and lid retraction, whereas myasthenia produces ptosis. The presence of lid retraction in a patient with myasthenia raises the possibility of thyroid eye disease. The presence of ptosis in a patient with thyroid eye disease raises the possibility of myasthenia.

Myasthenia tends to preferentially affect those extraocular muscles innervated by branches of the third nerve (e.g., the levator palpebrae and the medial rectus), often manifesting with ptosis and exotropia, whereas thyroid eye disease preferentially affects the inferior and medial recti muscles, commonly manifesting with a restrictive hypotropia and esotropia.

When myasthenia and thyroid eye disease coexist, both diseases are treated simultaneously. Most patients respond to pyridostigmine and prednisone (▶ Fig. 13.66).

13.5.3 The Lesion Involves a Cranial Nerve

The diagnosis and management of ocular motor cranial nerve dysfunction vary according to the age of the patient, characteristics of the cranial nerve palsy, and presence of associated symptoms and signs.

Sixth Cranial Nerve (Abducens Nerve) Palsies

A sixth nerve palsy results in paresis of abduction of the ipsilateral eye and gives binocular horizontal diplopia. Patients with a sixth nerve palsy describe binocular horizontal diplopia that is worse looking toward the side of the sixth nerve palsy. The sixth nerve originates in the pons, close to the facial nerve nucleus. It is often affected by meningeal processes and raised intracranial pressure.

A sixth nerve palsy results in paresis of abduction of the ipsilateral eye (▶ Fig. 13.67).

Anatomy of the Sixth Cranial Nerve (▶ Fig. 13.68)

The sixth cranial nerve has a long intracranial course:
- The nucleus is located at the medial dorsal pontomedullary junction, near the genu of the seventh (facial) nerve (facial colliculus area).
- From the sixth nerve nucleus, motor neuron axons traverse anteriorly within the sixth nerve fascicle, whereas interneurons cross over to ascend within the contralateral medial longitudinal fasciculus (MLF) to the medial rectus subnucleus of the third nerve.
- Motor neuron axons exit the pons anteriorly as the sixth nerve.
- The sixth nerve then ascends along the ventral aspect of the brainstem in the subarachnoid space.
- It passes through the Dorello canal beneath the petroclinoid (Gruber) ligament.
- The nerve then enters the cavernous sinus where it is freely situated, lateral to the internal carotid artery. There, it is in close relationship with the sympathetic fibers.
- It enters the orbit through the superior orbital fissure and annulus of Zinn.
- It then innervates the ipsilateral lateral rectus muscle.

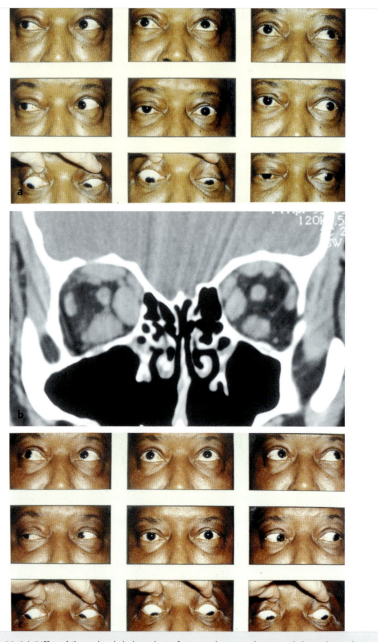

Fig. 13.66 (a) Diffuse bilateral ophthalmoplegia from ocular myasthenia and thyroid eye disease. Note the right ptosis, but also periorbital swelling and left lid retraction. There is mild bilateral proptosis. (b) Coronal computed tomographic scan of the orbits without contrast showing enlarged extraocular muscles (right worse than left) consistent with thyroid eye disease. (c) Same patient after treatment. The ptosis has resolved and the extraocular movements are full.

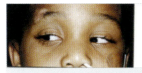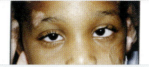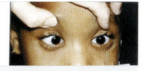

Fig. 13.67 Left sixth nerve palsy with no abduction of the left eye when looking to the left.

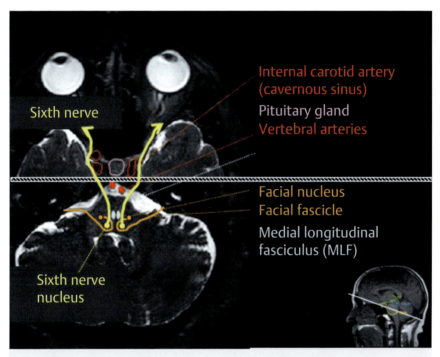

Fig. 13.68 Anatomical course of the sixth nerve (abducens). The top part of the picture is above (more rostral) the level of the bottom part to show the whole course of the sixth nerve.

Causes of Sixth Cranial Nerve Palsies (▶ Table 13.3)

- A sixth nerve nuclear lesion causes an ipsilateral horizontal gaze palsy (neither eye can look in the direction of the lesion). Because the genu of the facial nerve (seventh cranial nerve) passes around the sixth nerve nucleus in the facial colliculus, lesions in this area usually result in an ipsilateral peripheral seventh nerve palsy in addition to the conjugate gaze palsy (facial colliculus syndrome). The inability to move the eyes past the midline horizontally cannot be overcome by the oculocephalic (doll's head) maneuver or caloric testing (▶ Fig. 13.69)
- Because the sixth nerve lies freely within the cavernous sinus, rather than residing within the lateral wall, it may be particularly susceptible to compression in this location by tumor or aneurysm.

Table 13.3 Most Common causes of acquired sixth nerve lesions by anatomical location

Location of the lesion	Associated symptoms/signs	Most common causes
Nucleus (pons)	Ipsilateral horizontal conjugate gaze palsy Ipsilateral facial weakness	Infarction Hemorrhage (cavernoma) Neoplasm (metastasis) Congenital
Fascicle (pons)	Ipsilateral abduction paresis of one eye With associated neurologic symptoms/signs: Contralateral hemiparesis (Raymond syndrome) Ipsilateral seventh nerve palsy and contralateral hemiparesis (Millard–Gubler syndrome) Ipsilateral seventh nerve palsy, deafness, facial hypoesthesia, Horner, contralateral pain and thermal hypoesthesia, ataxia (Foville syndrome)	Infarction Hemorrhage Neoplasm Demyelination
Subarachnoid space	Typically isolated May present with headaches and papilledema	Microvascular Meningitis Trauma Tumors Infections (petrous apex) Raised intracranial pressure Low intracranial pressure Chiari malformation Vertebral/basilar aneurysm or ectasia
Cavernous sinus	Third, fourth, V1, (V2) Oculosympathetic dysfunction Pain may be prominent	Neoplasm Inflammation Carotid aneurysm Microvascular Carotid-cavernous fistula Cavernous sinus thrombosis
Orbital apex	Third, fourth, V1, V2 Oculosympathetic dysfunction Visual loss (optic nerve)	Neoplasm Inflammation Infection (fungus)

- Unilateral or bilateral sixth nerve palsies occur as false localizing signs of supratentorial mass lesions, edema, hemorrhage, or other causes of increased intracranial pressure. Within the subarachnoid space, the nerve is particularly vulnerable to downward pressure on the brainstem as it ascends the ventral aspect of the pons, passes beneath the petroclinoid ligament, and travels over the edge of the tentorium. This appears to be the mechanism of sixth nerve palsies resulting from increased intracranial pressure. For the same reason, hypotension of the cerebrospinal fluid (CSF) (after trauma with CSF leakage, postlumbar puncture, or spontaneous occurrence) can also cause a unilateral or bilateral sixth nerve palsy. All causes of meningitis (infectious, inflammatory, neoplastic) are frequently associated with a unilateral or bilateral sixth nerve palsy.

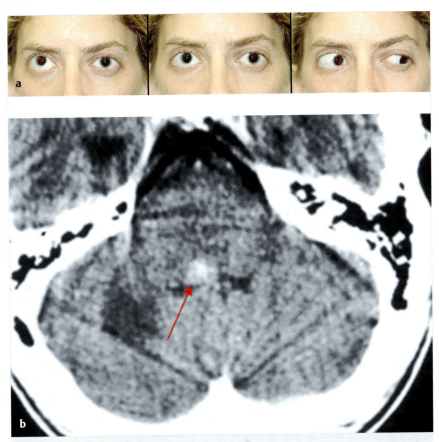

Fig. 13.69 (a) Right nuclear sixth nerve palsy with conjugate right gaze palsy (neither eye looks to the right). There is also a right peripheral facial palsy (deviation of the mouth to the left and difficulty closing the right eye with poor Bell phenomenon). (b) Axial computed tomographic scan of the brain without contrast showing a hyperdense lesion at the level of the right sixth nerve nucleus (*arrow*).

- Lesions of the petrous apex are a classic cause of ipsilateral sixth nerve palsy, most often associated with pain. Because of its relationship with the mastoid, infections are common causes (Gradenigo syndrome). Cerebral venous thrombosis extending to the petrosal sinuses can also produce a sixth nerve palsy. Skull base and cavernous sinus lesions commonly involve the sixth nerve. They may be difficult to see on routine brain MRI and will be easily missed if the MRI scan is performed without contrast (▶ Fig. 13.70 and ▶ Fig. 13.71).
- An isolated sixth nerve palsy occurring in a patient older than 50 and with atheromatous vascular risk factors is often a microvascular sixth nerve palsy.

Microvascular sixth nerve palsies are secondary to ischemia of the sixth cranial nerve (fascicle or subarachnoid space).
- The onset is acute or rapidly progressive.
- The sixth nerve palsy is isolated.

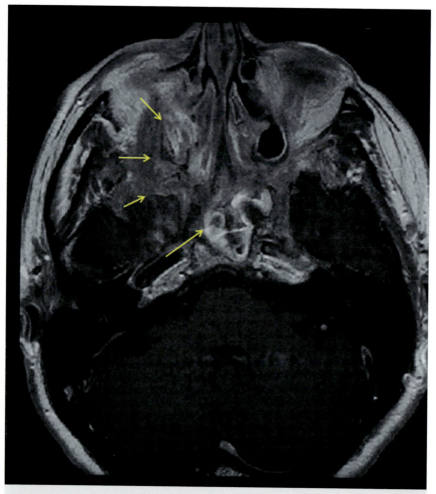

Fig. 13.70 Axial T1-weighted magnetic resonance imaging of the brain with contrast showing an infiltrative process of the skull base and facial sinuses (*arrows*) presenting with a painful right sixth nerve palsy. Biopsy showed lymphoma.

- Moderate pain over the brow or of the ipsilateral face or head is common.
- The sixth nerve palsy almost always resolves completely within 3 to 6 months (▶ Fig. 13.72).

Pearls

- ○ Microvascular sixth nerve palsies are most often nonarteritic, but giant cell arteritis should always be considered.
- ○ A microvascular sixth nerve palsy should resolve within 3 to 6 months. Persistent abduction deficit should prompt an extensive workup.

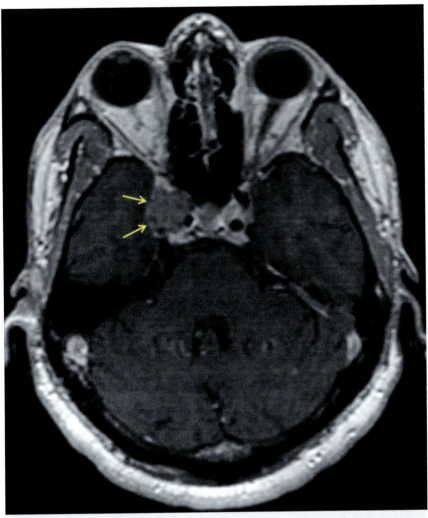

Fig. 13.71 Axial T1-weighted magnetic resonance imaging of the brain with contrast showing enlargement and enhancement of the right cavernous sinus (*arrows*) secondary to breast cancer metastasis. The patient presented with a painful right sixth nerve palsy.

Rarely, a microvascular sixth nerve palsy may be arteritic, related to vasculitis (especially giant cell arteritis) (▶ Fig. 13.73).

Diplopia in a patient over 50 should raise the possibility of giant cell arteritis.

- Always look for other symptoms or signs of giant cell arteritis.
- Obtain complete blood count (CBC), platelets, C-reactive protein (CRP), and erythrocyte sedimentation rate (ESR).
- The sixth nerve palsy may be subtle with apparently full ductions. The cross-cover test (or the red glass or Maddox rod test) shows an esotropia, which may be comitant. This is particularly common with raised intracranial pressure or Chiari malformations (▶ Fig. 13.74).

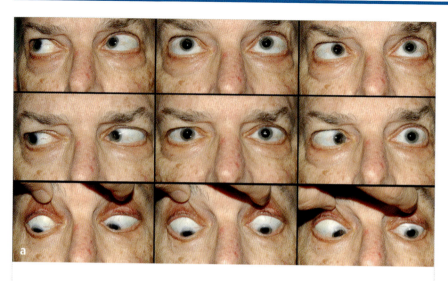

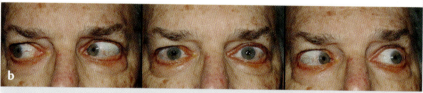

Fig. 13.72 (a) Left microvascular sixth nerve palsy. (b) Two months later, the sixth nerve palsy has spontaneously resolved.

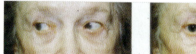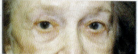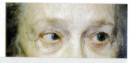

Fig. 13.73 Left abduction deficit in a patient with giant cell arteritis.

Chiari malformations often produce neuro-ophthalmic symptoms and signs (▶ Fig. 13.75):
- Headache (often with exercise)
- Dizziness
- Diplopia from unilateral or bilateral sixth nerve palsy or from "divergence insufficiency"
- Downbeat nystagmus
- Raised intracranial pressure with papilledema (rare)

Congenital Sixth Cranial Nerve Palsies

Duane Syndrome

- There is marked limitation of abduction and variable limitation of adduction.
- This is explained by congenital agenesis of the sixth nerve with resultant abnormal innervation of the lateral rectus muscle by branches from the third nerve.

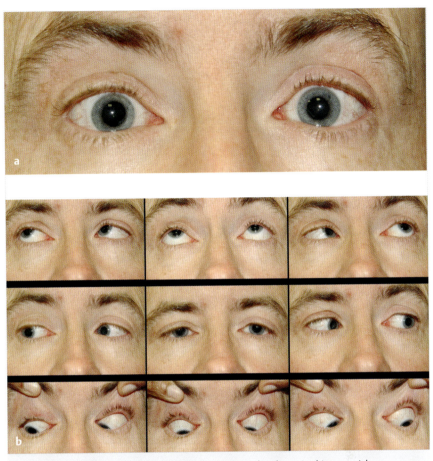

Fig. 13.74 (a) Corneal reflex showing a small esotropia related to raised intracranial pressure (obstructive hydrocephalus from a mass in the posterior fossa). (b) Subtle bilateral sixth nerve palsy with esotropia in a patient with headaches and bilateral papilledema.

- There is globe retraction and narrowing of the palpebral fissure on attempted adduction secondary to co-contraction of the medial and lateral rectus muscles.
- Duane syndrome can be unilateral or bilateral.
- It occurs more commonly in women and in the left eye.
- Most cases are sporadic.
- Patients usually do not complain of diplopia and are not amblyopic.
- There are systemic associations in 30 to 50% (deafness and Goldenhar syndrome are the most common).

There are three types of Duane syndrome:
- Type I: Limited abduction (most common; patient appears esotropic) (▶ Fig. 13.76)
- Type II: Limited adduction (patient appears exotropic)
- Type III: Limited abduction and adduction

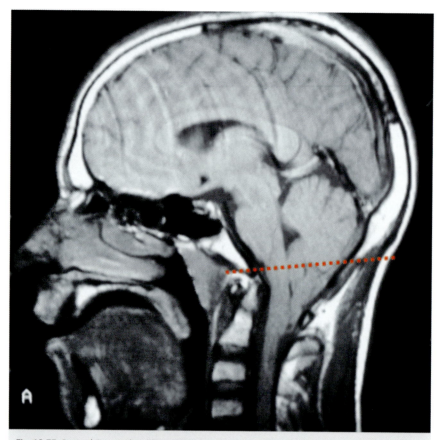

Fig. 13.75 Sagittal T1-weighted brain magnetic resonance imaging showing herniation of the cerebellar tonsils (below the red line).

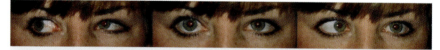

Fig. 13.76 Congenital Duane syndrome type I in the left eye: there is abduction deficit of the left eye and the left palpebral fissure is narrowed when she looks to the right.

Möbius Syndrome

- Congenital agenesis of the sixth and seventh nerve nuclei
- Congenital facial diplegia associated with bilateral horizontal gaze palsy
- May be accompanied by atrophy of the tongue, deformities of the head and face, endocrine abnormalities, and malformations of the chest, great vessels, and extremities
- Sporadic

Horizontal Gaze Paresis and Progressive Scoliosis (HGPPS)

- Autosomal recessive
- Congenital absence of horizontal conjugate eye movements with progressive scoliosis during early childhood

Causes of Sixth Cranial Nerve Palsies in Children

Cranial nerve palsies in children differ in frequency from what is classically observed in adults:

- Congenital sixth nerve palsies are common.
  - Cycloplegic refraction is important in children with esotropia: uncorrected hyperopia often results in accommodative esotropia.
  - Congenital esotropia is also common.
  - Duane syndrome is common.
- Acquired sixth nerve palsies are most commonly due to the following:
  - Trauma
  - Posterior fossa tumors
  - Meningitis
  - Raised intracranial pressure (hydrocephalus)

Mimickers of Sixth Cranial Nerve Palsies

Pearls

Not all patients with an abduction deficit have a sixth nerve palsy (disorders of the muscle and myasthenia can also give an isolated abduction deficit).

Thalamic Esotropia

- Thalamic lesions can rarely induce convergence of one or both eyes (a contralateral decrease in the normal inhibition of the medial rectus muscle), thereby mimicking unilateral or bilateral sixth nerve palsy.
- Thalamic esotropia is usually associated with up gaze deficits (▶ Fig. 13.77).

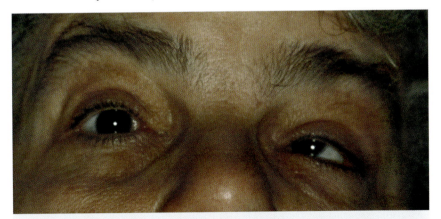

Fig. 13.77 Thalamic esotropia from a right thalamic hemorrhage. The left eye is deviated toward the nose, mimicking a left sixth nerve palsy.

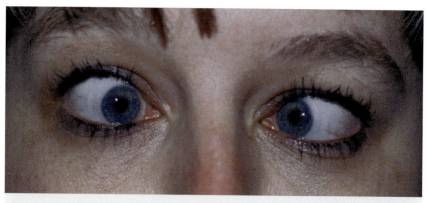

Fig. 13.78 Spasm of the near triad, with convergence, accommodation, and pupillary constriction.

Convergence Spasm

- Convergence spasm is often misinterpreted as unilateral or bilateral sixth nerve palsy.
- Both eyes are converged toward the nose, and there is pupillary constriction and lens accommodation (so-called spasm of the near triad).
- When the patient is asked to look to each side, the eyes do not move.
- Ductions should then be tested with each eye covered. Usually, the patient is able to move the eye laterally, and disruption of the near triad will be associated with pupillary dilation as the near triad is released; the pupils constrict again when the patient converges (▶ Fig. 13.78).

Evaluation of the Patient with Suspected Sixth Cranial Nerve Palsy

- Based on other illnesses and age
- Neurological evaluation looking for other symptoms or signs
- Ophthalmological evaluation looking for orbital syndrome, optic neuropathy, papilledema, other ocular motor cranial nerve involvement
- Systemic evaluation looking for giant cell arteritis (if over 50 years of age), fever, systemic inflammatory disorder, atheromatous vascular risk factors
- Could it be myasthenia?
- Is the sixth nerve palsy isolated, or not?
- Is the sixth nerve palsy painful, or not?

Patients with Isolated sixth nerve palsy may need the following evaluation:
- Patient older than 50 years: CBC, platelets, CRP, ESR, glucose, lipid profile
- MRI of brain and orbits with fat suppression and gadolinium with special attention to the course of the sixth nerve: pons, clivus, petrous area, cavernous sinus, pituitary gland, facial sinus, mastoid, orbital apex, and orbit (rectus muscles and superior orbital vein)
- Magnetic resonance angiography (MRA) or computed tomographic angiography
- (CTA) of the circle of Willis only if a vascular process (aneurysm or carotid cavernous fistula) is suspected

- Lumbar puncture with CSF opening pressure and CSF analysis if MRI is normal and raised intracranial pressure (headache and/or papilledema) or a meningeal process are suspected
- Bilateral sixth nerve palsies with normal MRI should have a lumbar puncture with CSF opening pressure and CSF analysis. Beware of the possibility of low CSF pressure (spontaneous CSF hypotension).

Although it is not always necessary to obtain an MRI scan in patients with suspected microvascular sixth nerve palsy, most patients undergo imaging. It is, however, also reasonable to observe such patients for recovery, and to obtain imaging only if their abduction deficit persists after 3 months.

Fourth Cranial Nerve (Trochlear Nerve) Palsies

Patients with a fourth nerve palsy have a superior oblique weakness. A fourth nerve palsy results in difficulty looking down when the eye is positioned in toward the nose. Patients complain of binocular vertical (or oblique) diplopia, especially when going down the stairs and reading. They have an ipsilateral hypertropia that is worse when they look to the other side and worse when they tilt their head toward the same side. They spontaneously tilt their head to the contralateral side to compensate for their diplopia.

Right superior oblique paresis (▶ Fig. 13.79) has the following characteristics:
- Decreased depression
- Right hypertropia
- Hypertropia worsens in left gaze
- Worse with right head tilt

A fourth nerve palsy also results in decreased intorsion, and some patients mention that one image is tilted (▶ Fig. 13.80).

When there is also a third nerve palsy, the eye cannot adduct (▶ Fig. 13.81).

To check that the fourth nerve functions normally when there is a third cranial nerve palsy, check that intorsion of the eye is preserved, a function that is best seen in abduction.
1. Ask the patient to abduct the eye with the third nerve palsy (left eye in this example).
2. Once the eye is in abduction, ask the patient to look down, and look carefully for intorsion by focusing on a scleral vessel.
3. Intact intorsion confirms that the fourth nerve is functional.

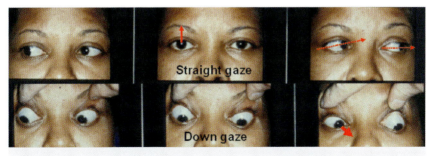

Fig. 13.79 Right superior oblique paresis.

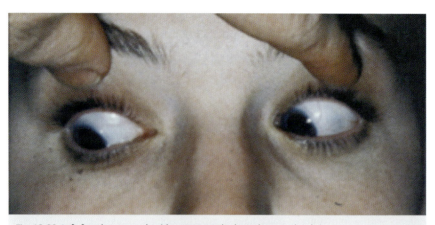

Fig. 13.80 Left fourth nerve palsy (the patient is looking down and right).

Pearls

Not all patients with a superior oblique paresis have a fourth nerve palsy (disorders of the muscle and myasthenia can also give a superior oblique weakness). Fourth nerve palsies may be difficult to differentiate from skew deviation.

The upright-supine test helps differentiate a skew deviation from trochlear nerve palsy: a vertical deviation that decreases by ≥ 50% from the upright to supine position suggests a skew deviation.

Anatomy of the Fourth Cranial Nerve (▶ Fig. 13.82)

The fourth nerve is unique in its dorsal exit from the midbrain, posterior crossover within the subarachnoid space, and innervation of the superior oblique muscle contralateral to its nucleus. Because of these anatomical features and the resultant long course from midbrain to muscle, the fourth nerve is particularly vulnerable to injury in the setting of head trauma.

- The nucleus is located at the ventral border of the periaqueductal gray matter, at the level of the inferior colliculus, and lies immediately next to the descending sympathetic pathways.
- The fascicle exits posteriorly and crosses over to the contralateral side of the midbrain.
- The nerve travels ventrally within the subarachnoid space (longest intracranial course of all cranial nerves, measuring 75 mm).
- It then curves around the upper pons where it passes between the superior cerebellar artery and the posterior cerebral artery to reach the prepontine cistern.
- The nerve then enters the lateral wall of the cavernous sinus and lies below the third nerve and above the ophthalmic division of the fifth nerve (V1).
- It reaches the orbital apex.
- The nerve enters the superior orbit outside of the annulus of Zinn to innervate the superior oblique muscle.

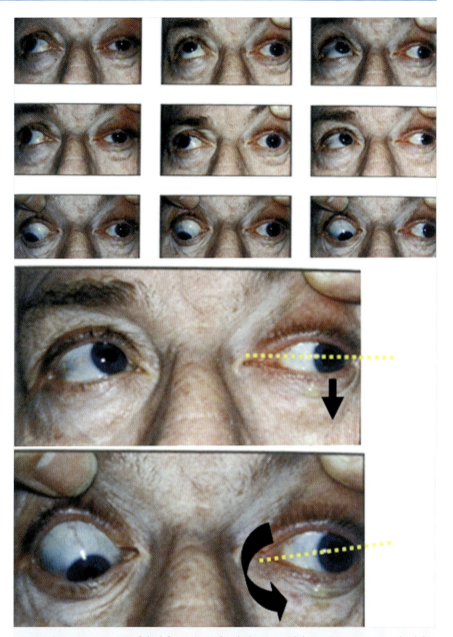

Fig. 13.81 Intact intorsion of the left eye (tested with the eye in abduction) in a patient with a left third nerve palsy.

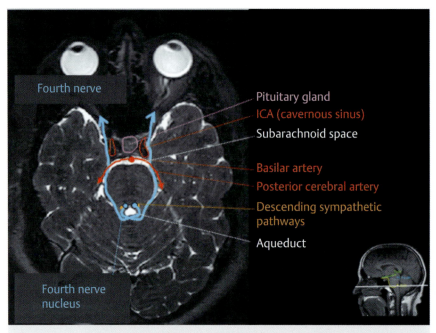

Fig. 13.82 Anatomical course of the fourth nerve (trochlear). ICA, internal carotid artery.

Causes of Fourth Cranial Nerve Palsies (▶ Table 13.4)

- A fourth nerve nuclear lesion causes a superior oblique palsy clinically similar to a fourth nerve lesion. However, the superior oblique weakness is contralateral to the nuclear lesion because of the fourth nerve's decussation after its dorsal emergence from the midbrain.
- A fourth nerve nuclear lesion is often associated with a Horner syndrome because the descending sympathetic pathway is very close to the fourth nerve nucleus (the Horner syndrome is on the side of the nuclear lesion, whereas the superior oblique paresis will involve the opposite eye).
- The two most common causes of fourth nerve palsy are trauma (unilateral or bilateral fourth nerve palsy) and decompensation of a congenital fourth nerve palsy.
- An isolated fourth nerve palsy occurring in a patient older than 50 and with atheromatous vascular risk factors is often a microvascular fourth nerve palsy. Mild brow pain is common. The fourth nerve palsy almost always resolves completely within 3 to 6 months. Rarely, a microvascular fourth nerve palsy may be arteritic, related to vasculitis (especially giant cell arteritis).

Pearls

- ○ Microvascular fourth nerve palsies are most often nonarteritic, but giant cell arteritis should always be considered.
- ○ A microvascular fourth nerve palsy should resolve within 3 to 6 months.
- ○ Persistent deficit should prompt imaging, if not performed initially.

Table 13.4 Most common causes of acquired fourth nerve lesions by anatomical location

Location of the lesion	Associated symptoms/signs	Most common causes
Nucleus (midbrain)	Contralateral superior oblique weakness Ipsilateral Horner syndrome	Trauma Infarction Hemorrhage (cavernoma) Neoplasm (metastasis)
Fascicle (midbrain)	Rare Contralateral dysmetria (superior cerebellar peduncle)	Trauma Infarction Hemorrhage Neoplasm Demyelination
Subarachnoid space	Typically isolated May present with headaches	Trauma Microvascular Meningitis Tumors
Cavernous sinus	Third, sixth, V1, (V2) Oculosympathetic dysfunction Pain may be prominent	Neoplasm Inflammation Carotid aneurysm Microvascular Carotid cavernous fistula Cavernous sinus thrombosis
Orbital apex	Third, sixth, V1 Oculosympathetic dysfunction Visual loss (optic nerve)	Neoplasm Inflammation Infection (fungus)

Rarely, an isolated fourth nerve palsy is secondary to a small tumor of the nerve in the subarachnoid space. In most cases, these tumors are schwannomas. Their prognosis is good, and symptomatic treatment of diplopia, such as prisms or even strabismus surgery if stable ocular deviation, is offered (▶ Fig. 13.83).

Congenital Fourth Cranial Nerve Palsy

Congenital fourth cranial nerve palsy is common and may decompensate at any age.
- Decompensated congenital fourth nerve palsy presents as intermittent diplopia in a patient with a long-standing head tilt (obvious on old photographs).
- There is evidence of chronicity as shown by the following:
  - Overaction of the ipsilateral inferior oblique in adduction (the eye shoots up in adduction)
  - Large vertical fusional amplitude, up to 10 or 15 prism diopters (patient's ability to fuse vertically separated images despite the placement of progressively larger amounts of vertical prism over one eye; normal vertical fusional amplitude is between 2 and 3 prism diopters) (▶ Fig. 13.84)

Causes of Fourth Cranial Nerve Palsies in Children

Fourth nerve palsies are less common in children than sixth and third nerve palsies. Trauma represents the most common cause. Congenital fourth nerve palsies are often not diagnosed in childhood.

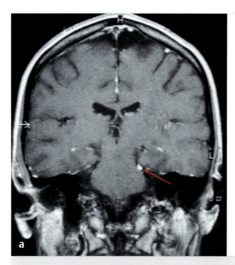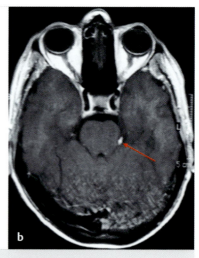

Fig. 13.83 (a) Coronal T1-weighted magnetic resonance imaging (MRI) of the brain with contrast showing a small enhancing mass along the left fourth nerve, suggestive of a fourth nerve schwannoma (*arrow*). (b) Axial T1-weighted MRI of the brain with contrast showing a small enhancing mass along the left fourth nerve, suggestive of a fourth nerve schwannoma (*arrow*).

Evaluation of the Patient with Suspected Fourth Cranial Nerve Palsy

- Based on other illnesses and age
- Neurological evaluation looking for other symptoms or signs
- Ophthalmological evaluation looking for orbital syndrome, optic neuropathy, papilledema, other ocular motor cranial nerve involvement
- Systemic evaluation looking for giant cell arteritis (if over 50), fever, systemic inflammatory disorder, atheromatous vascular risk factors
- Could it be myasthenia?
- Is the fourth nerve palsy isolated, or not?
- Is the fourth nerve palsy painful, or not?
- Is the fourth nerve palsy chronic?
  - Review old photos for head tilt.
  - Look for inferior oblique overaction.
  - Look for large vertical fusion amplitude.

Patients with isolated fourth nerve palsy need to be evaluated as follows:
- If posttraumatic or decompensation of congenital fourth nerve palsy, no further workup
- Patient older than 50 years: CBC, platelets, CRP, ESR, glucose, lipid profile
- If acquired and no precipitating trauma
  - MRI brain and orbits with fat suppression and gadolinium with special attention to the course of the fourth nerve: midbrain, cavernous sinus, pituitary gland, orbital apex, and orbit (trochlea)

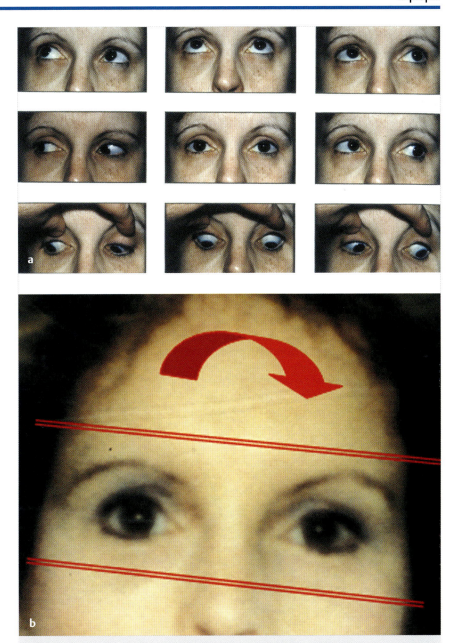

Fig. 13.84 (a) Right fourth nerve palsy. Note the upward overshoot of the right eye in adduction (when the patient looks to the left). (b) Left head tilt on the driver's license picture taken 5 years prior to onset of diplopia.

Third Cranial Nerve (Oculomotor Nerve) Palsies

A third nerve palsy results in ipsilateral paresis of the following:
- Adduction (medial rectus)
- Elevation (superior rectus and inferior oblique)
- Depression (inferior rectus)

The following also occur:
- Ptosis (levator palpebrae)
- Pupillary dilation (parasympathetics)
- Accommodation paralysis (parasympathetics)

The classic presenting symptoms of a patient with a third nerve palsy are binocular vertical and horizontal diplopia, droopy lid, or, less frequently, awareness of an enlarged pupil or blurred monocular vision at near. Associated symptoms are of extreme importance in the evaluation of the third cranial nerve (▶ Fig. 13.85).

Anatomy of the Third Cranial Nerve

The third nerve originates in the midbrain and is in close relationship with the internal carotid artery in its subarachnoid course (▶ Fig. 13.86); an acute third nerve palsy always raises the possibility of an intracranial aneurysm.
- The nucleus is a cluster of subnuclei in the dorsal midbrain (see Anatomy of the Third Nerve Nucleus for description).
- From the third nerve nucleus and motor and parasympathetic neuron axons traverse anteriorly within the third nerve fascicle.
- The third nerve then exits the midbrain near the medial aspect of the cerebral peduncle.

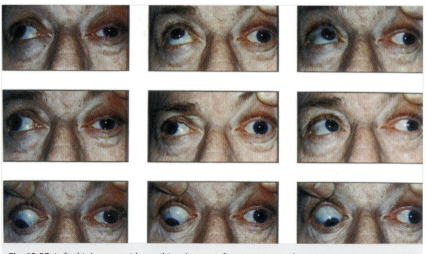

Fig. 13.85 Left third nerve with pupil involvement from a mass in the cavernous sinus.

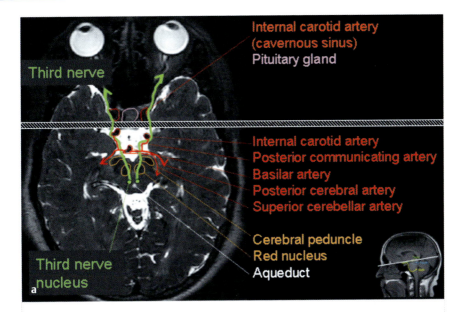

Internal carotid artery
(cavernous sinus)
Pituitary gland

Third nerve

Internal carotid artery
Posterior communicating artery
Basilar artery
Posterior cerebral artery
Superior cerebellar artery

Cerebral peduncle
Red nucleus
Aqueduct

Third nerve
nucleus

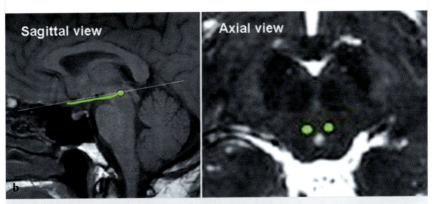

Sagittal view

Axial view

Fig. 13.86 Anatomical course of the third nerve (in green). (a) Axial view: the top part of the picture is below (more caudal) the level of the bottom part to show the whole course of the third nerve. (b) Sagittal (left) and axial (right) views of the third nerve nuclei.

- It enters the subarachnoid space, where it travels between the superior cerebellar artery and the posterior cerebral artery next to the tip of the basilar artery, then travels medially along the posterior communicating artery and lateral to the internal carotid artery.
- It enters the cavernous sinus where it is enclosed within the lateral wall, superior to the fourth nerve.
- It then enters the orbit through the superior orbital fissure and annulus of Zinn, at which point it divides into the following:
  - Superior division (innervates levator, superior rectus)
  - Inferior division (innervates the ciliary ganglion in the orbit (parasympathetics), medial rectus, inferior rectus, inferior oblique)

403

P: Parasympathetic (Edinger Westphal nucleus)
LP: Levator palpebrae (central caudal nucleus)
IO: Inferior oblique
IR: Inferior rectus
SR: Superior rectus
MR: Medial rectus

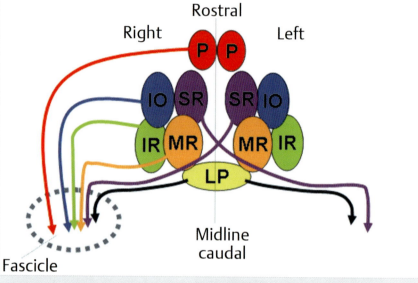

Fig. 13.87 Representation of both third nerve nuclear complexes.

Anatomy of the Third Nerve Nucleus (▶ Fig. 13.87)

The third nerve nucleus is a complex of small subnuclei: each muscle innervated by the third nerve is subserved by an individual subnucleus. Exceptionally, individual nuclei can be affected by a lesion, explaining the rare central partial third nerve palsies (in which not all extraocular muscles innervated by the third nerve are affected).

Each extraocular muscle innervated by the third nerve is subserved by an individual subnucleus located in the midbrain third nerve nuclear complex.

- The inferior oblique, inferior rectus, and medial rectus muscles are subserved by their ipsilateral subnuclei.
- The superior rectus muscle is subserved by the contralateral subnucleus (fibers cross the midline).
- Both levator palpebrae muscles are subserved by one single subnucleus (the central caudal nucleus).
- The pupillary constrictor and accommodation muscles are under the control of a parasympathetic pathway subserved by an ipsilateral subnucleus (Edinger–Westphal nucleus).

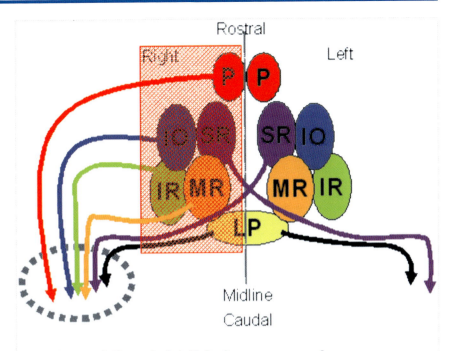

Lesion of the right third nerve nucleus:
.Complete ipsilateral (right) third nerve palsy
.Bilateral ptosis
.Bilateral elevation deficit

Fig. 13.88 Nuclear lesion of the right third nerve. P, parasympathetic; LP, levator palpebrae; IO, inferior oblique; IR, inferior rectus; SR, superior rectus; MR, medial rectus.

Because of these anatomical characteristics of the third nerve nuclear complex, specific clinical syndromes can be observed when there is a lesion at the level of the midbrain (► Fig. 13.88, ► Fig. 13.89, ► Fig. 13.90, ► Fig. 13.91, ► Fig. 13.92).

Partial lesions of one or both third nerve nuclei are possible and may produce a unilateral or bilateral incomplete (partial) third nerve palsy (► Fig. 13.93). For example, the pupils may be spared and there may be no ptosis. However, an isolated unilateral mydriasis or isolated unilateral or bilateral adduction deficit (medial rectus palsy) is almost never related to a third nerve palsy.

Classification of Third Cranial Nerve Palsies

Third nerve palsies may be classified as follows:
- *Partial:* when not all muscles innervated by the third nerve are involved or when there is only moderate paresis of the muscles
- *Complete:* when all the muscles innervated by the third nerve are involved *and* when the paresis is complete

- *With pupil involvement:* when there is anisocoria, with the larger pupil being on the side of the third nerve palsy and when the larger pupil does not react well to light
- *Pupil-sparing:* when the pupils are symmetric and briskly reactive to light

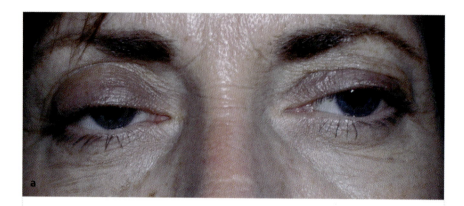

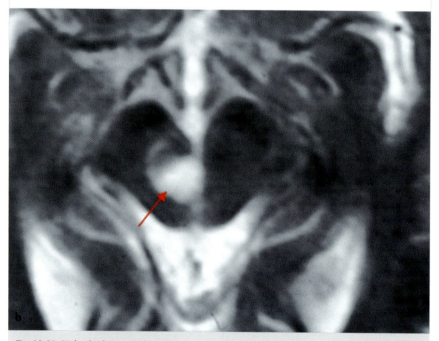

Fig. 13.89 Right third nerve palsy related to an inflammatory lesion involving the right third nerve nucleus. (a) There is bilateral ptosis, worse on the right, and decreased elevation, depression, and adduction of the right eye. The left eye does not elevate either. The right pupil is larger than the left and is poorly reactive to light. (b) Axial T2-weighted magnetic resonance imaging of the midbrain showing a lesion (*arrow*) involving the right third nerve nucleus.

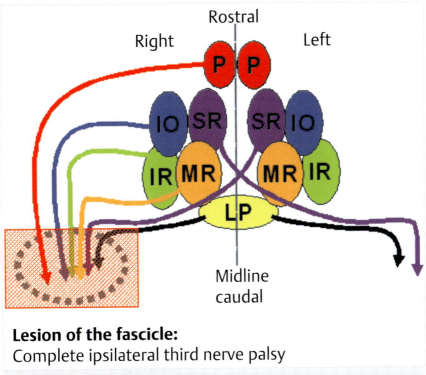

Lesion of the fascicle:
Complete ipsilateral third nerve palsy

Fig. 13.90 Fascicular lesion of the right third nerve producing an ipsilateral complete third nerve palsy. P, parasympathetic; LP, levator palpebrae; IO, inferior oblique; IR, inferior rectus; SR, superior rectus; MR, medial rectus.

Third Nerve Palsy with Pupillary Involvement

Because of the dorsal and peripheral location of the pupillary fibers, a dilated pupil associated with a third nerve palsy may be the first sign of a compressive lesion in the subarachnoid space (▶ Fig. 13.94).

In the subarachnoid space, the pupillary fibers are located at the surface of the third nerve, whereas the fibers subserving the extraocular muscles are located deeper in the nerve.

Isolated oculomotor nerve palsy with pupillary involvement in adults is usually related to compression of the third nerve either by an intracranial aneurysm, typically originating at the junction of the posterior communicating and the internal carotid arteries, or by a pituitary tumor (such as in pituitary apoplexy). Both disorders are life-threatening conditions.

Pupil-Sparing Third Nerve Palsy

Ischemia of the nerve usually involves only the very central part of the nerve itself, at the most distal end of the circulation. Therefore, occlusion of these small vessels (vasa-nervorum), as seen in diabetic patients, will present with abnormal eye movements but often normal pupils.

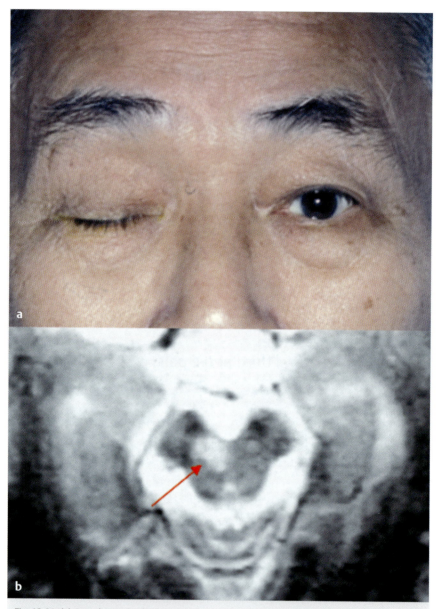

Fig. 13.91 (a) Complete right third nerve palsy related to a lacunar infarction involving the fascicle of the right third nerve. (b) Axial T2-weighted magnetic resonance imaging of the midbrain, showing a lesion (*arrow*) involving the right third nerve fascicle.

Pupil-sparing third nerve palsy refers only to *complete* third nerve palsies in which the pupil remains of normal size and reactivity. Third nerve palsies without dysfunction of *all* of the muscles innervated by the third nerve that also do not involve the pupil are not pupillary sparing. The distinction becomes very important in

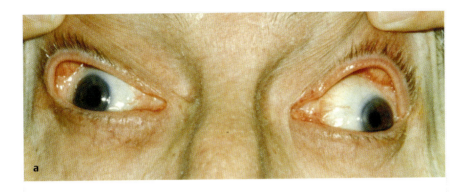

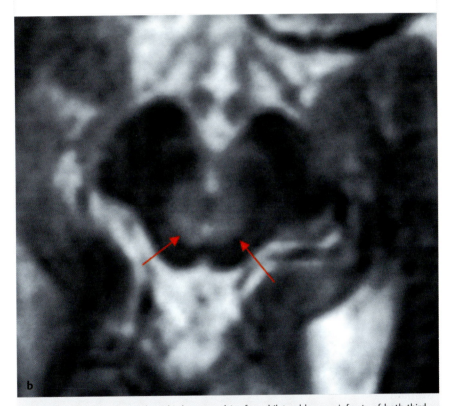

Fig. 13.92 (a) Bilateral complete third nerve palsies from bilateral lacunar infarcts of both third nerve nuclei in the midbrain. (b) Axial T2-weighted magnetic resonance imaging of the midbrain showing bilateral lesions (*arrows*) of the two third nerve nuclei.

management (to be discussed). The cause of most isolated pupil-sparing third nerve palsies is believed to be microvascular ischemia, frequently associated with diabetes mellitus or other vascular risk factors. Microvascular third nerve palsies may be quite painful but usually resolve after 3 to 4 months.

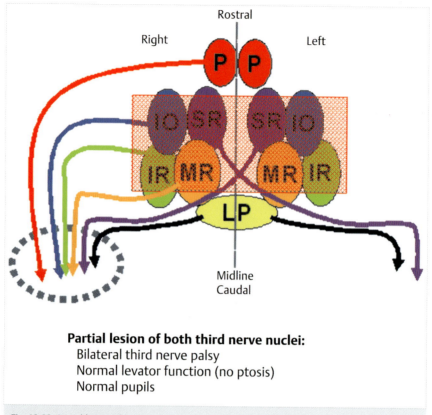

Partial lesion of both third nerve nuclei:
  Bilateral third nerve palsy
  Normal levator function (no ptosis)
  Normal pupils

Fig. 13.93 Partial lesion of both third nerve nuclei. P, parasympathetic; LP, levator palpebrae; IO, inferior oblique; IR, inferior rectus; SR, superior rectus; MR, medial rectus.

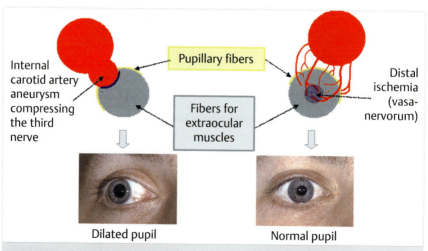

Fig. 13.94 Mechanism of pupillary involvement in lesions of the third nerve. External compression of the third nerve will present with dilation of the pupil in addition to ophthalmoplegia.

Evaluation of the Patient with Suspected Third Nerve Palsy (▶ Fig. 13.95)

- Based on other illnesses and age
- Neurological evaluation looking for other symptoms or signs
- Ophthalmological evaluation looking for orbital syndrome, optic neuropathy, papilledema, other ocular motor cranial nerve involvement
- Systemic evaluation looking for giant cell arteritis (if over 50), fever, systemic inflammatory disorder, atheromatous vascular risk factors
- Could it be myasthenia? (definitely not if the pupil is involved)
- Is the third nerve palsy
  ○ isolated, or not?
  ○ painful, or not?
  ○ complete, or not?
  ○ pupil-sparing, or not (only relevant if complete third nerve palsy)?

Causes of Third Nerve Palsy

Localization of the lesion producing a third nerve palsy is the first step of the diagnosis (▶ Table 13.5).

The sudden onset of a painful third nerve palsy with associated meningeal signs suggests subarachnoid hemorrhage from aneurysmal rupture. Pituitary apoplexy may also present similarly but is usually easily diagnosed on brain imaging.

These are a life-threatening emergency requiring immediate workup:

- Head CT without intravenous contrast (looking for blood in the subarachnoid space) and with contrast (looking for an intracranial aneurysm or alternate cause of oculomotor nerve palsy) and/or MRI of the brain with contrast is obtained.
- If a subarachnoid hemorrhage is diagnosed, a CT angiogram (CTA) and usually an emergent catheter angiogram are obtained.
- If there is no subarachnoid hemorrhage on imaging, and the patient has severe headaches, then a lumbar puncture should be performed looking for blood or xanthochromia (in cases of subarachnoid hemorrhage of more than 8 hours).
- Emergent noninvasive vascular imaging should be obtained in all patients with a third nerve palsy. When interpreted by experienced neuroradiologists, CTA and magnetic resonance angiography (MRA) are very sensitive, especially for aneurysms measuring at least 3 to 5 mm. However, smaller aneurysms can also rupture, and the consequences of missing an intracranial aneurysm are potentially grave; interpretation of CTA and MRA is difficult, and the clinician must make sure that the interpreting radiologist knows that the test is obtained to look for an aneurysm in a patient with a third nerve palsy. A catheter angiogram is sometimes obtained if there is still a high suspicion of aneurysm, or if there is doubt concerning the CTA or MRA results.

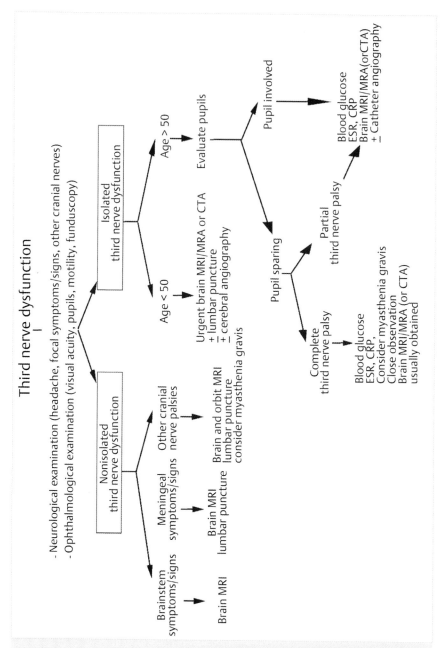

Fig. 13.95 Evaluation of a third nerve palsy (in adults). MRI: magnetic resonance imaging; CTA: computed tomography angiogram; ESR: erythrocyte sedimentation rate; CRP: c-reactive protein.

Table 13.5 Most common causes of acquired third nerve lesions by anatomical location of the lesion

Location of the lesion	Associated symptoms/signs	Most common causes
Nucleus	Complete ipsilateral third with contralateral ptosis and contralateral superior rectus weakness	Infarction Hemorrhage (cavernoma) Neoplasm (metastasis)
Fascicle	Contralateral hemiparesis (Weber syndrome) Contralateral tremor (Benedikt syndrome) Contralateral tremor and ataxia (Claude syndrome) Ipsilateral ataxia (Nothnagel syndrome)	Infarction Hemorrhage Neoplasm Demyelination
Subarachnoid space	Typically isolated May present with headaches or orbital pain	ICA/Pcom A/Basilar/PCA aneurysm Microvascular Neoplasm Meningitis Herniation Trauma
Cavernous sinus	Fourth, sixth, V1, (V2) Oculosympathetic dysfunction Pain may be prominent	Neoplasm Inflammation Carotid aneurysm Microvascular Carotid cavernous thrombosis Carotid cavernous fistula
Orbital apex	Fourth, sixth, V1 Oculosympathetic dysfunction Visual loss (optic nerve)	Trauma Neoplasm Inflammation Infection (fungus)

Abbreviations: ICA, internal carotid artery; Pcom A, posterior communicating artery; PCA, posterior cerebral artery.

Although most aneurysms responsible for a third nerve palsy involve the ipsilateral carotid circulation, the basilar circulation must also be studied to exclude a more posterior location. The contralateral carotid circulation should also be evaluated because ~ 20% of patients have more than one aneurysm.

All patients under the age of 50 who present with an isolated third nerve palsy of any extent should also have complete neurologic evaluation, including brain MRI, MRA, and CTA (if MRI and MRA are normal). A catheter angiogram may also be obtained in selected patients with normal noninvasive imaging (▶ Fig. 13.96 and ▶ Fig. 13.97).

Patients over the age of 50 who present with an isolated, pupil-sparing, but otherwise complete third nerve palsy, even in the presence of pain, can usually be assumed to have a microvascular third nerve palsy. However, brain imaging with noninvasive vascular imaging (CTA or MRA) is always obtained in patients with third nerve palsies. These patients must be observed closely for the next week for evidence of pupillary involvement.

The patient over age 50 with an isolated complete oculomotor nerve palsy with some pupillary involvement or a partial third nerve palsy should have at least MRI, MRA, and CTA scans.

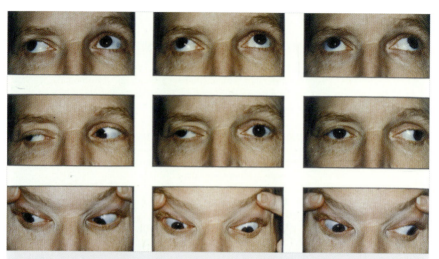

Fig. 13.96 Partial right third nerve palsy associated with right eyebrow pain. There is incomplete palsy of the extraocular muscles innervated by the third nerve. The right pupil is dilated.

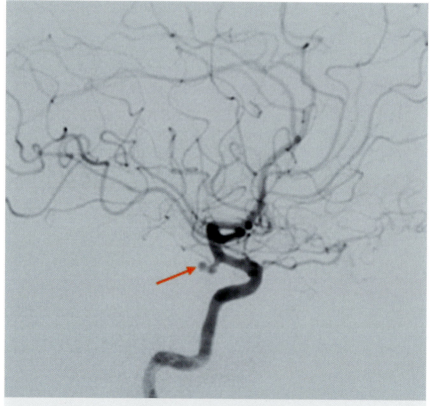

Fig. 13.97 Lateral view of cerebral catheter angiography showing a large aneurysm (*arrow*) at the junction of the right internal carotid artery and posterior communicating artery.

Although aneurysms are life threatening and need to be ruled out by vascular imaging, it is very important to obtain an MRI scan with contrast to rule out a mass or an infiltrative process as the cause of the third nerve palsy when vascular imaging is normal.

Third nerve palsies sometimes precede aneurysmal rupture and subarachnoid hemorrhage. Prompt recognition allows emergent diagnosis and treatment before the aneurysm ruptures. In these cases, the aneurysm is either treated by endovascular approach or surgically clipped, and the prognosis is usually excellent. On the other hand, the prognosis of ruptured aneurysms is poor, with a high, acute mortality rate. Devastating neurologic sequelae are common in survivors (▶ Fig. 13.98).

Intracranial aneurysms may be missed on noninvasive imaging such as CTA or MRA. Interpretation of these tests is difficult; the clinician must communicate with the interpreting radiologist, who should know that an aneurysm is suspected, and who should be aware of the patient's clinical presentation.

Causes of Third Nerve Palsies in Children

Causes of third nerve palsies in children are different from those classically observed in adults:
- Congenital
- Acquired, most commonly due to the following:
  - Trauma
  - Posterior fossa tumors
  - Meningitis

Children with an isolated third nerve palsy should be evaluated with brain MRI (with contrast). A lumbar puncture is usually performed only in children with acquired, acute third nerve palsies with normal imaging. Vascular imaging is usually not obtained in children younger than 10 years.

Congenital Third Nerve Palsies

Most have pupillary involvement, aberrant regeneration, and amblyopia.

Aberrant Regeneration of the Third Nerve

Aberrant regeneration of the third nerve (synkinesis) occurs after trauma or with compression of the third nerve. Branches of the third nerve originally destined for one muscle aberrantly regenerate to innervate a different muscle, including even the pupillary sphincter (▶ Fig. 13.99).

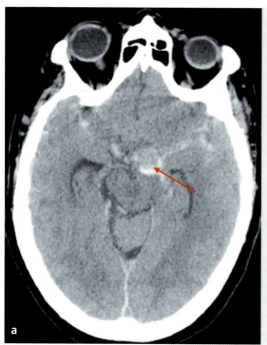

Fig. 13.98 (a) Axial computed tomographic scan of the brain without contrast showing a subarachnoid hemorrhage (spontaneous hyperdensity in the subarachnoid space) with a large aneurysm (*arrow*). The patient had a complete left third nerve palsy with pupil involvement and sudden headache. (b) Lateral view of cerebral catheter angiography showing a large aneurysm (*arrow*) at the level of the left posterior communicating artery.

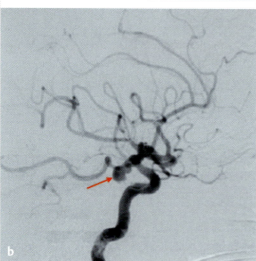

Pearls

In the absence of trauma, the presence of aberrant regeneration of the third nerve makes a compressive cause of the third nerve palsy very likely.

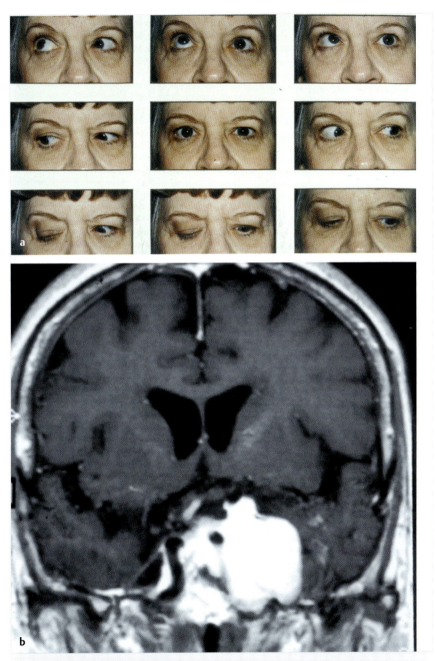

Fig. 13.99 (a) Aberrant regeneration of the left third nerve. The ptotic left eyelid elevates in down gaze. (b) Coronal T1-weighted magnetic resonance imaging of the brain with contrast showing enhancement of the left cavernous sinus related to a large left cavernous sinus meningioma.

The majority of third nerve palsies of ischemic etiology resolve within 3 months.

Compressive or traumatic oculomotor nerve palsies may take longer to improve, and incomplete recovery with or without aberrant regeneration is more likely.

13.5.4 The Lesion Involves Multiple Cranial Nerves

Lesions involving more than one cranial nerve often produce unilateral or bilateral ophthalmoplegia. Associated signs (such as Horner syndrome, optic neuropathy, chiasmal visual field defect, pain, skin lesions, and other neurologic findings) help localize the lesion.

Classic locations and causes of unilateral or bilateral ophthalmoplegia related to multiple cranial nerve palsies include the following:
- *Orbital apex syndrome:* third, fourth, sixth, and fifth (first branch) nerve palsies with optic neuropathy, sometimes with Horner syndrome. Causes include mostly neoplasms and fungal infections (aspergillosis and mucormycosis).
- *Cavernous sinus lesion:* third, fourth, sixth, and often fifth (first branch and sometimes second branch) nerve palsies, sometimes with Horner syndrome. Causes include numerous neoplasms, inflammations, and infections. Aneurysms and carotid-cavernous fistulas are also common.
- *Pituitary mass:* with expansion into, or compression of, cavernous sinuses (chiasm or optic nerve compression often associated)
- *Meningeal process:* such as infectious, inflammatory, or neoplastic meningitis
- *Skull base lesions:* such as infiltrating neoplasms
- *Perineural spread:* from skin cancers
- *Zoster:* involving the trigeminal territory
- *Brainstem lesions:* can rarely produce multiple cranial nerve palsies (almost always associated with other neurologic symptoms and signs).
- *Systemic disorders affecting the cranial nerves:*
  ○ Miller Fisher syndrome
  ○ Guillain–Barré syndrome
  ○ Botulism
  ○ Wernicke encephalopathy
  ○ Other peripheral neuropathies (e.g., chronic inflammatory demyelinating peripheral neuropathy)

Pearls

Always consider ocular myasthenia in patients with unilateral or bilateral ophthalmoplegia and normal pupils presumed to result from "multiple cranial neuropathies."

Orbital Apex Syndrome

Orbital apex syndrome (▶ Fig. 13.100) consists of combinations of the following:
- Ophthalmoplegia (multiple cranial nerve palsies)
- Horner syndrome
- Pain and V1 sensory loss (trigeminal nerve)
- Visual loss (optic neuropathy)

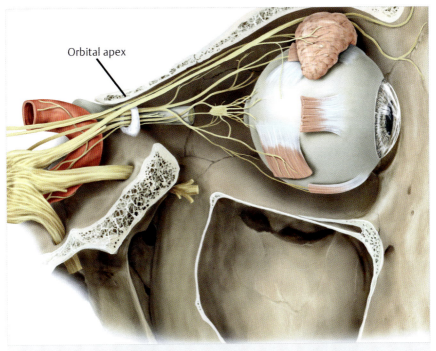

Fig. 13.100 Anatomy of the orbital apex. (From Schuenke M, Schulte E, Schumacher U, Ross LM, Lamperti ED, Voll M. THIEME Atlas of Anatomy, Head and Neuroanatomy. Stuttgart, Germany: Thieme; 2007. Illustration by Karl Wesker.)

Classic causes include the following:
- Neoplasms (metastases, lymphoma)
- Infections (aspergillus, mucormycosis)

Orbital apex lesions are usually very small and are difficult to see on imaging.

The adjacent sinuses are often abnormal, making it even more difficult to see a subtle enhancement on orbital CT or MRI. The appropriate imaging is either a CT scan of the orbits, the cavernous sinus, and the facial sinuses with contrast, or, preferably, a brain MRI scan with dedicated orbital views, fat suppression, and contrast.

A biopsy (often through the nose and the adjacent sinuses) is often necessary to ensure a proper diagnosis.

Diabetic patients have a higher risk of fungal infections, which often originate in or near the facial sinuses. These patients are particularly at risk for a rare, but devastating, infection by mucormycosis.

The sphenoid and the ethmoid sinuses are in very close relation to the orbital apex. Identification of a "sinusitis" on the side of an orbital apex syndrome is highly suspicious for fungal infection. Biopsy for pathology and specific cultures is mandatory (▶ Fig. 13.101).

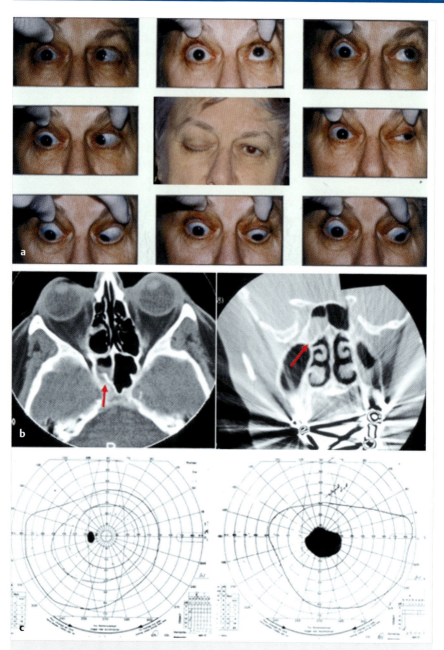

Fig. 13.101 (a) Painful right complete ophthalmoplegia in a diabetic patient. (b) Computed tomographic scan of the orbits (axial on the left and coronal on the right) showing a subtle sphenoid sinusitis on the side of the orbital syndrome (*arrow*). Biopsy of the sinus demonstrated mucormycosis. (c) Right optic neuropathy with central scotoma on Goldmann visual field. The fundus was normal acutely.

- A painful orbital apex syndrome in a diabetic patient should be presumed caused by a local infection by mucormycosis until proven otherwise.
- Normal imaging does not rule out an orbital apex lesion.

Cavernous Sinus Syndrome

Cavernous sinus syndrome involves combinations of the following:
- Ophthalmoplegia (multiple ocular motor cranial nerve palsies)
- Horner syndrome
- Pain and V1 (sometimes also V2) sensory loss

If there is venous hypertension (carotid-cavernous fistula or cavernous sinus thrombosis), there may be proptosis and periorbital edema from orbital venous congestion.

Anatomy of the Cavernous Sinus

The cavernous sinuses are triangular interconnecting structures that flank the lateral sides of the sella turcica (where the pituitary gland resides; ▶ Fig. 13.102). Each cavernous sinus contains a plexus of veins draining the orbits and some of the intracranial veins. The carotid artery (surrounded by sympathetic fibers) passes through the cavernous sinus. All ocular motor cranial nerves traverse the cavernous sinus before entering the orbit.

Tumors and vascular lesions of the cavernous sinus are common and typically present with ophthalmoplegia from ipsilateral third, fourth, and sixth nerve paresis.

Pain is common because the first division of the fifth nerve (trigeminal nerve) is also commonly affected (▶ Fig. 13.103).

- The third, fourth, and fifth nerves (V1 and V2) are enclosed in the lateral wall of the cavernous sinus (made of dura).
- The sixth nerve is free within the cavernous sinus and in close relation with the internal carotid artery. This is why cavernous carotid artery aneurysms often present with an isolated sixth nerve palsy.
- The internal carotid artery is covered by sympathetic fibers in the cavernous sinus. A lesion of the carotid artery compressing the sixth nerve usually also gives rise to an ipsilateral Horner syndrome.

Causes of Cavernous Sinus Syndrome

Common causes of cavernous sinus syndrome include the following:
- Neoplasms:
  - Meningioma
  - Pituitary tumor
  - Lymphoma
  - Metastasis
  - Other neoplasms

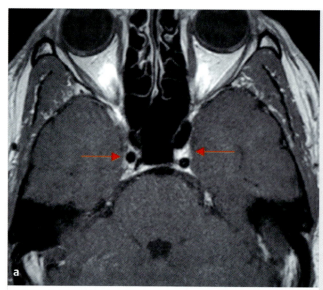

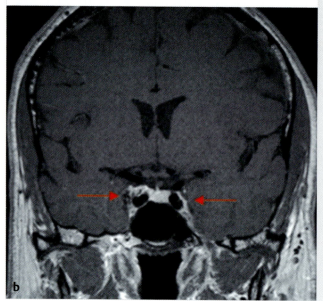

Fig. 13.102 Normal cavernous sinuses (*arrows*). (a) Axial T1-weighted magnetic resonance imaging (MRI) postcontrast. (b) Coronal T1-weighted MRI postcontrast. A normal cavernous sinus lateral wall usually appears concave.

- Carotid-cavernous aneurysm
- Carotid-cavernous fistula
- Abscess
- Fungal infection
- Inflammation:
  - Sarcoidosis
  - Wegener granulomatosis
  - Nonspecific (so-called Tolosa–Hunt syndrome)

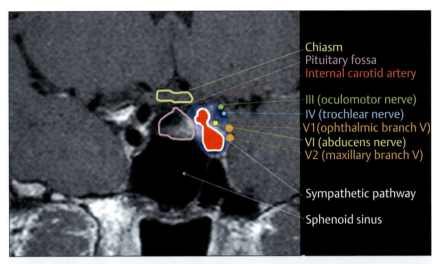

Chiasm
Pituitary fossa
Internal carotid artery

III (oculomotor nerve)
IV (trochlear nerve)
V1 (ophthalmic branch V)
VI (abducens nerve)
V2 (maxillary branch V)

Sympathetic pathway

Sphenoid sinus

Fig. 13.103 Coronal view of the left cavernous sinus.

Cavernous sinus *meningiomas* represent the most common cause of cavernous sinus lesions. There is little pain unless the trigeminal nerve is involved (▶ Fig. 13.104).

Lesions of the cavernous sinus cannot be easily biopsied, and the diagnosis is sometimes difficult to confirm.

The term *Tolosa–Hunt syndrome* is sometimes used to describe painful ophthalmoplegia with enhancement of the cavernous sinus. The pain and ophthalmoplegia are exquisitely responsive to treatment with steroids, and the presumed mechanism of the lesion is nonspecific inflammation. However, patients with malignant neoplasms (such as metastasis or lymphoma) or infection (such as aspergillosis or mucormycosis) may have a similar clinical and radiologic presentation and similar response to steroids, making the diagnosis of Tolosa–Hunt syndrome often misleading, erroneously reassuring, and frequently wrong (▶ Fig. 13.105).

Cavernous sinus aneurysms are relatively common and classically present with isolated unilateral sixth nerve palsy associated with an ipsilateral Horner syndrome. When the aneurysm enlarges, complete ophthalmoplegia may develop.

These aneurysms are usually not life threatening. Their rupture rate is low, and when they do rupture, they do not result in subarachnoid hemorrhage (they rupture inside the cavernous sinus, which is an enclosed space), but rather the rupture causes a direct carotid-cavernous fistula (▶ Fig. 13.106).

Pituitary Tumors and Pituitary Apoplexy

Pituitary masses compressing or invading the cavernous sinus are a common cause of unilateral or bilateral ophthalmoplegia (the pituitary gland is located between the two cavernous sinuses).

Pituitary apoplexy (acute pituitary hemorrhage or infarction, usually in a preexisting, although often unrecognized, pituitary tumor) classically results in sudden unilateral or bilateral ophthalmoplegia, headache, and often visual loss (from compression of the optic nerves and chiasm) (▶ Fig. 13.107).

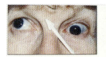

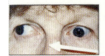
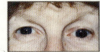

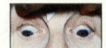

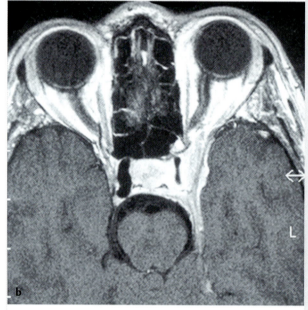

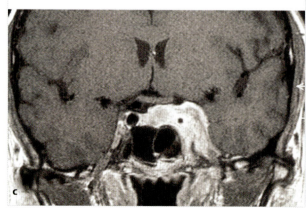

Fig. 13.104 (a) Left third, fourth, and sixth nerve palsies secondary to a left cavernous sinus meningioma in a 57-year-old woman. There is mild left ptosis and downward displacement of the left eye (left hypotropia). The left eye has no elevation, relatively good depression, decreased adduction and abduction. There is no intortion of the left eye. The left pupil is only sluggishly reactive to light. The visual acuity is normal. The ophthalmoplegia was progressive over a few months, and there is no pain. (b) Axial and (c) coronal T1-weighted magnetic resonance imaging with contrast showing enhancement and enlargement of the left cavernous sinus suggesting a left cavernous sinus meningioma. The left internal carotid artery is constricted. Note the convex appearance of the abnormal cavernous sinus.

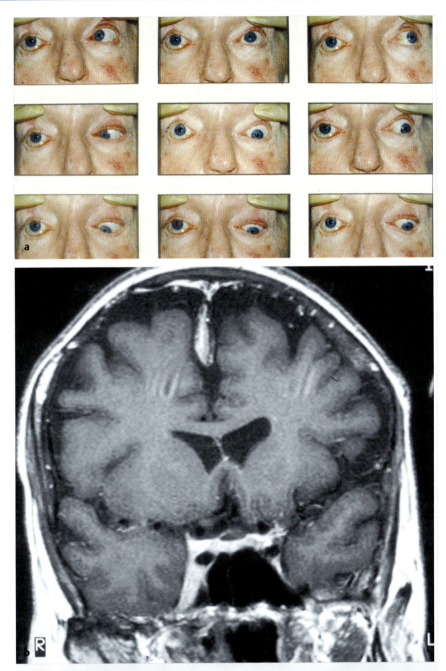

Fig. 13.105 (a) Complete right ophthalmoplegia associated with severe ipsilateral pain. Biopsy of the lesion seen on magnetic resonance imaging (MRI) was consistent with lymphoma. (b) Coronal T1-weighted MRI with contrast showing enhancement and enlargement of the right cavernous sinus.

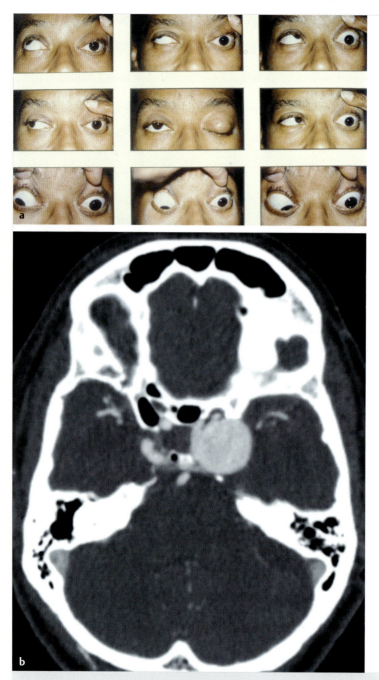

Fig. 13.106 (a) Left complete ophthalmoplegia secondary to a large left cavernous sinus aneurysm. (b) Computed tomographic angiogram with contrast showing a large left carotid cavernous aneurysm.

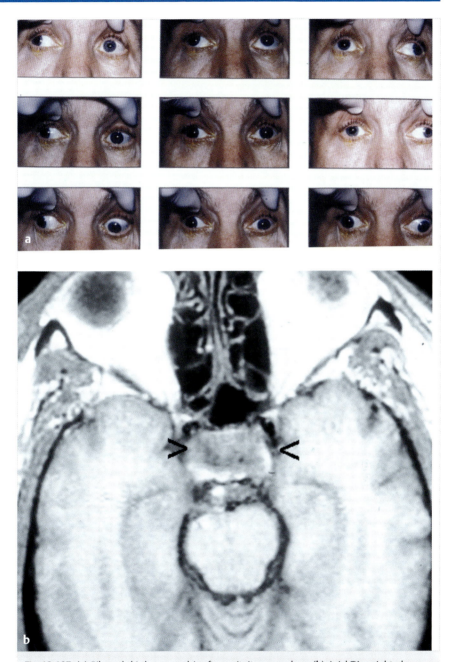

Fig. 13.107 (a) Bilateral third nerve palsies from pituitary apoplexy. (b) Axial T1-weighted magnetic resonance imaging with contrast showing enlargement of the pituitary gland compressing both cavernous sinuses laterally (*arrows*).

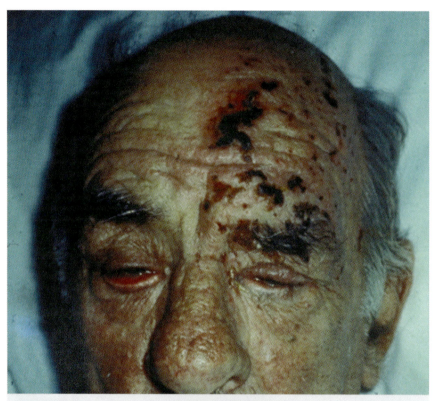

Fig. 13.108 Skin lesions of zoster involving the frontal branch of the left trigeminal nerve (V1). There is complete left ophthalmoplegia.

Trigeminal Zoster

Trigeminal zoster is a rare cause of ophthalmoplegia (▶ Fig. 13.108). Severe varicella zoster virus infection involving the V1 territory can rarely produce a single or multiple cranial nerve palsy on the same side. The presumed mechanism is extension of the inflammatory reaction into the cavernous sinus. However, orbital myositis is sometimes seen on imaging. These patients often require prolonged treatment with IV antiviral agents and corticosteroids.

Cutaneous Squamous Cell Carcinomas or Basal Cell Carcinomas

Cutaneous squamous cell carcinomas or basal cell carcinomas located on the face can spread to the perineural space along the cranial nerves. They produce progressive painful ophthalmoplegia, which is often misdiagnosed for months or even years (▶ Fig. 13.109).

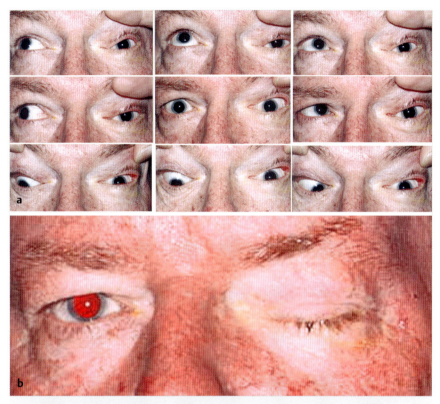

Fig. 13.109 a–d (a) Complete left painful ophthalmoplegia from squamous cell carcinoma perineural spread. (b) The patient had multiple small skin lesions (squamous and basal cell carcinomas) previously removed. (*continued*)

Miller Fisher Syndrome and Guillain–Barré Syndrome

Demyelinating polyradiculopathies can be associated with multiple cranial nerve palsies and bilateral ophthalmoplegia.

Miller Fisher syndrome presents with a classic triad:

- Ataxia
- Areflexia
- Ophthalmoplegia (bilateral third, fourth, and sixth nerve palsies; the pupils are often involved)

Bilateral facial weakness is common, but there is no limb weakness. The diagnosis is suspected clinically and is confirmed by CSF analysis (elevated protein and few or no cells) and by electromyography. Serum antibodies for *Campylobacter jejuni* or anti-GQ1b gangliosides may be positive. Prognosis is usually good with supportive

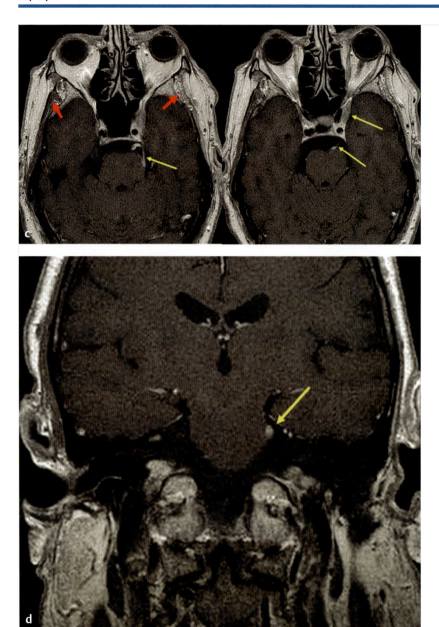

Fig. 13.109 (*continued*) (**c**) Axial T1-weighted magnetic resonance imaging (MRI) of the orbits with contrast demonstrating enhancement of the left cavernous sinus and of cranial nerves III and V (*yellow arrows*). The red arrows show the normal temporalis muscle on the right and the atrophic temporalis muscle on the left (this muscle is innervated by the motor branch of the trigeminal nerve). (**d**) Coronal T1-weighted MRI of the orbits with contrast demonstrating enhancement of the left trigeminal nerve (*yellow arrow*).

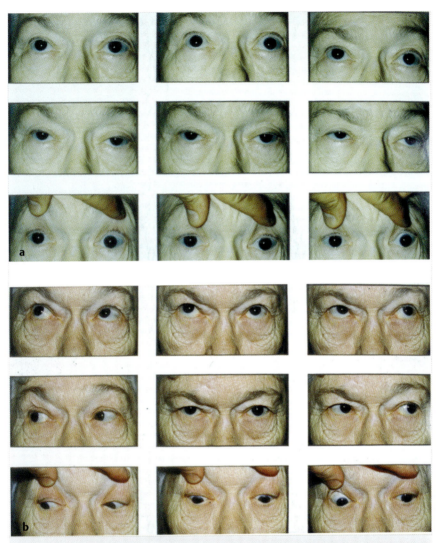

Fig. 13.110 (a) Bilateral ophthalmoplegia and mydriasis from Miller Fisher syndrome. The patient had bilateral facial weakness, ataxia, and areflexia. (b) Normal extraocular movements a few weeks later.

measures; treatment with intravenous immunoglobulins or plasmapheresis is usually performed (▶ Fig. 13.110).

Guillain–Barré syndrome may have the same clinical presentation as Miller Fisher syndrome but also includes progressive ascending symmetric limb weakness (no sensory loss), which may be complicated by respiratory paralysis.

Wernicke Encephalopathy

Thiamine deficiency usually occurs as a result of chronic alcoholism and severe chronic malnutrition, especially after bariatric surgery. It should be suspected in any patient presenting with the following:
- Confusion
- Ataxia
- Ophthalmoplegia (any pattern is possible, including sixth nerve palsy, horizontal or vertical gaze palsy, internuclear ophthalmoplegia)
- Nystagmus (common)

Brain MRI often shows symmetric increased T2 signal intensity in the mammillary bodies, the medial thalami, the tectal plate, and the periaqueductal area. Treatment with vitamin B1, hydration, and appropriate nutrition is urgent to prevent irreversible dementia.

Pearls

Thiamine deficiency can mimic any extraocular movement disorder; nystagmus is commonly associated.

Botulism

Clostridium botulinum poisoning (from contaminated canned food or contaminated wounds) causes systemic signs (nausea, vomiting, dysphagia, proximal extremity weakness) associated with bilateral diffuse ophthalmoplegia, ptosis, and bilateral mydriasis.

Botulinum toxins interfere with the release of acetylcholine vesicles in the synapse and block neuromuscular transmission.

This life-threatening disorder requires immediate life-support measures and treatment with specific antitoxins.

13.5.5 The Lesion Is Internuclear or Supranuclear

Internuclear and supranuclear ocular motor disorders are caused by damage to those parts of the brain proximal to the ocular motor nuclei that include pathways controlling eye movement.

They include lesions in the following:
- Brainstem (medulla, pons, and midbrain)
- Cerebellum
- Hemispheres (thalamus, basal ganglia, cerebral hemispheres)

There are separate final common pathways for control of horizontal eye movements (▶ Fig. 13.111) and control of vertical eye movements.

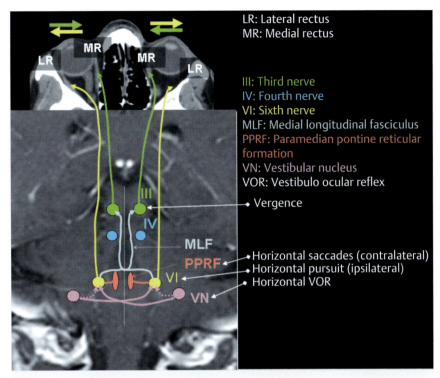

Fig. 13.111 Anatomy of conjugate horizontal gaze.

Control of Horizontal Eye Movements

- The sixth nerve nucleus (also known as the horizontal gaze center) has interneurons that connect to the contralateral third nerve nucleus via the MLF. This allows both eyes to move in the same direction at the same time (e.g., activation of the right sixth nerve nucleus will activate the right lateral rectus innervated by the right sixth nerve, and the left medial rectus innervated by the left third nerve).
- The paramedian pontine reticular formation (PPRF) contains burst neurons responsible for horizontal saccades only.
- Each vestibular nuclear complex sends axons to the ipsilateral (inhibitory) and contralateral (excitatory) sixth nerve nuclei to stabilize the conjugate gaze.

Horizontal Eye Movement Abnormalities

Abnormal horizontal eye movements include the following:

Horizontal Gaze Paresis

A lesion in the pons is the most common location for a horizontal gaze deficit.
- Lesion of the sixth nerve nucleus (▶ Fig. 13.112 and ▶ Fig. 13.113)

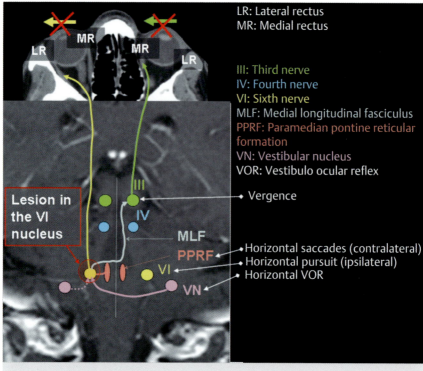

LR: Lateral rectus
MR: Medial rectus

III: Third nerve
IV: Fourth nerve
VI: Sixth nerve
MLF: Medial longitudinal fasciculus
PPRF: Paramedian pontine reticular formation
VN: Vestibular nucleus
VOR: Vestibulo ocular reflex

Vergence

Horizontal saccades (contralateral)
Horizontal pursuit (ipsilateral)
Horizontal VOR

Fig. 13.112 Lesion of the right sixth nerve nucleus.

- Loss of all ipsilateral voluntary and reflexive conjugate eye movements
- Ipsilateral facial weakness
- Lesion of the PPRF
  - Loss of all ipsilateral horizontal rapid eye movements (saccades)
  - Vestibulo-ocular reflexes and pursuit eye movements are spared with lesions of the PPRF

Classic causes of horizontal gaze paresis include the following:
- Lesions of the pons
  - Infarction (anterior cerebellar artery syndrome)
  - Hemorrhage (vascular malformations)
  - Multiple sclerosis
  - Tumor (glioma, metastasis)
  - Abscess
  - Central pontine myelinolysis
- Wernicke encephalopathy
- Gaucher disease

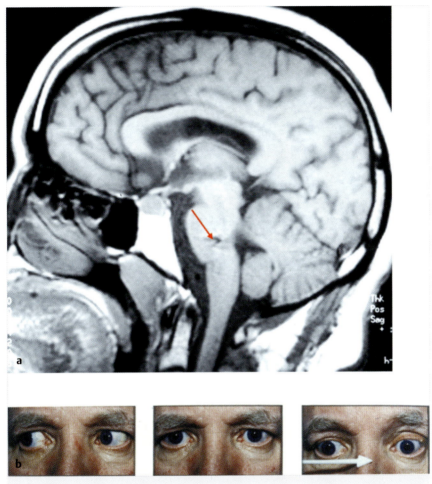

Fig. 13.113 (a) Sagittal T1-weighted magnetic resonance imaging of the brain showing a small cavernoma in the pons (*arrow*). (b) Left horizontal gaze palsy from a sixth nerve nucleus lesion. The gaze is normal to the right, and neither eye moves when the patient tries to look to the left or when the vestibulo-ocular reflex is tested. Vertical eye movements are normal.

- Congenital diseases:
  - Bilateral Duane syndrome
  - Möbius syndrome
  - HGPPS

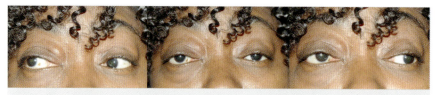

Fig. 13.114 Right internuclear ophthalmoplegia. Gaze is straight in primary position (center). Adduction of the right eye is decreased and there is nystagmus of the left eye in abduction. Also note the skew deviation, with the left eye being lower than the right eye.

Internuclear Ophthalmoplegia

A lesion of the MLF causes an internuclear ophthalmoplegia (INO).
Unilateral INO (▶ Fig. 13.114 and ▶ Fig. 13.115) consists of the following:
- Ipsilesional deficit of adduction (slowing of adducting saccades)
- Nystagmus of the contralateral abducting eye
- Skew deviation
- Convergence may overcome the adduction deficit

Bilateral Internuclear Ophthalmoplegia (▶ Fig. 13.116)

Bilateral internuclear ophthalmoplegia includes the following:
- No adduction of either eye (or slow adducting saccades bilaterally)
- Nystagmus of abducting eyes
- Convergence may overcome the adduction deficits.
- Walleyed bilateral INO (WEBINO): same as already described, but the patient is exotropic and there is loss of convergence

Classic causes of unilateral or bilateral ophthalmoplegia include the following:
- Lesions involving the MLF
  - Multiple sclerosis
  - Infarction (lacune)
  - Hemorrhage (vascular malformations)
  - Tumor (glioma, metastasis)
  - Abscess
  - Central pontine myelinolysis
- Wernicke encephalopathy

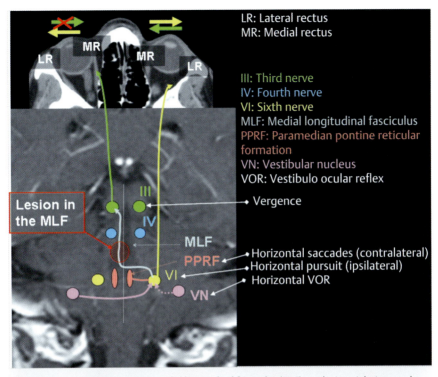

LR: Lateral rectus
MR: Medial rectus

III: Third nerve
IV: Fourth nerve
VI: Sixth nerve
MLF: Medial longitudinal fasciculus
PPRF: Paramedian pontine reticular formation
VN: Vestibular nucleus
VOR: Vestibulo ocular reflex

Vergence

Horizontal saccades (contralateral)
Horizontal pursuit (ipsilateral)
Horizontal VOR

Fig. 13.115 A lesion of the right medial longitudinal fasciculus (MLF) results in a right internuclear ophthalmoplegia: ipsilateral adduction deficit (right medial rectus weakness) during conjugate horizontal eye movements, often manifesting as a slowing of adducting saccades ("adduction lag"). Adduction may be intact during convergence. There is abducting nystagmus of the contralateral eye (left eye). Skew deviation due to interruption of the otolithic pathway (hypotropia in contralesional eye [left eye]) is common.

Pearls

Bilateral internuclear ophthalmoplegia is a classic finding in patients with multiple sclerosis.

One-and-a-Half Syndrome

Lesions involving both the abducens nucleus and the MLF cause a "one-and-a-half" syndrome (▶ Fig. 13.117 and ▶ Fig. 13.118):
- The "one" is an ipsilateral conjugate gaze palsy (lesion of the abducens nucleus)
- The "half" is an ipsilateral internuclear ophthalmoplegia (lesion of the MLF)

Classic causes of one-and-a-half syndrome are as follows:
- Lesions involving the pons
  - Infarction (lacuna)
  - Hemorrhage (vascular malformations)

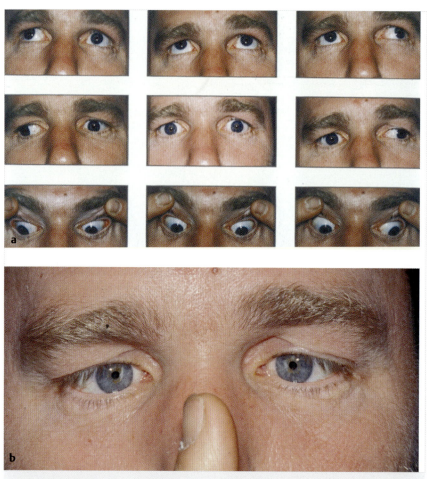

Fig. 13.116 (a) Bilateral internuclear ophthalmoplegia in a patient with multiple sclerosis. Neither eye adducts and there is nystagmus of the abducting eye. Vertical eye movements are full. (b) Convergence is normal.

- ○ Multiple sclerosis
- ○ Tumor (glioma, metastasis)
- ○ Abscess
- ○ Central pontine myelinosis
- • Wernicke encephalopathy

438

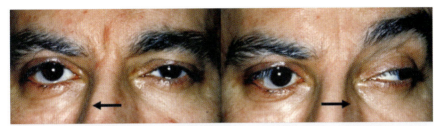

Fig. 13.117 Right one-and-a-half syndrome. Neither eye looks to the right, and there is impaired adduction of the right eye and nystagmus of the left eye in abduction. The patient also has a right facial palsy (explaining why the right palpebral fissure is wider—lagophthalmos).

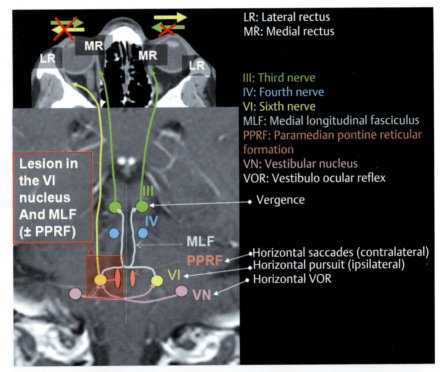

Fig. 13.118 Right one-and-a half syndrome: lesion of the right sixth nerve nucleus and right medial longitudinal fasciculus. The only intact horizontal eye movement is the abduction of the contralateral eye (which also has abducting nystagmus).

Congenital Ocular Motor Apraxia

- It affects young children.
- Defective or absence of voluntary horizontal saccades to visual stimuli: they cannot move their eyes horizontally to look at a target. Instead they turn their head briskly (head thrust) to shift fixation.

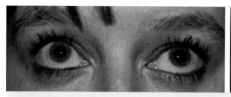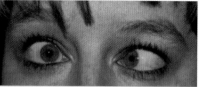

Fig. 13.119 Looking straight ahead (left), the pupils are midsized. With voluntary convergence (right), there is esotropia, accommodation, and miosis.

- Smooth pursuit and vertical eye movements are usually preserved.
- Eye movements are usually bilateral and symmetric in the horizontal plane.
- It is often idiopathic, but it has also been associated with several cerebral malformations and genetic disorders.

Acquired Ocular Motor Apraxia

- Occurs in older children
- Associated with mostly metabolic disorders (Gaucher disease, ataxia-telangiectasia, spinocerebellar ataxias, Niemann–Pick disease)

Convergence Spasm

Also called spasm of the near triad (▸ Fig. 13.119)

- Intermittent convergence
- Always with accommodation and pupillary constriction

Classic causes of convergence spasm include the following:
- Most often nonorganic
- Excessive accommodation from uncorrected refractive error
- Lesions at the diencephalic–mesencephalic junction (very rare)

Convergence Insufficiency

Convergence insufficiency is a very common condition, characterized by the following:
- Exotropia greater at near than at distance (at least 10 prism diopters difference)
- Causes symptoms of "asthenopia" (fatigue with reading, diplopia at near, intermittent blurred vision when reading)
- Usually benign; may improve with orthoptic exercises
- Sometimes requires prisms in reading glasses or strabismus surgery

Classic causes of convergence insufficiency include the following:
- Idiopathic most often (in children or young adults)
- Head trauma
- Parkinson disease
- Progressive supranuclear palsy

The ability to converge can be measured (▸ Fig. 13.120). A near card is brought toward the patient's nose until the patient sees double. The distance at which diplopia occurs is noted (near point of convergence).

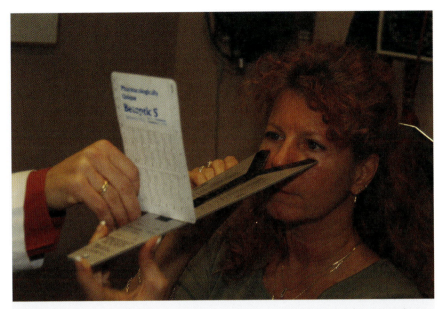

Fig. 13.120 Measurement of the near point of convergence (must be done with correction).

A similar technique is used for rehabilitation: the patient is instructed to do "push-up exercises" (looking at an object intermittently moved in and out from the bridge of the nose) daily at home to decrease the near point of convergence.

Divergence Insufficiency

Divergence insufficiency is characterized as follows:
- Comitant esotropia is present at distance but not at near.
- Ductions and versions are full.
- It is most often related to raised intracranial pressure or Chiari malformation.

Classic causes of divergence insufficiency include the following:
- Raised intracranial pressure
- Chiari malformation
- Head trauma
- Intracranial hypotension (low CSF pressure syndrome)
- Cerebellar lesions
- Midbrain mass

Abnormal Horizontal Conjugate Deviations

Gaze deviations are relatively common in large cerebral and pontine lesions (▶ Fig. 13.121).

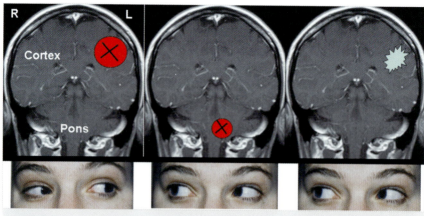

Fig. 13.121 Gaze deviations in cerebral lesions and seizures: the eyes deviate horizontally toward a cortical lesion (left); the eyes deviate horizontally away from a pontine lesion (center); the eyes deviate horizontally away from a cortical seizure focus (right).

Control of Vertical Eye Movements (▶ Fig. 13.122 and ▶ Fig. 13.123)

Control of vertical eye movements include the following:
- Critical supranuclear structures mediating vertical gaze are located in the rostral midbrain at the level of the pretectum (just rostral to the superior and inferior colliculi).
- The four most important pretectal areas are the rostral interstitial nucleus of the MLF (riMLF), the interstitial nucleus of Cajal (INC), the nucleus of the posterior commissure, and the posterior commissure.
- The paramedian riMLF contains burst neurons responsible for vertical saccades.
- The riMLF controls upward saccades via the elevator muscles (projections to the superior rectus and inferior oblique subnuclei) and downward saccades via the depressor muscles (projections to the inferior rectus subnucleus and to the fourth nerve nucleus).
- The INC serves as the neural integrator for vertical gaze and torsion (coordinates signals from the saccadic burst neurons in the riMLF, vestibular projections coming from the vestibular nuclei via the MLF, and descending pursuit fibers).
- Some fibers cross from one side to another at the level of the pretectum via the posterior commissure.

There is still some uncertainty about projections involved in vertical eye movements, and only clinically relevant pathways are included in these simplified anatomical diagrams.

The following are shown for upward eye movement (▶ Fig. 13.123a):
- Neurons from the riMLF (and nucleus of the posterior commissure), which contains burst neurons for vertical saccades, project both ipsilaterally and contralaterally to the oculomotor nuclear complexes, innervating the superior rectus and the inferior oblique subnuclei bilaterally.

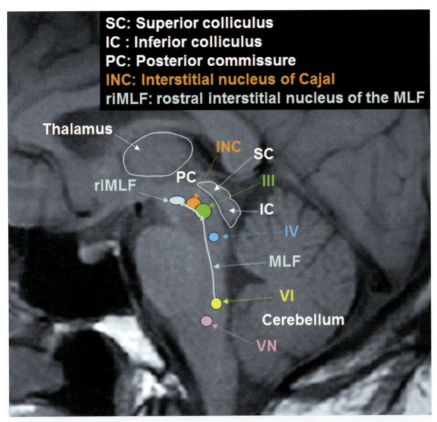

SC: Superior colliculus
IC : Inferior colliculus
PC: Posterior commissure
INC: Interstitial nucleus of Cajal
riMLF: rostral interstitial nucleus of the MLF

Thalamus
INC SC
riMLF PC III
IC
IV
MLF
VI
Cerebellum
VN

Fig. 13.122 Anatomy of conjugate vertical gaze shown on a sagittal view of the posterior fossa. VN: vestibular nucleus; IV: IVth nerve nucleus; VI: VIth nerve nucleus; III: third nerve nucleus.

- Axons from the INC, the neural integrator for vertical gaze, cross within the posterior commissure before reaching the oculomotor nuclear complexes and the superior rectus and inferior oblique subnuclei.

The following are shown for downward eye movement (▶ Fig. 13.123b):
- For down gaze, each riMLF supplies the ipsilateral inferior rectus subnucleus and the ipsilateral fourth nerve nucleus (which innervates the contralateral superior oblique muscle).
- Axons from the INC innervate the ipsilateral inferior rectus subnucleus and fourth nerve nucleus.

Vertical Eye Movement Abnormalities

Up Gaze Paresis

Dorsal Midbrain Syndrome(▶ Fig. 13.124 and ▶ Fig. 13.125) (Parinaud syndrome or pretectal syndrome) classically includes the following:
- Supranuclear vertical up gaze paresis
- Convergence retraction nystagmus with attempted up gaze

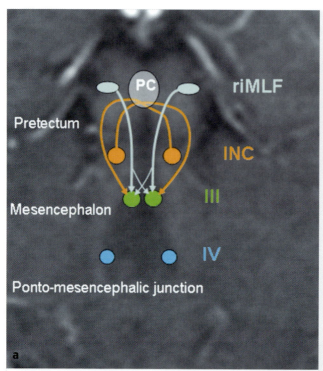

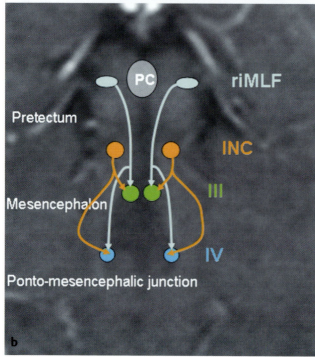

Fig. 13.123 (a) Major pathways subserving upward eye movements (coronal view). (b) Major pathways subserving downward eye movements (coronal view). INC, interstitial nucleus of Cajal; riMLF, rostral interstitial nucleus of the medial longitudinal fasciculus; III, third nerve nucleus; IV, IVth nerve nucleus; PC, posterior chamber.

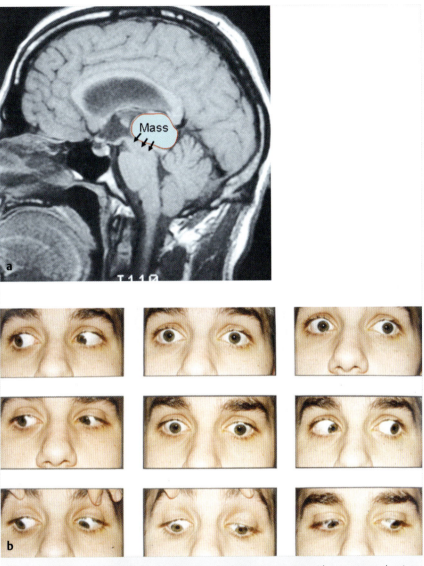

Fig. 13.124 (a) Sagittal T1-weighted brain magnetic resonance imaging without contrast showing a mass compressing the posterior commissure (*arrows*) and responsible for obstructive hydrocephalus. (b) Up gaze palsy (Parinaud or dorsal midbrain syndrome) secondary to compression of the posterior commissure disrupting the crossing fibers subserving up gaze. There is also lid retraction (Collier sign) and convergence-retraction nystagmus with attempted up gaze. There is light-near dissociation of the pupils.

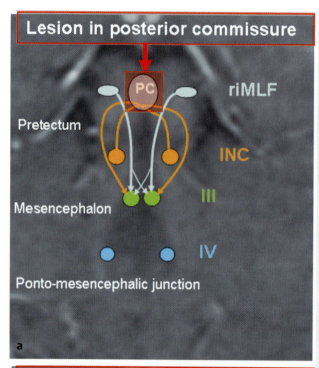

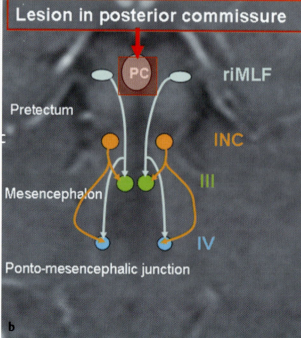

Fig. 13.125 Diagram showing why lesions of the posterior commissure (PC) (and nucleus of the posterior commissure) limit upward eye movements (**a**), whereas downward eye movements remain intact (**b**). riMLF, rostral interstitial nucleus of the medial longitudinal fasciculus; INC, interstitial nucleus of Cajal; III, third nerve; IV, fourth nerve.

- Lid retraction (Collier sign)
- Pupillary light-near dissociation

It may be associated with any of the following:

- Pseudoabducens palsy (thalamic esotropia)
- Convergence insufficiency
- Accommodative insufficiency
- Skew deviation
- Third nerve palsy
- Internuclear ophthalmoplegia
- See-saw nystagmus

Lesions of the posterior commissure (and of the nucleus of the posterior commissure) limit upward eye movements. Convergence–retraction nystagmus with attempted up gaze results from asynchronous convergent saccades.

Lesions may also damage the pretectal (light) fibers entering the Edinger–Westphal nucleus, sparing fibers for the near response (accommodation) that enter the Edinger–Westphal nucleus more ventrally. This results in light-near dissociation of the pupils (▸ Fig. 13.126).

Pearls

Obstructive hydrocephalus is a common cause of dorsal midbrain syndrome, and patients with vertical gaze deficits should have urgent neuroimaging (▸ Fig. 13.127).

Thalamic hemorrhages classically present with sudden headache and contralateral hemisensory loss. Hemiparesis (internal capsule) and homonymous hemianopia (optic tract) may occur. Large hemorrhages can result in vertical and horizontal ocular deviations (▸ Fig. 13.128).

Down Gaze Paresis

Isolated down gaze paresis due to a midbrain lesion is much less common than isolated up gaze paresis or combined up- and down gaze paresis (▸ Fig. 13.125 and ▸ Fig. 13.129).

- A unilateral lesion of one riMLF or its descending fibers will affect downward saccades more than upward saccades (due to the duplication of riMLF input into the oculomotor subnuclei for up gaze, but not down gaze).
- A unilateral lesion of the riMLF may cause defective torsion of the ipsilateral eye, thereby producing torsional nystagmus beating contralateral to the side of the lesion.
- Bilateral lesions of the riMLF or its descending fibers will result in a more severe defect of vertical gaze than that due to unilateral lesions. Downward saccades are typically affected more than upward saccades, but a complete vertical gaze palsy also occurs.
- Bilateral lesions are common, with small infarctions involving the paramedian arteries (arteries of Percheron) at the top of the basilar artery (one medial artery often vascularizes both riMLF) (▸ Fig. 13.129 and ▸ Fig. 13.130).

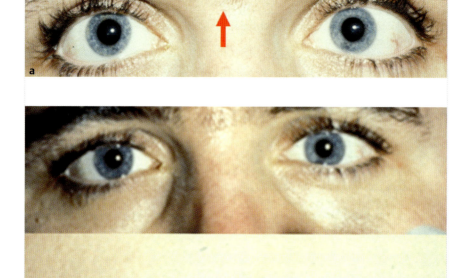

Fig. 13.126 (a) Selective up gaze deficit with normal down gaze and normal horizontal movements secondary to compression of the dorsal midbrain and posterior commissure by a pineal germinoma. (b) Light-near dissociation from dorsal midbrain syndrome. The pupils are mildly dilated in both eyes and are not reactive to light (top). They constrict at near (bottom).

Causes of Vertical Gaze Palsy

- Lesions of the upper midbrain, pretectum, posterior commissure
    - Infarction (paramedian, thalamic, top of the basilar syndrome)
    - Hemorrhage (upper midbrain, thalamic) (hypertensive, vascular malformations)
    - Obstructive hydrocephalus
    - Pineal region tumors
        - Germinoma, pineoblastoma, pineal cysts, tectal glioma

- ○ Basal ganglia abscess
- ○ Multiple sclerosis
- Progressive supranuclear palsy
- Huntington disease
- Whipple disease
- Wernicke encephalopathy
- Niemann–Pick disease
- Gaucher disease
- Tay–Sachs disease
- Wilson disease
- Paraneoplastic syndromes

Up gaze is often limited to some degree in otherwise healthy elderly patients and may be a normal finding.

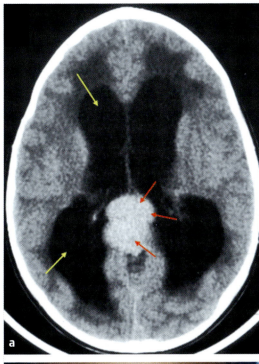

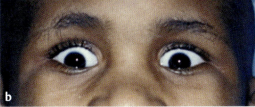

Fig. 13.127 (a) Axial computed tomographic scan of the brain with contrast showing a pineal mass (*red arrows*) pressing on the posterior commissure and causing obstructive hydrocephalus (*yellow arrows*). (b) Dorsal midbrain syndrome with bilateral lid retraction (Collier sign) and downward displacement of the eyes with up gaze paresis. There is convergence-retraction nystagmus with attempted up gaze.

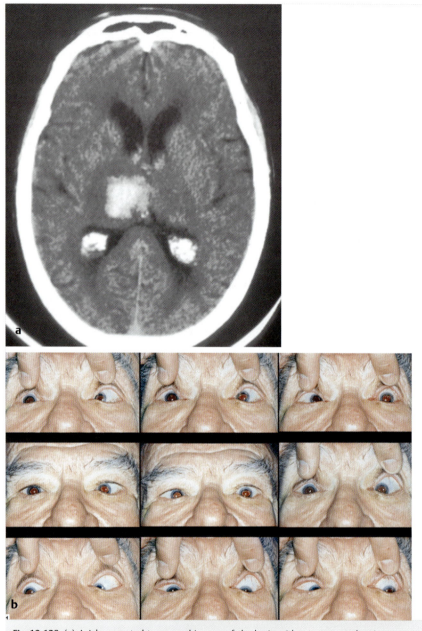

Fig. 13.128 (a) Axial computed tomographic scan of the brain without contrast showing a spontaneous hyperdensity in both thalami (right greater than left) consistent with a thalamic hemorrhage. (b) Bilateral abduction deficits (thalamic esotropia) and downward deviation of both eyes with complete up gaze palsy. (The pupils are pharmacologically dilated).

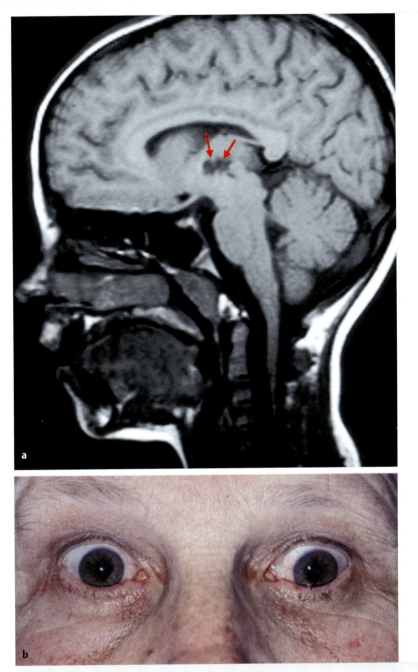

Fig. 13.129 (a) Sagittal T1-weighted magnetic resonance imaging of the brain showing a lesion of the pretectum (*arrows*). (b) Down gaze paresis with inability to move either eye downward. Upward saccades were very slow. Note also the lid retraction (Collier sign).

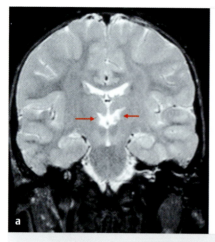
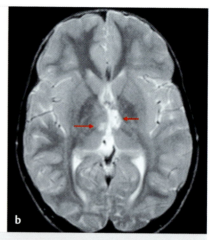

Fig. 13.130 **(a)** Coronal T2-weighted magnetic resonance imaging (MRI) of the brain showing bilateral paramedian infarctions (*arrows*). The patient was unable to look down. **(b)** Axial T2-weighted MRI of the brain showing bilateral paramedian infarctions (*arrows*).

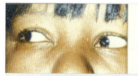
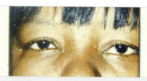
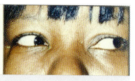

Fig. 13.131 Alternating skew deviation in a patient with raised intracranial pressure. There is a right hypertropia in right gaze and a left hypertropia in left gaze.

Skew Deviation and the Ocular Tilt Reaction

Skew deviation (▶ Fig. 13.131) consists of the following:
- Vertical misalignment of the eyes commonly results from acute brainstem dysfunction.
- Patients complain of vertical diplopia, sometimes with a torsional component.
- There are usually other neurologic symptoms.
- The hypertropia of a skew deviation may be comitant (deviation is the same in all positions of gaze) or noncomitant (deviation varies with gaze position). When a skew deviation is noncomitant, it may be difficult to distinguish from a third nerve palsy or a fourth nerve palsy.

Ocular tilt reaction (OTR) (▶ Fig. 13.132) is a combination of the following:
- Skew deviation
- Ocular torsion (*both* eyes are tilted toward the hypotropic eye) (It is easy to see the ocular torsion on funduscopic examination: the imaginary line drawn between the optic nerve and the fovea appears tilted.)
- Head tilt (toward the hypotropic eye)

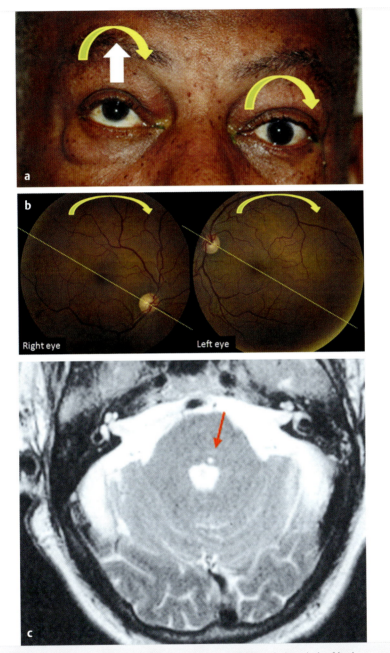

Fig. 13.132 (a) Ocular tilt reaction. Right hypertropia with left head tilt and tilt of both eyes toward the hypotropic eye (the left eye). (b) On funduscopic examination, the optic nerve and fovea are not aligned horizontally, as they should be, because of the tilt toward the hypotropic eye. (c) Small pontine lesion (*arrow*).

- Common with lesions of the pontomedullary junction or the paramedian thalamic–mesencephalic region
- Results from dysfunction of the utricular pathways that begin in the labyrinths and terminate in the rostral brainstem at the INC
- The OTR will be
  - ipsiversive with peripheral and pontomedullary lesions
  - contraversive with pontomesencephalic lesions

Skew deviation and the ocular tilt reaction occur when there is disruption of the otolith–ocular pathway in the vestibular nerves, the brainstem, or the cerebellum.
    Classic causes of skew deviation and ocular tilt reaction include the following:
- Acute peripheral vestibulopathy
  - Lesion of the vestibular organ or its nerve
  - Tullio phenomenon: sound-induced vestibular symptoms caused by a perilymph
  - Fistula or abnormalities of the ossicular chain in the ear
- Lesion in the vestibular nuclei (e.g., part of the lateral medullary syndrome)
- Lesion in the cerebellum
- Lesion in the MLF
- Lesion in the midbrain and INC
- Raised intracranial pressure

Control of the Saccade System

Saccadic eye movements (fast conjugate eye movements to a fixed target) are initiated in the frontal and parietal lobes (frontal and parietal eye fields).
- The *horizontal* saccadic pathway is a crossed pathway. Pathways from the frontal and parietal eye fields descend via the superior colliculus into the brainstem and cross at the level of the midbrain–pontine junction to synapse on the contralateral PPRF.
- The PPRF projects to the ipsilateral sixth nerve nucleus. From the sixth nerve nucleus, axons of abducens motor neurons travel to the ipsilateral lateral rectus muscle, whereas axons of sixth nerve interneurons cross over and ascend in the contralateral MLF to the medial rectus subnucleus of the third nerve.
- This internuclear connection between the sixth nerve nucleus and the contralateral third nerve nucleus via the MLF is responsible for conjugate horizontal gaze.
- Each frontal eye field, therefore, generates a conjugate movement of the eyes toward the *contralateral* side of the body.
- Brainstem pathways for *vertical saccades* involve the riMLF, the posterior commissure (PC) and nucleus of the PC, and the INC.

Slow Saccades

Differential diagnosis of slow saccades includes the following:
- Lesions in the pons and the cerebellum
  - Spinocerebellar ataxias
  - Lesions of the PPRF
  - Internuclear ophthalmoplegia
  - Paraneoplastic syndrome
- Lesions in the midbrain
  - Progressive supranuclear palsy
  - Whipple disease

- Lesions in the basal ganglia
  - Parkinson syndromes
  - Huntington disease
  - Creutzfeldt–Jakob disease
- Miscellaneous
  - Medications (anticonvulsants, benzodiazepines)
  - Wilson disease
  - Lipid storage diseases

Control of the Pursuit System

Smooth pursuit eye movements (conjugate maintenance of fixation of the eyes while following a moving target) are generated in higher cortical centers, especially the parieto–occipital–temporal junction.

Inputs are sent from each parieto–occipital–temporal junction to the superior colliculi (SC), which mediate control of horizontal and vertical pursuit eye movements.

Descending horizontal gaze pursuit fibers synapse on the sixth nerve nucleus directly without synapsing in the PPRF.

Unlike the saccadic system, in which each hemisphere (frontal eye fields and other centers) produces conjugate horizontal eye movements toward the contralateral direction because of crossing of the saccadic pathways in the brainstem, the pursuit system is designed such that each hemisphere controls conjugate pursuit eye movements to the *ipsilateral* visual space.

Vestibulo-ocular System

Conjugate gaze in both the vertical and horizontal planes is stabilized through inputs from the vestibular nuclei.

- From each vestibular nuclear complex, axons subserving horizontal gaze-holding send an excitatory connection to the contralateral sixth nerve nucleus and an inhibitory projection to the ipsilateral abducens nucleus; motor neurons from the sixth nerve nucleus innervate the lateral rectus, whereas interneurons cross over to ascend in the MLF to the third nerve nucleus. Stimulatory input from each vestibular nucleus, therefore, produces conjugate horizontal gaze toward the contralateral side of the body.
- Inputs from the vestibular nuclei also influence vertical gaze-holding through inputs (some via the MLFs) to the contralateral fourth nerve nucleus, third nerve nucleus, INC, and riMLF. The maintenance of ocular alignment in the vertical plane is controlled by the existence of balanced inputs from the vestibular nuclei to the fourth nerve nucleus (which innervates the contralateral superior oblique muscle), the superior rectus subnucleus (innervates the contralateral superior rectus), and the inferior oblique and inferior rectus subnuclei (innervate the ipsilateral inferior oblique and inferior rectus). An imbalance between these inputs to the various subnuclei results in skew deviation.

13.5.6 Other Eye Movement Abnormalities

Locked-in Syndrome

Large bilateral lesions (essentially transecting the pons) may cause a neurologic state characterized by the combination of the following:

- Quadriplegia
- Absence of horizontal eye movements

- Mutism
- Preservation of vertical eye movements
- Normal blinking
- Normal consciousness

These patients are able to communicate only by using blinking and vertical eye movements.

Ocular Neuromyotonia

In ocular neuromyotonia, tonic spasms of the extraocular muscles innervated by a specific ocular motor nerve (e.g., third or sixth cranial nerve) occur during sustained eccentric gaze (hyperaction of the muscle).

Affected patients complain of episodic diplopia lasting seconds or minutes and occurring after they look in a specific direction for a few seconds. Some patients feel that the eye is pulled in the orbit. The examination is usually normal between episodes.

This rare disorder classically develops months or years after radiation involving the ocular motor nerves (usually for pituitary tumor or skull base tumor). Carbamazepine is sometimes helpful.

Ocular Motility Deficits in High Myopia

Adults with high axial myopia (associated with a long globe) may develop an esotropia, abduction deficit, or vertical misalignment.

Various explanations have been proposed, including the following:
- Elongated globe (compromising free movements of the eye in the orbit)
- Heavy globe
- Lateral rectus (or its tendon) abnormalities
- Defective orbital connective tissue
- Abnormal insertions of the extraocular muscles

Diplopia after Ocular Surgery

Numerous processes may explain diplopia after ocular surgery.
- Monocular diplopia is common after refractive surgery, cataract surgery, and retinal surgery resulting from any of the following unwanted outcomes:
  - Irregular cornea
  - Incision-induced astigmatism
  - Decentered, tilted intraocular lens
  - Cracked lens
  - Problem (fold, tear, opacity) of the posterior capsule
  - Eccentric pupil
  - Iridectomy creating multiple pupils
- Binocular diplopia suggests ocular misalignment, which can occur as a result of the following:
  - Disrupted fusion secondary to
    - anisometropia
    - surgical pupil changes
    - altered brightness sense between the eyes
    - prolonged decreased vision in the eye with cataract
    - sensory exotropia

- Decentered or tilted intraocular lens with induced prism
- Extraocular muscle trauma from local anesthesia (peri- or retrobulbar block)
- Unmasking of preexisting tropia (the patient sees double because the vision has improved)
- Impaired eye movement after scleral buckle (retinal detachment repair)
- Bridle suture sometimes placed on a rectus muscle during surgery

Isolated ptosis after ocular surgery is common, usually related to damage to the levator palpebrae from the speculum used to keep the eye open during surgery.

13.6 Evaluation of the Patient with Binocular Diplopia: Practical Tips

13.6.1 Assessment of Diplopia

- Is the diplopia binocular or monocular?
- If monocular, you are done! Send the patient to an ophthalmologist.
- If binocular:
  - Is it horizontal or vertical?
  - Is it worse at distance or at near?
  - In which direction of gaze is the diplopia worse?

Pearls

Esotropia (e.g., an abduction deficit) gives diplopia worse at distance (the eyes normally converge at near). Exotropia (e.g., an adduction deficit) gives diplopia worse at near (the eyes normally diverge when looking at distance). The diplopia is worse in the direction of the paretic muscle.

Example: A patient with a right sixth nerve palsy complains of the following (▶ Fig. 13.133):
- Binocular diplopia
- Horizontal diplopia
- Worse at distance (the eyes need to diverge at distance)
- Worse when looking to the right

Example: A patient with a complete ptosis and abnormal eye movements may not complain of diplopia until the ptotic eyelid is raised by the examiner (▶ Fig. 13.134).

13.6.2 Further Assessment of the Diplopic Patient

- Is there a head tilt? (important in vertical diplopia) or a face turn?
- Review of old photographs to look for head tilt, face turn, or old strabismus.

Patients and families are often not aware of head tilt. A long-standing head tilt is best revealed by reviewing old pictures.

Example: In a patient with binocular vertical diplopia, a long-standing head tilt is highly suggestive of decompensation of a congenital fourth nerve palsy (patients tilt their head to the opposite side to compensate for the diplopia) (▶ Fig. 13.135).

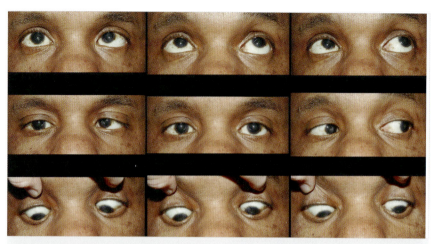

Fig. 13.133 Right abduction deficit secondary to a right sixth nerve palsy.

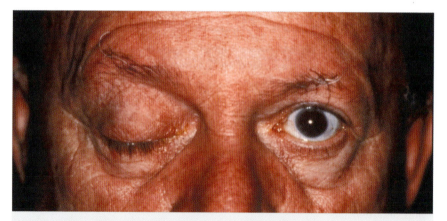

Fig. 13.134 Right third nerve palsy with complete ptosis on the right.

Pearls

Patients often compensate for their diplopia by turning their face or tilting their head (giving the appearance of torticollis). This is particularly common in young children. Eye movements should be evaluated in children with torticollis.

13.6.3 Look at the Patient

There may be an obvious orbital problem, with red eye or proptosis, alleviating the need for a neurologic evaluation.

Example: The finding of an orbital syndrome (proptosis, periorbital edema, periorbital redness, visual loss) in a patient complaining of diplopia localizes the process to the

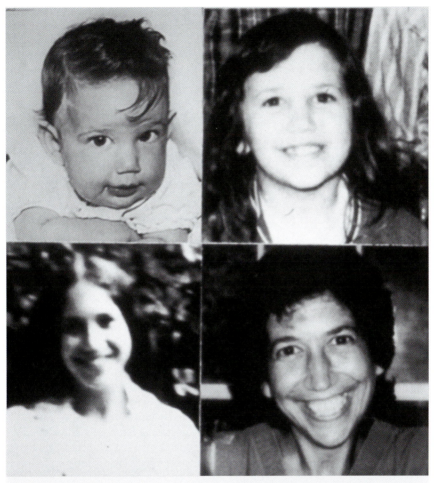

Fig. 13.135 Long-standing right head tilt from a congenital left fourth nerve palsy. Note the overaction of the left inferior oblique muscle in the picture taken at age 6 months (upper left).

orbit itself. In this case, the diplopia is usually secondary to dysfunction of the extra-ocular muscles (▶ Fig. 13.136).

13.6.4 Visual Acuity, Pupils, and Fundus Also Need to Be Carefully Examined

- Decreased vision suggests an orbital or an orbital apex process (the visual acuity and visual fields are normal with lesions of the cavernous sinus).
- Bilateral disc edema in the setting of good visual acuity and sixth nerve palsy suggests papilledema secondary to raised intracranial pressure.
- In the evaluation of a third nerve palsy, it is essential to carefully evaluate the pupil.
- A Horner syndrome on the side of a sixth nerve palsy localizes to the cavernous sinus.

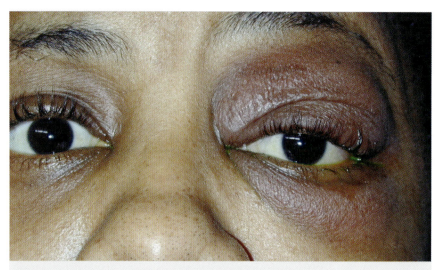

Fig. 13.136 Left proptosis, periorbital edema, and redness from orbital inflammation.

Example: A classic cause of unilateral or bilateral sixth nerve palsy is raised intracranial pressure. These patients may have headaches in addition to the binocular horizontal diplopia.

Funduscopic examination needs to be systematically performed in all patients complaining of diplopia. Finding papilledema in the setting of an abduction deficit suggests a sixth nerve palsy from raised intracranial pressure (▶ Fig. 13.137).

Example: The cavernous sinus is the only place where the sixth nerve is very close to the sympathetic pathway. Therefore, a cavernous sinus lesion can produce a sixth nerve palsy and an ipsilateral Horner syndrome, with no other neurologic signs.

Lesions of the intracavernous carotid artery (such as aneurysm) are particularly common with such a clinical presentation (▶ Fig. 13.138).

Example: The pupils are always normal when the extraocular muscles are affected directly (lesion localizing to the muscles), or when the neuromuscular junction is affected (myasthenia gravis).

Lesions of the third cranial nerve may produce a mydriasis that reacts poorly to light. Therefore, finding anisocoria, worse in the light, with the large pupil being on the side of a ptosis and abnormal eye movements, is highly suggestive of a third nerve palsy (▶ Fig. 13.139).

Pearls

Third nerve palsies with pupil involvement need to be evaluated emergently. The two main causes are intracranial aneurysm and pituitary apoplexy.

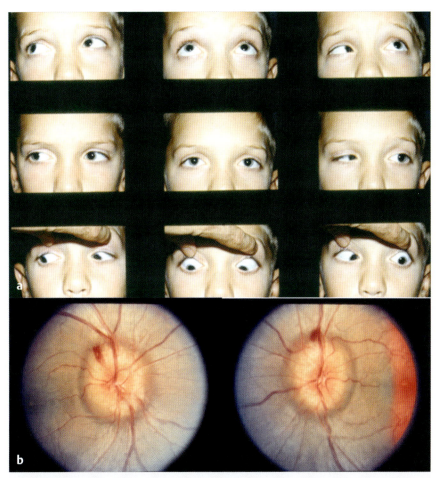

Fig. 13.137 (a) Left sixth nerve palsy with (b) bilateral papilledema from raised intracranial pressure (cerebral venous thrombosis).

Pearls

Localization of the lesion is the most important step when evaluating a patient with binocular diplopia. A patient with an isolated abduction deficit of one eye does not necessarily have a sixth nerve palsy. An isolated paresis of the lateral rectus could be due to a disease of the muscle itself, to deficient transmission at the level of the neuromuscular junction (myasthenia), or to a lesion of the cranial nerve (sixth nerve palsy). Associated symptoms and signs often allow localization of the pathological process.

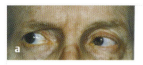
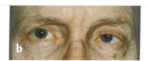
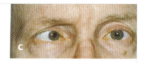
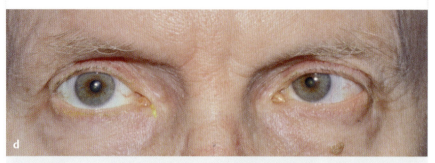

Fig. 13.138 (a–c) Left abduction deficit with ipsilateral Horner syndrome (mild left ptosis and anisocoria, with the left pupil being smaller than the right pupil in dim light) from a left carotid cavernous aneurysm. (d) In primary position, the left esotropia and left Horner syndrome are well seen.

13.7 Specific Syndromes

Associated neurologic symptoms and signs localize the diplopia to the brainstem.

Specific syndromes need to be known because of their highly localizing value (▶ Table 13.6).

13.8 Treatment of Diplopia

Binocular diplopia resolves when the patient closes one eye. Most patients realize this spontaneously and patch one eye to suppress diplopia. This is an acceptable temporary treatment, either until the diplopia resolves by itself or until other treatments are decided on.

Many simple, commonsense measures can improve the vision of diplopic patients.

For example, if a patient complains of diplopia only when looking down, then avoiding looking down may be the best treatment. This can be accomplished by recommending correction of presbyopia with single-vision reading glasses instead of bifocal or progressive lenses (which require that the patient look down to read); patients can also be advised to read sitting up with the book on a table or on a book (or music) stand instead of reading lying down in bed.

13.8.1 Patching

Any patch works. A nonsticky, removable patch is more comfortable.

Many patients prefer semiopaque tape placed over one lens (on their regular glasses or on sunglasses). It suppresses diplopia as well as an opaque patch but still allows them to see shadows and use their peripheral vision while ambulating (▶ Fig. 13.140).

In adults, patching one eye, even for a long period of time, does not alter visual function. Alternating the patch is not necessary, and patients can choose which eye

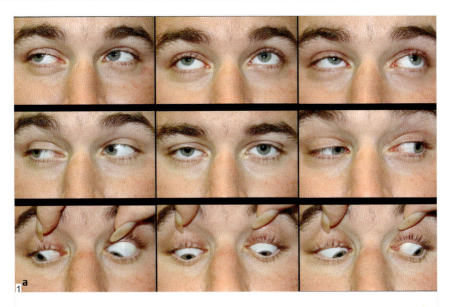

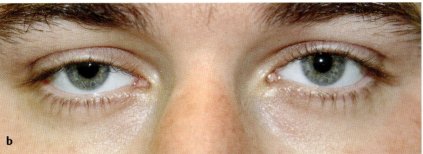

Fig. 13.139 (a) Partial right third nerve palsy due to a right posterior communicating aneurysm. (b) There is mild right ptosis and an elevation deficit responsible for binocular vertical diplopia in up gaze. The right pupil is larger than the left and poorly reactive to light.

to patch (they usually prefer not to patch the dominant eye or the eye that sees or moves best).

In young children (< 10 years old), prolonged patching may induce amblyopia. This is why it is usually recommended to alternate patching in children.

Patching is usually the best acute solution for sick patients, patients in the hospital or in rehabilitation, and older patients who are at risk of falling.

13.8.2 Prisms

Diplopia can be corrected by placing a prism of appropriate power in front of one eye (the power of the prism is equivalent to the amount of ocular deviation measured with prisms).

Table 13.6 Specific syndromes

Clinical syndrome	Lesion location
Horizontal gaze palsy with ipsilateral facial palsy	Pons (sixth nerve nucleus)
Sixth nerve palsy with contralateral hemiparesis (*Raymond syndrome*)	Pons (sixth nerve fascicle and corticospinal tract)
Sixth nerve palsy with ipsilateral seventh nerve palsy and contralateral hemiparesis (*Millard-Gubler syndrome*)	Pons (sixth nerve fascicle, seventh nerve fascicle, and corticospinal tract)
Sixth nerve palsy with ipsilateral seventh nerve palsy, deafness, facial hypoesthesia, Horner, contralateral pain, and thermal hypoesthesia (*Foville syndrome*)	Pons (sixth nerve fascicle or nucleus, ipsilateral seventh nerve fascicle or nucleus, auditory nerve, descending tract of fifth nerve, cerebellar peduncle, spinothalamic tract)
Sixth nerve palsy with ipsilateral Horner syndrome	Cavernous sinus
Nystagmus, skew deviation, ocular tilt reaction, vertigo, lateropulsion, ipsilateral Horner syndrome, cerebellar syndrome, facial hypoesthesia, cranial nerves IX and X, and contralateral pain and thermal hypoesthesia (*Wallenberg syndrome*)	Lateral medullary (descending tract of fifth nerve, cerebellar peduncle, spinothalamic tract, cranial nerves IX and X, sympathetic pathway, vestibular nuclei)
Fourth nerve palsy with contralateral Horner syndrome	Midbrain–pontine junction (fourth nerve nucleus on the side of the Horner syndrome)
Third nerve palsy with contralateral ptosis and contralateral superior rectus weakness	Midbrain (third nerve nucleus)
Third nerve palsy with contralateral hemiparesis (*Weber syndrome*)	Ventral midbrain (third nerve fascicle and cerebral peduncle)
Third nerve palsy and ipsilateral cerebellar ataxia (*Nothnagel syndrome*)	Midbrain (third nerve fascicle and superior cerebellar peduncle)
Third nerve palsy and contralateral tremor (*Benedikt syndrome*)	Midbrain (third nerve fascicle and red nucleus)
Third nerve palsy and contralateral ataxia with tremor (*Claude syndrome*)	Midbrain (third nerve fascicle, red nucleus, and cerebellar peduncle)
Third nerve palsy with vertical gaze palsy, lid retraction, skew deviation, and convergence nystagmus	Dorsal midbrain (top of the basilar syndrome)
Third nerve palsy with depressed mental status	Transtentorial uncal herniation

This is usually a very good way to correct diplopia as long as the ocular deviation is not too large (usually < 20 or 30 prism diopters) and is relatively stable (prisms are not a good solution for myasthenic patients whose diplopia fluctuates during the day).

Prisms are either temporary (Fresnel prisms are thin, soft plastic sheets than can be taped to the patient's glasses and are easily removed) or permanent (prisms are ground invisibly into permanent glasses). Permanent prisms can be expensive and should be prescribed only when the diplopia has been stable for several months.

Prisms are not perfect because they correct incomitant diplopia in only one direction of gaze and because they degrade visual acuity and can induce distortion. They may not be tolerated in older patients with difficulty walking and with balance disorders.

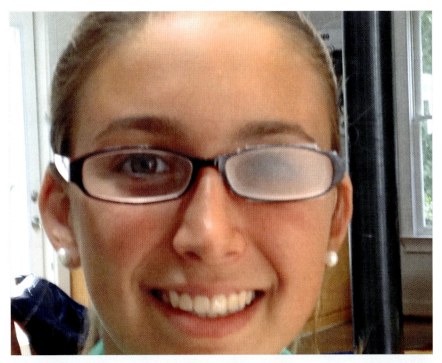

Fig. 13.140 Semiopaque tape over one lens suppresses diplopia.

13.8.3 Strabismus Surgery

Surgery on one or more extraocular muscles is a very effective way to definitively correct ocular misalignment. Surgery is performed only for relatively large deviations once they have been documented to be stable (it is usually recommended to wait at least 6 months after an injury resulting in diplopia before performing strabismus surgery). Surgery is highly successful for simple ocular deviations such as from a sixth nerve palsy or superior oblique paresis. It can be more difficult after a third nerve palsy.

13.8.4 Botulinum Toxin Injection

Injection of botulinum toxin into an extraocular muscle results in temporary (several weeks) paralysis of the muscle. This technique is used to temporarily straighten an eye in rare cases of severe ocular deviation from paralysis of a rectus muscle (e.g., some patients with trauma and a sixth nerve palsy may have a severe deviation of the affected eye toward the nose; injection of botulinum toxin in the medial rectus will weaken the medial rectus, and the eye will straighten for several weeks while recovering its normal function).

14 Orbital Syndrome

Orbital disorders usually manifest with symptoms and signs that include proptosis, periocular swelling, decreased vision, and diplopia.

14.1 Clinical Anatomy of the Orbit

All orbital structures can be involved in orbital lesions (▶ Fig. 14.1). Because the orbit is an enclosed space surrounded by bones, any orbital process will result in proptosis (exophthalmos).

14.2 Causes of Acute or Subacute Orbital Syndrome

Acute orbital syndromes are most often vascular or inflammatory, whereas subacute presentations are most likely secondary to tumors.

Vascular abnormalities
- Carotid–cavernous sinus fistula
- Cavernous sinus thrombosis
- Superior ophthalmic vein thrombosis
- Orbital varix
- Orbital arteriovenous malformation

Inflammatory processes
- Infectious
  - Bacterial orbital cellulitis
  - Fungal infections
  - Orbital tuberculosis
- Noninfectious
  - Thyroid-related orbitopathy
  - Idiopathic orbital inflammation (inflammatory orbital pseudotumor)
  - Immunoglobulin G4 (IgG4) related disease
  - Sarcoidosis
  - Wegener granulomatosis
  - Giant cell arteritis
  - Polyarteritis nodosa

Tumors (only the most classic tumors in each age group are listed, in order of decreasing frequency)
- Primary
  - Adults
    - Cavernous hemangioma
    - Lymphangioma
    - Schwannoma
    - Lymphoma
    - Optic nerve sheath meningioma
  - Children
    - Rhabdomyosarcoma
    - Lymphangioma
    - Capillary hemangioma

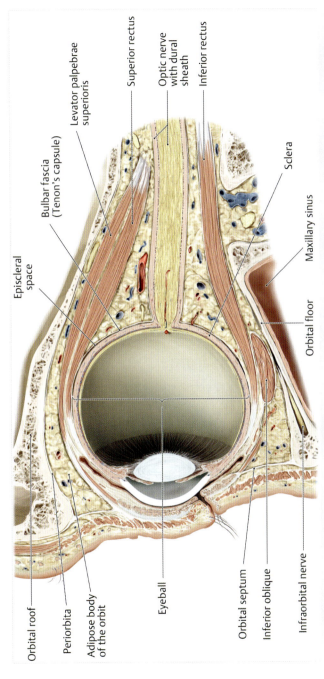

Fig. 14.1 Anatomy of the orbit (sagittal view through the eye and the optic canal). (From Schuenke M, Schulte E, Schumacher U, Ross LM, Lamperti ED, Voll M. THIEME Atlas of Anatomy, Head and Neuroanatomy. Stuttgart, Germany: Thieme; 2007. Illustration by Karl Wesker.)

- Optic nerve glioma
- Cysts, including mucocele
- Secondary/invasive
  - Sinonasal tumors
  - Brain tumors
  - Perineural spread of cutaneous tumors
- Metastatic
  - Adults
    - Breast carcinoma
    - Bronchogenic carcinoma
    - Prostate carcinoma
  - Children
    - Neuroblastoma
    - Leukemia

Trauma
- Orbital wall fractures
- Retrobulbar hematoma

The clinical examination may help further differentiate among the possible etiologies, but imaging studies are imperative to ascertain the ultimate diagnosis. In the absence of diagnostic imaging findings, tissue biopsy is usually the next step in determining the cause of an orbital syndrome.

14.3 Features of Orbital Syndrome

The following symptoms and signs can reveal an orbitopathy:
- Proptosis (exophthalmos)
- Eyelid malposition
  - Retraction
  - Ptosis
- Globe displacement
- Ocular pulsations or orbital bruit
- Vision loss
  - Optic neuropathy from
    - compression
    - infiltration
    - ischemia
    - Elevated intraocular pressure
  - Venous stasis causing
    - retinal hemorrhages
    - macular edema
    - serous retinal detachment
- Diplopia
  - Extraocular muscle restriction
    - Venous engorgement
    - Mechanical limitation secondary to mass effect
  - Cranial neuropathy (secondary to nerve ischemia or direct compression)
- Enophthalmos rarely (secondary to scarring with tissue retraction or bony orbital wall destruction)

14.3.1 Causes of Proptosis

Orbital space occupying lesions induce proptosis:
- Thyroid eye disease
- Orbital tumors
- Orbital inflammatory pseudotumor
- Orbital infection (cellulitis)
- Orbital vascular malformations
  - Arteriovenous malformations
  - Orbital varix
- Orbital venous congestion
  - Cavernous sinus fistula
  - Cavernous sinus thrombosis
  - Superior orbital vein thrombosis
  - Orbital hemorrhage
- Bony deformations of the orbit
  - Fibrous dysplasia
  - Sphenoid wing hypoplasia
- Trauma to the orbit
- Pseudoproptosis
  - High myopia
  - Racial (common in blacks)

Pearls

The most common cause of unilateral or bilateral proptosis is thyroid eye disease
(▶ Fig. 14.2).
  Orbital tumors often produce proptosis with displacement of the globe (▶ Fig. 14.3).
  Orbital metastases from breast cancer are classically associated with atrophy of fat,
resulting in enophthalmos rather than proptosis (exophthalmos) (▶ Fig. 14.4).

14.4 Evaluation of a Patient with Orbital Syndrome

Because of the risk of visual loss, patients with suspected orbital syndrome must be
evaluated urgently.
- Clinical:
  - Unilateral or bilateral
  - Tempo of onset and duration of symptoms
  - History of trauma
  - Pain
  - Prognostic:
    - Visual loss
    - Elevated intraocular pressure
- Orbital imaging:
  - Computed tomography (CT) of the orbits with contrast
  - Magnetic resonance imaging (MRI) of the orbits with fat suppression and contrast

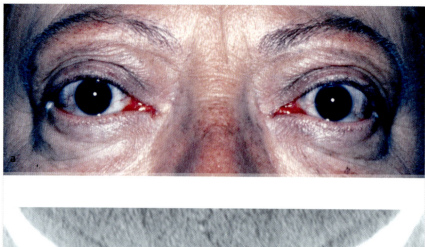

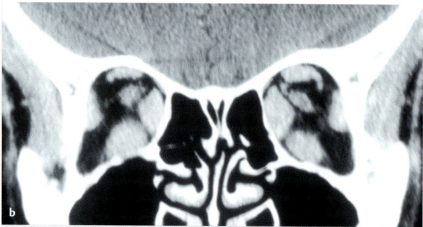

Fig. 14.2 (a) Bilateral proptosis with periorbital swelling from thyroid eye disease. (b) Coronal computed tomography (CT) of the orbits showing enlarged extraocular muscles in both orbits from thyroid eye disease.

○ Orbital ultrasound (to detect enlarged extraocular muscles and superior ophthalmic vein)
• Orbital biopsy often necessary

An orbital syndrome is suspected clinically and is confirmed by imaging of the orbits with contrast (CT or MRI). Brain imaging often misses orbital processes.

Orbital biopsy is often necessary.

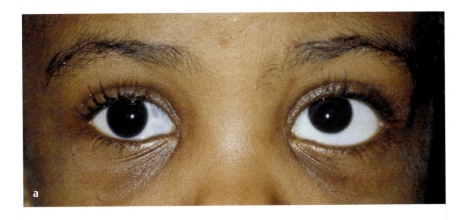

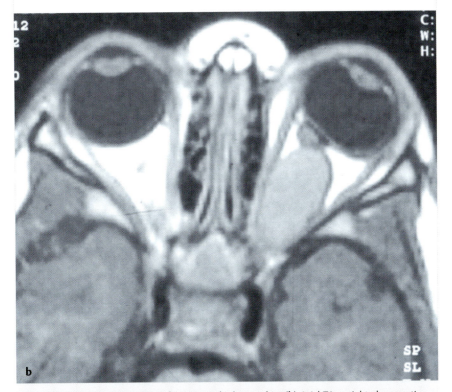

Fig. 14.3 (a) Left proptosis. The left eye is pushed up and in. (b) Axial T1-weighted magnetic resonance imaging (MRI) without contrast showing a left optic nerve glioma.

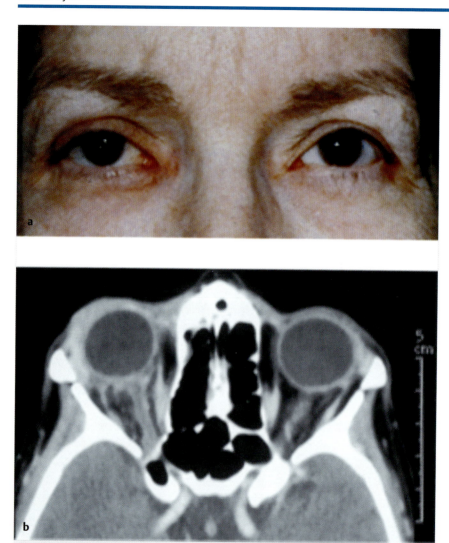

Fig. 14.4 (a) Enophthalmos of the right eye with visual loss, ophthalmoplegia, and pain related to a right orbital metastasis from breast cancer. (b) Axial computed tomography of the orbits with contrast showing enhancement of the right orbit but no proptosis.

15 Cavernous Sinus and Orbital Vascular Disorders

Cavernous sinus and orbital vascular disorders are commonly seen in neuro-ophthalmology. They include cavernous sinus aneurysms, carotid-cavernous fistulas, cavernous sinus thrombosis, and venous disorders of the orbit.

15.1 Vascular Drainage of the Orbit and Cavernous Sinus

Each cavernous sinus contains a plexus of veins draining the orbits and some of the intracranial veins (▶ Fig. 15.1). The carotid artery passes through the cavernous sinus. Vascular disorders are a common cause of cavernous sinus and orbital syndromes.

The major orbital veins include the superior and the inferior ophthalmic veins. The cavernous sinus is connected anteriorly to the superior and inferior ophthalmic veins

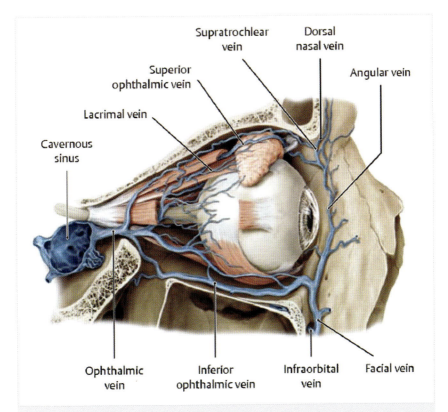

Fig. 15.1 Lateral view of the orbit showing the venous drainage of the orbit. (From Schuenke M, Schulte E, Schumacher U, Ross LM, Lamperti ED, Voll M. THIEME Atlas of Anatomy, Head and Neuroanatomy. Stuttgart, Germany: Thieme; 2007. Illustration by Karl Wesker.)

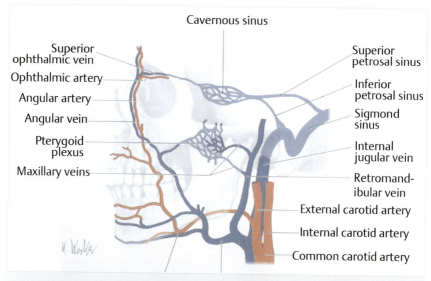

Fig. 15.2 Clinically important vascular relationships in the facial region. (From Schuenke M, Schulte E, Schumacher U, Ross LM, Lamperti ED, Voll M. THIEME Atlas of Anatomy, Head and Neuroanatomy. Stuttgart, Germany: Thieme; 2007. Illustration by Karl Wesker.)

and posteriorly to the superior and inferior petrosal sinuses (▶ Fig. 15.2). There are numerous communications between the facial veins and the orbital veins, explaining why facial infections are often complicated by orbital cellulitis and rarely by cavernous sinus thrombosis. Impaired venous drainage results in orbital congestion, which presents like an orbital syndrome.

15.2 Carotid-Cavernous Aneurysms

Aneurysms of the internal carotid artery may develop within the cavernous sinus (▶ Fig. 15.3 and ▶ Fig. 15.4). They are often asymptomatic until patients develop diplopia (ocular motor nerve compression) and ipsilateral pain (trigeminal nerve compression).

An ipsilateral third-order Horner syndrome may be present. There is usually no visual loss.

15.3 Carotid-Cavernous Fistulas

A carotid-cavernous fistula (CCF) is an abnormal communication between the carotid artery and the cavernous sinus, a venous plexus (▶ Fig. 15.5). The cavernous sinus fills with arterial blood, and the pressure increases. This results in impaired drainage of all veins normally draining into the cavernous sinus with resultant venous congestion (▶ Fig. 15.6).

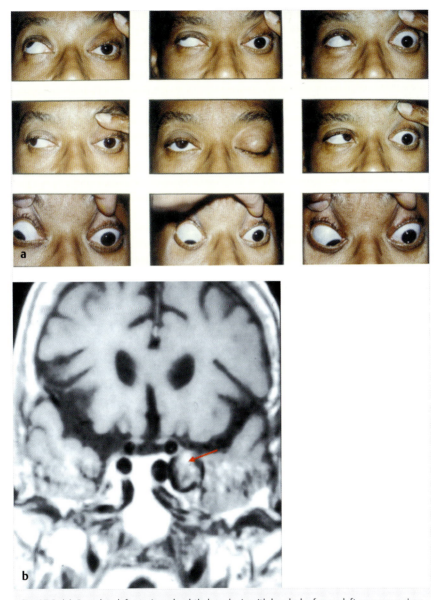

Fig. 15.3 (a) Complete left ptosis and ophthalmoplegia with headache from a left cavernous sinus aneurysm. (b) Coronal T1-weighted magnetic resonance imaging of the brain with contrast showing a round mass in the left cavernous sinus consistent with an aneurysm (*arrow*) of the left internal carotid artery in the cavernous sinus.

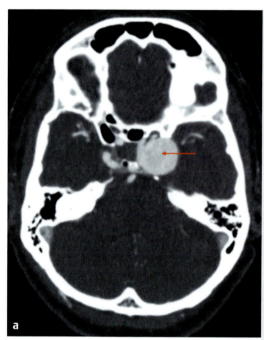

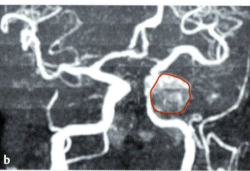

Fig. 15.4 (a) Source image of a computed tomographic angiogram (CTA) with contrast showing a left cavernous sinus aneurysm (*arrow*). (b) Angiographic reconstruction of the CTA showing a large aneurysm (*outlined*) of the left internal carotid artery within the cavernous sinus.

15.3.1 Classification

CCFs can be classified by four different schemes:
1. Etiologically (traumatic or spontaneous)
2. Hemodynamically (high flow or low flow)
3. Anatomically (direct or dural)
4. Angiographically:
   - *Type A fistulas are direct shunts* between the internal carotid artery and the cavernous sinus. They represent from 70 to 90% of all CCFs, are usually of the high-flow type, and most often are posttraumatic. They can also arise from rupture of an intracavernous carotid artery aneurysm or from complications of surgery or catheter angiography. Because of the high blood flow rate, direct CCFs usually manifest with acute and severe symptoms, and they rarely resolve spontaneously.

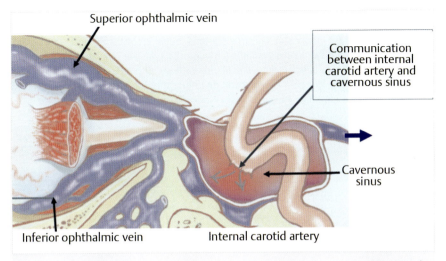

Fig. 15.5 Sagittal view of the cavernous sinus and posterior part of the orbit showing a carotid cavernous fistula.

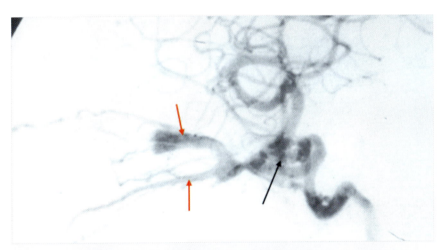

Fig. 15.6 Catheter angiogram (lateral view) showing a direct carotid cavernous fistula (*black arrow*). Note the dilated superior and inferior ophthalmic veins (*red arrows*).

- *Types B, C, and D are indirect or dural shunts.* They represent congenital arteriovenous connections between small arterial branches and the cavernous sinus that open spontaneously in older women or in the setting of hypertension, diabetes, atherosclerotic disease, childbirth, or collagen-vascular disease. Dural CCFs usually cause insidious and less severe symptoms. In contrast to direct fistulas, dural shunts are much more likely to be misdiagnosed initially and to resolve spontaneously.

15.3.2 Features

As a result of these abnormal communications between arteries and veins, and because of the baseline pressure gradient between the two, the affected veins become "arterialized," with a resultant elevation in intravenous pressure and changes in the hemodynamics of the involved vasculature, including rate and direction of blood flow (▶ Fig. 15.7, ▶ Fig. 15.8, ▶ Fig. 15.9).

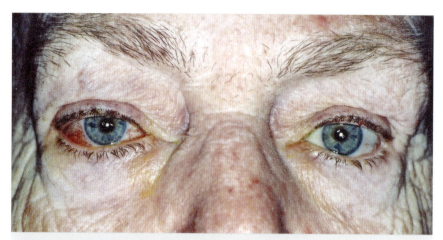

Fig. 15.7 Indirect right carotid-cavernous fistula with arterialization of the conjunctival vessels in the right eye, mistaken for months as chronic conjunctivitis.

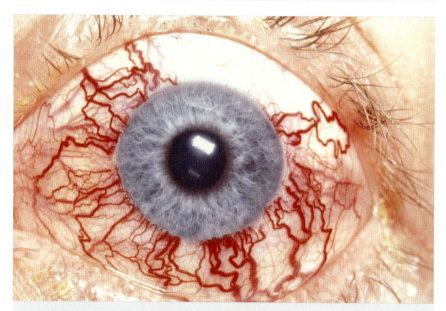

Fig. 15.8 Direct right traumatic carotid-cavernous fistula with arterialization of the conjunctival vessels in the left eye. Note the "corkscrew" dilation of the vessels.

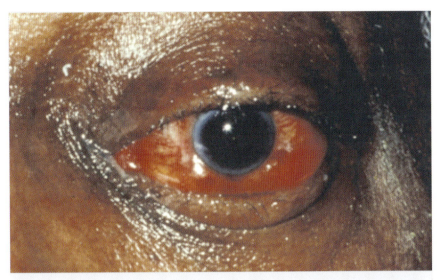

Fig. 15.9 Direct left carotid-cavernous fistula with hemorrhagic chemosis and proptosis of the left eye.

When arterial blood flow escapes posteriorly from the cavernous sinus through the petrosal sinuses, patients may not develop ocular symptoms or signs.

When arterial blood flows anteriorly into the superior and/or inferior ophthalmic veins, ocular manifestations occur from venous and arterial stasis within the eye and the orbit, increased episcleral venous pressure, and decreased arterial blood flow to the cranial nerves within the cavernous sinus. These manifestations are usually unilateral and ipsilateral to the fistula, but they may be bilateral or even contralateral because of the connections between the two cavernous sinuses.

Classic features in CCF include the following:

- Arterialization of the conjunctival vessels and conjunctival chemosis are a direct consequence of arterial blood flow into the orbital and conjunctival veins.
- Proptosis, from congestion of orbital tissues, is often one of the earliest findings. It is highly variable, commonly associated with eyelid swelling, and may produce exposure keratopathy.
- Elevated intraocular pressure results from increased episcleral venous pressure and orbital congestion, and rarely from neovascularization associated with chronic hypoxia or from angle closure glaucoma.
- There is usually a subjective or objective cranial bruit (detected by placing the bell of the stethoscope over the patient's temple or the orbit). The bruit can sometimes be heard without a stethoscope.
- Ophthalmoplegia is common in CCFs and results from direct damage to the ocular motor nerves by trauma (direct CCF), compression of the ocular motor nerves by a carotid-cavernous aneurysm, and the fistula itself causing ischemia and/or compression of the ocular motor nerves. The sixth cranial nerve is the most commonly affected nerve because of its free-floating location within the cavernous sinus. Mechanical restriction of the extraocular muscles results from venous stasis, orbital edema, and engorgement of the muscles.

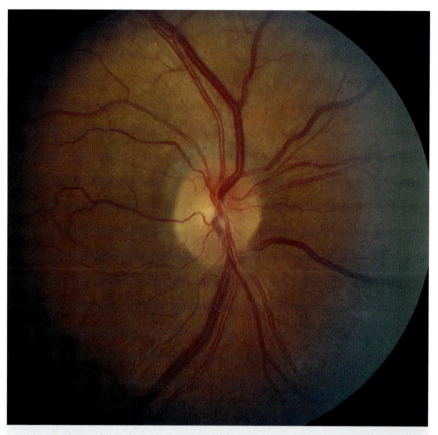

Fig. 15.10 Dilation of retinal veins in a patient with an indirect carotid-cavernous fistula. The optic nerve is slightly hyperemic.

Classic fundus findings in direct CCFs include the following (▶ Fig. 15.10 and ▶ Fig. 15.11):

- Ipsilateral optic disc swelling
- Dilation of retinal veins
- Intraretinal hemorrhages from venous stasis and impaired retinal blood flow
- Preretinal or intravitreous hemorrhages (rare)
- Choroidal thickening, choroidal detachment, and retinal serous detachment

Pearls

Consider the diagnosis of CCF in all patients with elevated intraocular pressure, mild headache, or a bruit accompanying a chronically red eye, especially in elderly women.

The diagnosis of CCF is based on imaging (▶ Fig. 15.12, ▶ Fig. 15.13, ▶ Fig. 15.14). Prominence of the superior ophthalmic vein and diffuse enlargement of all the extraocular muscles are frequently detected on computed tomographic (CT) scan or magnetic

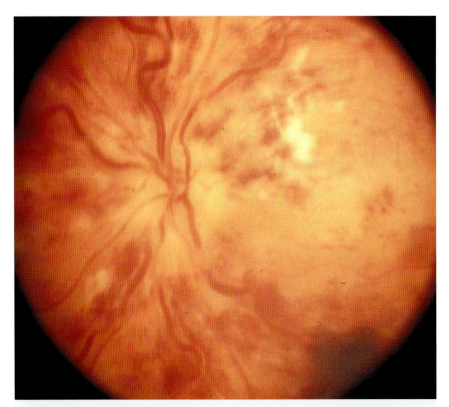

Fig. 15.11 Extensive retinal hemorrhages, exudates, and edema with dilation of the retinal veins in a patient with a direct carotid-cavernous fistula.

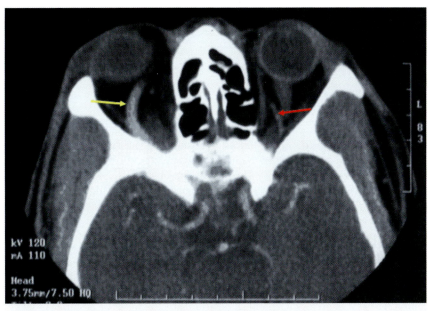

Fig. 15.12 Axial computed tomography with contrast showing dilation of the right superior ophthalmic vein (*yellow arrow*) in a patient with a right carotid-cavernous fistula. Note the normal left superior ophthalmic vein (*red arrow*).

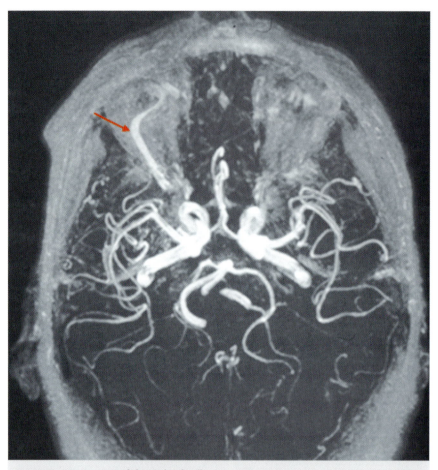

Fig. 15.13 Superior view of the circle of Willis on magnetic resonance angiography showing dilation of the right superior ophthalmic vein (*red arrow*) in a patient with a right carotid-cavernous fistula.

resonance imaging (MRI) or on orbital ultrasonography. Computed tomographic angiography (CTA) and magnetic resonance angiography (MRA) are not very useful, except for the source images.

Definitive diagnosis depends on catheter angiographic evaluation, with selective injection of both internal and external carotid arteries and the vertebral circulation.

15.3.3 Prognosis

Visual loss associated with CCF may be immediate, most often from coincident ocular or optic nerve damage at the time of the head injury, or delayed, caused by exposure keratopathy, elevated intraocular pressure, vitreous hemorrhage, retinal venous stasis, central retinal vein occlusion, choroidal detachment, or anterior or posterior ischemic optic neuropathy. Although CCFs are rarely a life-threatening condition, patients with

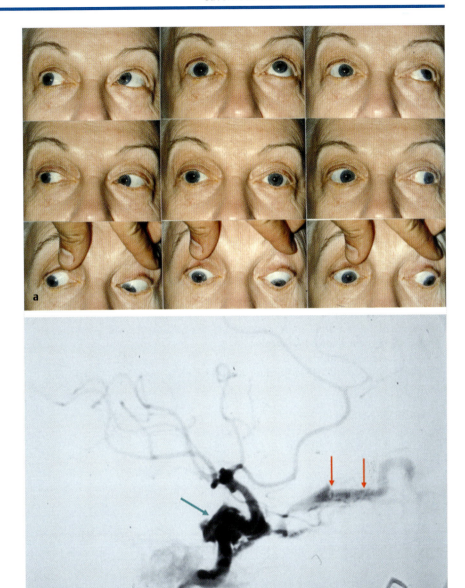

Fig. 15.14 (a) Partial right third nerve palsy from carotid-cavernous fistula. There is mild right ptosis, decreased elevation, adduction, and depression of the right eye, and the right pupil is dilated and poorly reactive to light. (b) Selective catheter angiogram of the right internal carotid artery (lateral view) showing abnormal filling of the cavernous sinus (*green arrow*). Note the dilated superior ophthalmic vein (*red arrows*).

direct CCFs may have venous infarction, massive epistaxis, intracranial hemorrhage, or subarachnoid hemorrhage from rupture of the fistula.

15.3.4 Treatment

Treatment is indicated in all cases of direct carotid fistula and in indirect fistula with visual loss or cortical vein drainage (which have a high risk of intracranial hemorrhage). The ideal result is closure of the fistula and normalization of orbital hemodynamics, while preserving internal carotid artery patency.

Occlusion of the fistula can be done by occlusion of the internal carotid artery (although there is a risk of ipsilateral cerebral infarction and ocular ischemic syndrome). Selective closure of the fistula without occlusion of the internal carotid artery can be done by endovascular approaches (embolization and detachable balloon occlusion) or, more rarely, by direct surgical approaches.

Secondary glaucoma and ischemic retinopathy may require specific treatments.

15.4 Carotid-Cavernous Thrombosis

15.4.1 Features and Causes

Thrombosis of the cavernous sinus produces an acute or subacute orbital syndrome (▶ Fig. 15.15), which includes the following:

- Pain (periorbital and headache)
- Proptosis with periorbital edema (often periorbital ecchymoses)
- Chemosis
- Visual loss
  - Optic neuropathy
  - Venous congestion with disc edema and retinal hemorrhages
  - Increased intraocular pressure
- Ophthalmoplegia
  - Multiple cranial nerve palsies in the cavernous sinus
  - Enlargement of extraocular muscles from venous congestion
- Systemic symptoms such as fever and altered mental status

Cavernous sinus thrombosis is usually a complication of a severe facial, sinus, or orbital infection. It is rarely secondary to a hypercoagulable state.

15.4.2 Prognosis and Treatment

There is a high rate of morbidity and mortality with risk of extension of the venous thrombosis to intracranial veins and cerebral infarction, as well as a high risk of permanent visual loss. The prognosis is mostly based on the cause of the cavernous sinus thrombosis: severe facial and sinus infections can be complicated by cerebral abscess, infectious meningitis, and spread of infection to the contralateral cavernous sinus and fellow orbit.

Treatment includes aggressive treatment of the underlying cause. If there is local infection, treatment would include drainage and administration of antibiotics, as well as anticoagulation therapy. Corticosteroids are sometimes started once the infection is controlled to reduce inflammation and edema.

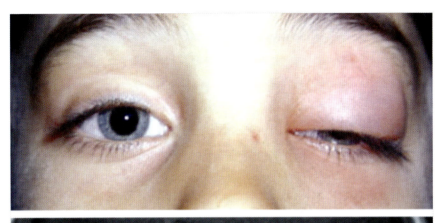

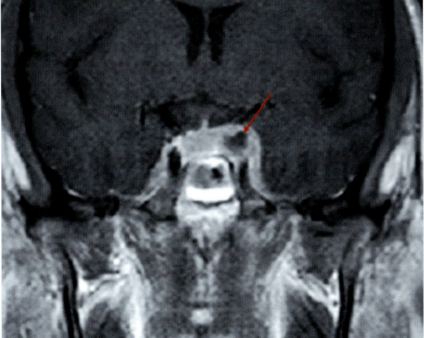

Fig. 15.15 (a) Left periorbital swelling, ptosis, proptosis, and ophthalmoplegia with headache secondary to left cavernous sinus thrombosis. (b) Coronal T1 weighted MRI with contract showing enlargement and enchancement of the left vacernous sinue (left cavernous sinus thrombosis) (*arrow*).

15.5 Superior Ophthalmic Vein Thrombosis

Thrombosis of the orbital veins produces a very acute and severe orbital syndrome (▶ Fig. 15.16). It is rare and usually occurs in the setting of sepsis or hypercoagulable state. It may also complicate a cavernous sinus thrombosis or a CCF.

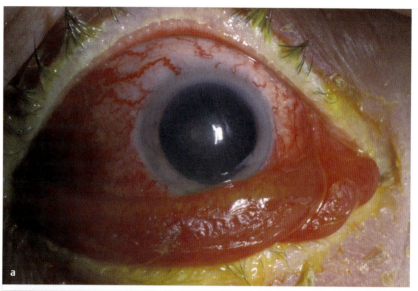

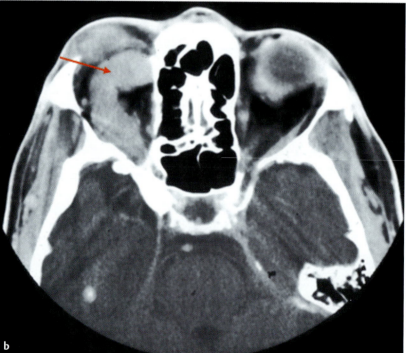

Fig. 15.16 (a) Severe chemosis and proptosis from superior ophthalmic vein thrombosis after orbital trauma. (b) Axial CT of the orbits with contrast showing a dilated superior ophthalmic vein in the right orbit (*red arrow*), suggesting a superior ophthalmic vein thrombosis. Note the major proptosis.

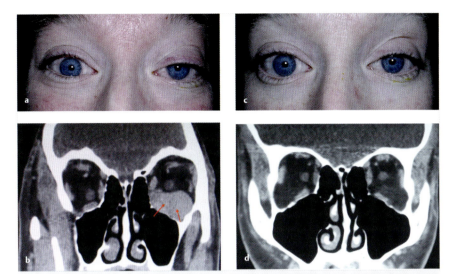

Fig. 15.17 (a) Left proptosis and periorbital fullness after Valsalva maneuver in a patient with a left orbital varix. (b) Coronal CT of the orbits after Valsalva maneuver shows a large varix (dilation of the inferior ophthalmic vein) in the left orbit *(red arrows)*. (c) After rest, the proptosis and fullness have resolved, but there is persistent mild left ptosis. (d) Coronal CT of the orbits after rest showing deflation of the varix.

15.6 Orbital Varix

Venous angiomas may occur in the orbit and are usually called orbital varices (▶ Fig. 15.17). Clinical presentation is characteristic and results from intermittent filling and emptying of the varix, resulting in variable proptosis.

Pearls

Consider orbital varix when there is eye bulging in a crying infant, proptosis during Valsalva maneuver, or orbital ecchymoses.

---

16 Nystagmus and Other Ocular Oscillations

Nystagmus is a rhythmic, repetitive oscillation of the eyes, initiated by a *slow* eye movement that drives the eye off target, followed by a fast movement that is corrective (jerk nystagmus) or another slow eye movement in the opposite direction (pendular nystagmus). Saccadic intrusions (opsoclonus and flutter) are abnormal rapid eye movements (saccades) that have no slow phase. All such eye movements disrupt fixation and may interfere with vision.

16.1 Nystagmus

Nystagmus may occur physiologically in response to an environmental stimulus or change in body position. It is also seen with diseases of the central nervous system or peripheral vestibular system and in some cases of visual loss.

Physiologic nystagmus or rapid gaze-evoked nystagmus is present only in extremes of horizontal gaze and dampens within seconds. It resolves when the eyes are in a slightly less eccentric position.

Pathologic nystagmus is characterized as jerk or pendular, and infantile (congenital) or acquired. In patients presenting with nystagmus and vertigo, it is essential to differentiate peripheral vestibular nystagmus from central nystagmus (▶ Table 16.1, ▶ Table 16.2, ▶ Table 16.3, ▶ Table 16.4).

Most patients with nystagmus complain of oscillopsia (oscillating vision with illusion that objects are moving), and in most cases, nystagmus can be recognized clinically without eye movement recording. However, eye movement recording allows far more

Table 16.1 Clinical description of nystagmus: jerk versus pendular

Jerk nystagmus	Pendular nystagmus
Alternation of slow phase drift followed by a rapid corrective saccade in the opposite direction	Sinusoidal oscillation with slow phases in both directions and no corrective saccades
Right- or left-beating horizontal nystagmus[a] Upbeat or downbeat nystagmus Torsional or rotary nystagmus (clockwise or counterclockwise)	May be horizontal or vertical but would not be characterized as right-, left-, up-, or downbeating because there is no fast phase

[a]Direction of jerk nystagmus = direction of the fast phase.

Table 16.2 Pendular nystagmus: acquired versus infantile (congenital)

	Acquired	Infantile (congenital)
Form	Pure sinusoidal	Variable waveforms
Different in the two eyes	Frequent	Rare
Direction	Omnidirectional (vertical, circular, elliptical)	Horizontal, uniplanar Rarely vertical or torsional
OKN reversal	Never	Frequent
Oscillopsia	Frequent	Mild (if any)

Abbreviation: OKN, optokinetic nystagmus.

Table 16.3 Peripheral versus central nystagmus

	Peripheral	Central
Feature	Unilateral[a] disease of vestibular organ or nerve Usually benign disease: Labyrinthitis Ménière disease	Disease of the brainstem and its connections with the vestibulocerebellum Any CNS disorder
Direction	Horizontal component[b] Mixed: horizontal/torsional, sometimes vertical component Fast phase away from lesion	Torsional pure Vertical pure Horizontal pure[c]
Visual fixation	Inhibits nystagmus	No inhibition
Frenzel goggles or darkness (inhibition of fixation)	Peripheral nystagmus increases in intensity	Central nystagmus is not changed
Severity of vertigo	Severe	Mild (except for Wallenberg syndrome)
Induced by head movements	Often	Rare
Associated eye movement deficits	None	May have pursuit or saccadic defects
Other findings	Hearing loss	May have cranial nerve or long tract signs No tinnitus or hearing loss

Abbreviation: CNS, central nervous system.
[a]Bilateral disease of vestibular organ and nerve (typically from drug toxicity) does not give nystagmus but produces loss of the vestibulo-ocular reflex.
[b]Intensity increases when the eyes are turned in the direction of the quick phase.
[c]Direction of nystagmus may change with gaze.

accurate characterization of the nystagmus by analyzing the slow phase (velocity, amplitude, and frequency) (▶ Fig. 16.1 and ▶ Fig. 16.2).

▶ Fig. 16.1 and ▶ Fig. 16.2 show the waveforms of horizontal jerk and pendular nystagmus.

16.1.1 Patient Evaluation

The goals of the evaluation are to decide whether there is a central or peripheral pattern of nystagmus and to determine if localization is possible based on the findings (▶ Table 16.3 and ▶ Table 16.4).

Symptoms include oscillopsia (absent in congenital nystagmus), decreased acuity, nausea or vomiting, and vertigo. There may be coexisting neurologic deficits.

Table 16.4 Differentiation of peripheral versus central nystagmus with the Dix–Hallpike maneuver

Findings	Peripheral	Central
Latency	Present	Absent
Duration	<1 min	>1 min
Fatigability	Yes	No
Reversal with upright position	Yes	No

Table 16.5 Localizing acquired central nystagmus

Jerk nystagmus	
Downbeat	Cervicomedullary junction Vestibulocerebellum[a] Medulla
Upbeat	Medulla Cerebellar vermis Midbrain
Periodic alternating	Cervicomedullary junction Cerebellum
Rebound	Cerebellum Medulla
Brun	Cerebellopontine angle
Dissociated jerk	Internuclear ophthalmoplegia (MLF in brainstem)
Pendular nystagmus	
Monocular (often vertical)	Visual loss
Seesaw	Parasellar lesions Septo-optic dysplasia
Oculopalatal myoclonus	Mollaret triangle (connecting red nucleus to inferior olive and dentate nucleus)
Oculomasticatory myorhythmia	Whipple disease

Abbreviation: MLF, medial longitudinal fasciculus.
[a]Vestibulocerebellum includes the flocculus, paraflocculus, nodulus, and uvula.

The examination (in primary position as well as all positions of gaze) differentiates jerk from pendular nystagmus. If the finding is jerk nystagmus, look for the direction of the fast phase—watch for a few minutes, as nystagmus may occasionally alternate directions. Look for coexisting head oscillations or head turns, the effect of convergence on nystagmus, the presence of a null point (eye position where nystagmus is least prominent), and subtle nystagmus or vestibular nystagmus that is suppressed by fixation. The last can be assessed by performing ophthalmoscopy in one eye while the patient fixates at distance, then covering the fixating eye. Nystagmus may then be viewed through the ophthalmoscope (the fast phase direction is the opposite of what it appears through the direct ophthalmoscope). Frenzel goggles may be used to assess nystagmus in the absence of fixation. Electronystagmography

(ENG) is another method of identifying nystagmus not present with eyes open. Finally, the Dix–Hallpike or Bárány maneuver can be done to look for positional nystagmus in patients who complain of positional vertigo (see ▶ Table 16.4; ▶ Fig. 16.3).

16.1.2 Infantile (Congenital) Nystagmus

Infantile (congenital) nystagmus is usually not noted at birth but becomes apparent during the first few months of life.

Characteristics

- Horizontal nystagmus (mixed pendular and jerk); may have a rotary component.
- There are bilateral conjugate movements of the eyes.

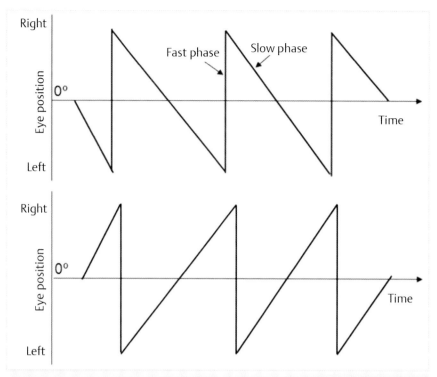

Fig. 16.1 Jerk nystagmus. (a) Right-beating nystagmus (fast phase beats to the right, slow phase drifts to the left). (b) Left-beating nystagmus (fast phase beats to the left, slow phase drifts to the right).

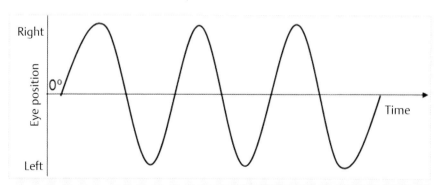

Fig. 16.2 Pendular nystagmus. Sinusoidal wave (there is no fast phase).

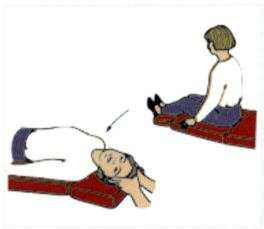

Fig. 16.3 Dix-Hallpike maneuver. The patient is brought suddenly from sitting to a supine position, while the head is turned 45 degrees to one side and extended about 20 degrees backward. The test is positive when the patient develops a burst of nystagmus. The test can be made more sensitive by having the patient wear Frenzel goggles, which suppress fixation and magnify the eyes, thereby making the nystagmus more obvious. (From Rohkamm R. Color Atlas of Neurology. New York, NY: Thieme; 2004:59. Reprinted by permission.)

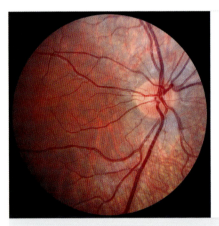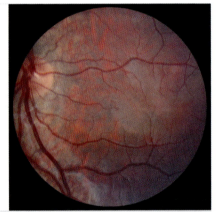

Fig. 16.4 Infantile nystagmus in a patient with albinism and bilateral foveal hypoplasia (no fovea can be seen).

- Nystagmus is not present during sleep.
- There may be associated latent nystagmus.
- Null point (the preferred eye position for the patient to fixate) usually results in a head turn.
- Convergence decreases the nystagmus, and fixation increases it.
- Patients may have a head tremor that in some cases improves visual acuity.
- Reverse response to optokinetic stimulus may be seen (fast phase in direction of moving optokinetic nystagmus [OKN] tape).
  - Nystagmus may be seen in isolation (also called congenital motor nystagmus), or it may be associated with strabismus or afferent visual system defects (e.g., albinism (see ▶ Fig. 16.4), congenital stationary night blindness, or optic nerve hypoplasia).
  - There is no oscillopsia, but there is decreased visual acuity (related to associated afferent conditions and to the nystagmus present in primary gaze).

> **Pearls**
>
> Children with nystagmus should undergo a thorough ophthalmologic examination because underlying visual loss from a variety of retinal, optic nerve, or cerebral etiologies is a common cause.

Treatment

Treatment of infantile nystagmus includes the following:
- Use base-out prisms to induce convergence (dampens the nystagmus and may improve visual acuity).
- Use prisms to shift the viewing position into the null region.
- Contact lenses may dampen the nystagmus.
- Gabapentin may dampen the nystagmus.
- Surgical procedures include moving the extraocular muscles to place the null zone in primary position (Kestenbaum procedure) and recessing all four horizontal rectus muscles to decrease their tension (large-recession procedure).

Other Types of Infantile Nystagmus

Latent Nystagmus

This is a variant of infantile nystagmus that is not evident during binocular fixation but appears when either eye is covered (uncovered eye beats away from the covered eye). It is often seen in infantile esotropia (most common), often with amblyopia, and with any lesion disrupting binocular development in the first 6 months of life. It is also common in Down syndrome.

Spasmus Nutans

Spasmus nutans involves a triad of symptoms:
- Very asymmetric and occasionally monocular nystagmus (rapid pendular eye movements)
- Head nodding
- Torticollis (head tilt or head turn)

Onset is usually in the first year of life, with the nystagmus typically lasting for several months. The condition is usually benign with no neurologic abnormalities.

Neuroimaging is recommended (anterior visual pathway gliomas may mimic spasmus nutans). Ophthalmologic evaluation and possibly electroretinogram are recommended (retinal disorders causing visual loss may mimic spasmus nutans).

Infantile Monocular Pendular Nystagmus

This is usually due to visual loss (often optic neuropathy or chiasmal glioma). In cases of bilateral visual loss, there is bilateral nystagmus, with nystagmus greater in the eye with the poorest vision.

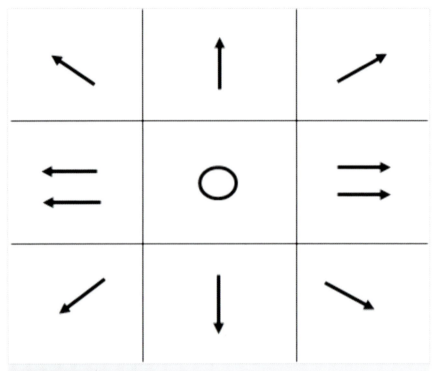

Fig. 16.5 Gaze-evoked nystagmus is upbeating in upgaze, right-beating in right gaze, and so on.

16.1.3 Acquired Nystagmus

Gaze-Evoked Nystagmus

Gaze-evoked is the most common type of nystagmus (see ▶ Fig. 16.5). It is absent in the primary position and is not visually disabling. Jerk nystagmus beats in the direction of gaze. It results from impairment in eccentric gaze-holding mechanisms, such as from sedative medications/anticonvulsants and brainstem and cerebellar lesions (central vestibular dysfunction).

Nystagmus with Positional Vertigo

Paroxysmal vertigo occurs only in certain positions. When the Dix–Hallpike maneuver (see ▶ Fig. 16.3) is performed, nystagmus is seen (see ▶ Table 16.4). Most patients have benign paroxysmal positional vertigo (BPPV) from a peripheral lesion, usually canalolithiasis or cupulolithiasis in the posterior semicircular canal. BPPV does not respond well to medications but may have a long-term favorable response to numerous maneuvers aimed at dislodging the debris from the posterior semicircular canal. Positional vertigo may also occur with central nervous system disease.

Acquired Central Nystagmus

The most important goal of the evaluation is to identify those patterns of nystagmus that have a localizing value.

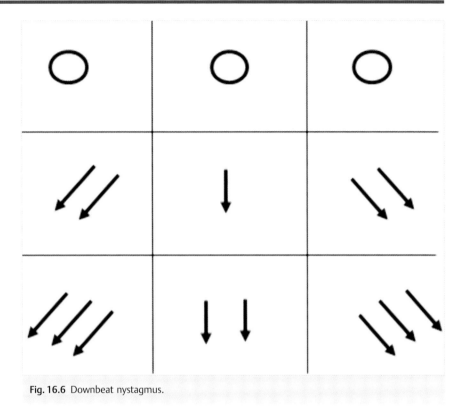

Fig. 16.6 Downbeat nystagmus.

Downbeat Nystagmus

Downbeat nystagmus is a type of jerk nystagmus, with the fast phase downward in the primary position (▶ Fig. 16.6). The nystagmus decreases in upgaze and worsens in downgaze; it is usually most prominent in lateral gaze and downgaze. Oscillopsia is usually prominent because the nystagmus is present in primary position and in downgaze, the preferred reading position.

Downbeat nystagmus is caused by lesions at the cervicomedullary junction, foramen magnum, vestibulocerebellum, and medulla. It is commonly seen in cerebellar degenerations; paraneoplastic syndromes; Chiari malformation (▶ Fig. 16.7); encephalitis; trauma; hypomagnesemia; thiamine deficiency; B12 deficiency; and toxicity with lithium, alcohol, amiodarone, toluene, phenytoin, and carbamazepine.

The treatment of downbeat nystagmus is limited. Removal of a toxic drug and treatment of vitamin deficiency way result in improvement. Aminopyridines, clonazepam, valproate, baclofen, and gabapentin may dampen downbeat nystagmus. Patients should be advised to avoid looking down and to not use glasses with bifocal or progressive lenses. Base-down prisms in reading glasses can be used to force the eyes upward.

Upbeat Nystagmus

Upbeat nystagmus is a type of jerk nystagmus with fast phase upward in primary position (▶ Fig. 16.8). It often worsens in upgaze.

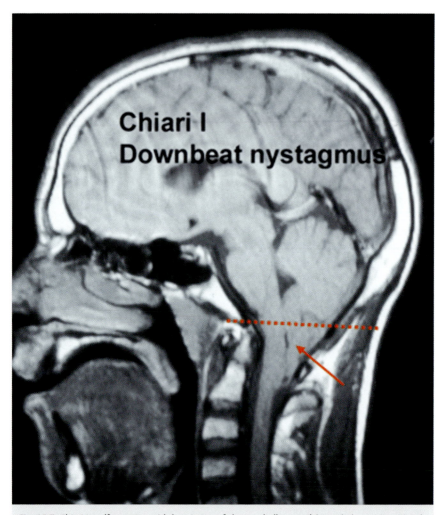

Fig. 16.7 Chiari I malformation with herniation of the cerebellar tonsil (*arrow*). (see ▶ Fig. 20.61).

It may be caused by lesions of the medulla, cerebellar vermis, and midbrain and is commonly seen in Wernicke encephalopathy and encephalitis.

Aminopyridines and baclofen may dampen upbeat nystagmus. Patients should avoid looking up and should not use glasses with progressive lenses. Base-up prisms in reading glasses can be used to force the eyes downward.

Periodic Alternating Nystagmus

Periodic alternating nystagmus (PAN) is a type of horizontal jerk nystagmus that alternates direction in primary position (i.e., jerk nystagmus to the right for about 60 to 90 seconds, which diminishes, only to begin beating to the left for another 60 to 90 seconds) (▶ Fig. 16.9). Patients may have a periodic alternating head turn to minimize the nystagmus, and oscillopsia is usually present.

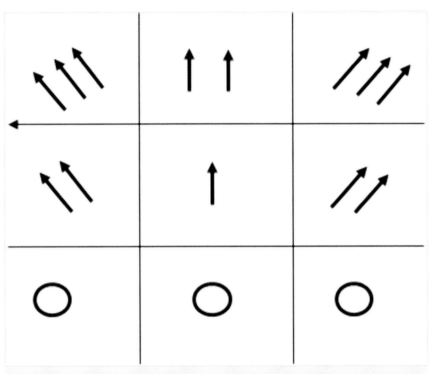

Fig. 16.8 Upbeat nystagmus.

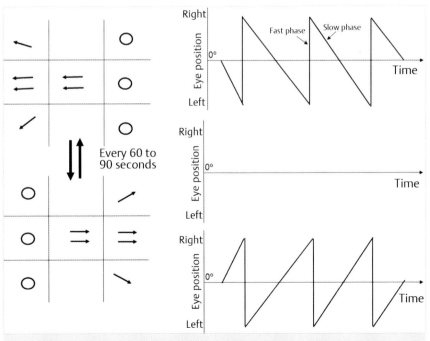

Fig. 16.9 Periodic alternating nystagmus (as seen by the examiner).

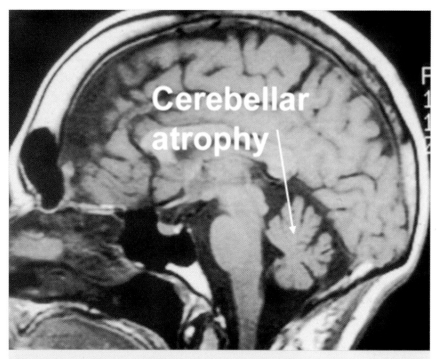

Fig. 16.10 Cerebellar atrophy related to spinocerebellar degeneration.

PAN is caused by lesions of the cerebellum, particularly the nodulus and uvula, and by lesions of the cervicomedullary junction. It is commonly seen in multiple sclerosis, cerebellar degenerations (▶ Fig. 16.10), Chiari malformations, trauma, hepatic encephalopathy, and albinism, as well as with use of anticonvulsants and lithium. It is responsive to baclofen.

Rebound Nystagmus

Rebound nystagmus is seen in some patients with gaze-evoked nystagmus. It is the reversal of jerk nystagmus direction after sustained eccentric gaze.

Rebound nystagmus is caused by cerebellar disorders and lesions of the medulla (in the region of the nucleus prepositus hypoglossi and medial vestibular nucleus).

Brun Nystagmus

Brun nystagmus is a combination of unilateral peripheral vestibular nystagmus from an eighth nerve tumor (▶ Fig. 16.11) and gaze-paretic central nystagmus as the tumor compresses the pons. It is characterized by high-frequency, low-amplitude nystagmus on looking away from the lesion, beating in the direction of gaze (due to the vestibular lesion), and low-frequency, high-amplitude horizontal nystagmus on looking toward the lesion, beating in the direction of gaze (due to defective gaze holding). Brun nystagmus is caused by large tumors in the cerebellopontine angle.

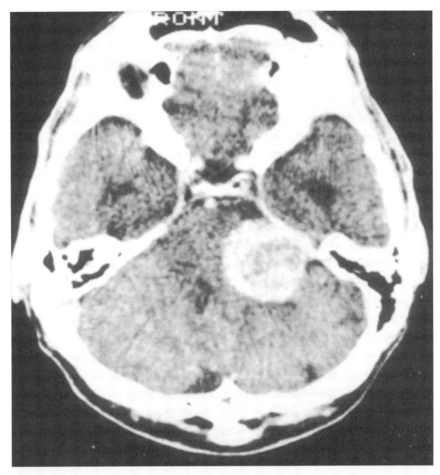

Fig. 16.11 Large left acoustic neuroma producing Brun nystagmus.

Dissociated Jerk Nystagmus

Dissociated jerk nystagmus refers to nystagmus that is different in the two eyes. The most common cause is internuclear ophthalmoplegia (adduction deficit associated with a contralateral abducting nystagmus) (▶ Fig. 16.12). The abducting nystagmus may be an adaptive mechanism to overcome the adduction paresis.

Acquired Pendular Nystagmus

One of the most common types of nystagmus is acquired pendular nystagmus, which is visually disabling because of severe oscillopsia (▶ Fig. 16.2).

It most commonly is caused by multiple sclerosis. Oscillopsia may improve with gabapentin, memantine, clonazepam, or valproate.

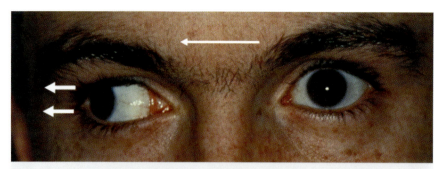

Fig. 16.12 Left internuclear ophthalmoplegia in multiple sclerosis. The patient looks to the right (*arrow*). The left eye does not adduct and there is nystagmus on the right abducting eye (*double arrow*).

Seesaw Nystagmus

Seesaw nystagmus (▶ Fig. 16.13) is defined as pendular nystagmus with elevation and intorsion of one eye simultaneous with depression and extorsion of the other eye, followed by a reversal of the cycle, so that the eyes move like a seesaw.

Seesaw nystagmus produces very disabling oscillopsia that responds poorly to any treatment. It is most often caused by parasellar lesions and may be seen with pituitary tumors (▶ Fig. 16.14), craniopharyngiomas, septo-optic dysplasia, and brainstem lesions (especially in the midbrain).

Oculopalatal Myoclonus (or Tremor)

Oculopalatal myoclonus is a type of vertical pendular nystagmus coexisting with a tremor of the palate and/or facial muscles, larynx, and diaphragm. It is present during sleep.

It usually develops months after an infarction or hemorrhage involving the Mollaret triangle (the region connecting the red nucleus to the inferior olive and the dentate nucleus; ▶ Fig. 16.15) but can also be delayed after trauma to this region.

The condition may improve with gabapentin, anticholinergic agents, or ceruletide.

Oculomasticatory Myorhythmia

Oculomasticatory myorhythmia is defined as pendular nystagmus with pendular convergence and divergence movements of the eyes, with occasional movements of the jaw, face, or limbs. It is often associated with a supranuclear vertical gaze palsy and is pathognomonic of Whipple disease.

> **Pearls**
>
> Wernicke encephalopathy (vitamin B1 deficiency—occurs most often in the setting of alcoholism and bariatric surgery) may produce any type of nystagmus. Intravenous thiamine should be given to any confused patient with nystagmus.

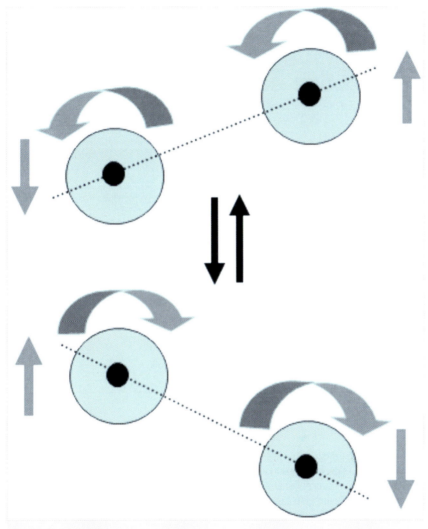

Fig. 16.13 Seesaw nystagmus.

16.1.4 Management of Nystagmus

The aim of management is to improve oscillopsia and/or visual blurring.

Drug therapy is often empirical; there are usually poor results, except for PAN and some cases of acquired pendular nystagmus. Commonly used medications include the following:

• Baclofen (periodic alternating nystagmus)
• Gabapentin (acquired pendular nystagmus)
• Memantine (acquired pendular nystagmus)
• Aminopyridines (downbeat and upbeat nystagmus)

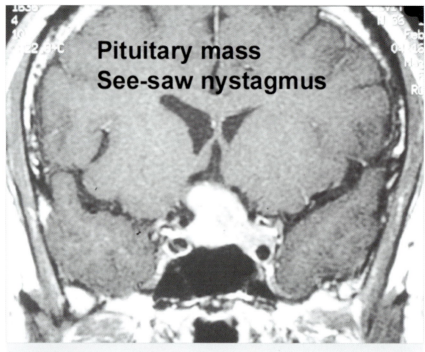

Fig. 16.14 Large pituitary tumor.

- Clonazepam
- Valproate
- Trihexyphenidyl or other anticholinergics

Other treatment possibilities are prisms to move the null point into primary position or away from a triggering gaze (i.e., move the eyes up in cases of downbeat nystagmus), or to induce convergence; contact lenses to dampen the nystagmus; eye muscle surgery (Kestenbaum procedure) to move the null point into primary position; and injection of botulinum toxin in the extraocular muscles to immobilize the eye (but this induces diplopia and often requires patching of one eye).

16.2 Other Nystagmoid Eye Movements

16.2.1 Convergence–Retraction Nystagmus

Convergence–retraction nystagmus (▶ Fig. 16.16a) is not truly nystagmus, but rather bilateral adducting saccades causing convergence of both eyes, without any slow phase. It is most often elicited by having the patient attempt to look up, at which time the eyes converge and retract in the orbit. The retraction is best seen by observing the patient from the side.

Convergence–retraction nystagmus is one of many signs of Parinaud dorsal midbrain syndrome (upgaze paresis, light-near dissociation of the pupils, and upper eyelid retraction). It is caused by midbrain/posterior commissure lesions (▶ Fig. 16.16b).

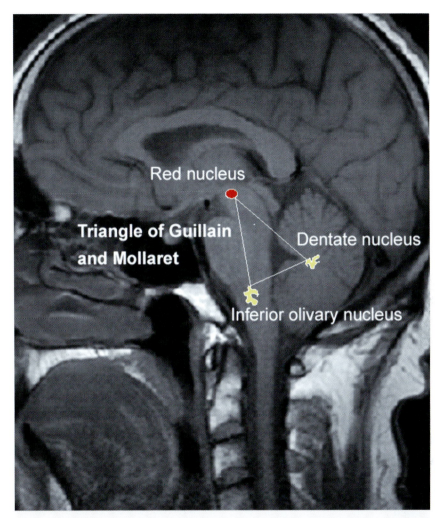

Fig. 16.15 Mollaret triangle.

16.2.2 Superior Oblique Myokymia

Superior oblique myokymia (▶ Fig. 16.17) is defined as oscillation of one eye due to intermittent firing of the superior oblique muscle (myokymia or tremor of the superior oblique muscle). It produces oscillopsia or intermittent diplopia, elicited by having the patient look in the direction of the superior oblique muscle, and is characterized by monocular, rapid, intorsional movements. It is best seen at the slit lamp or with an ophthalmoscope.

Superior oblique myokymia is usually benign, and no underlying etiology is found. However, neuroimaging is recommended, looking for posterior fossa tumors. Superior oblique myokymia is usually chronic with periods of remission.

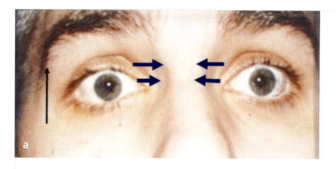

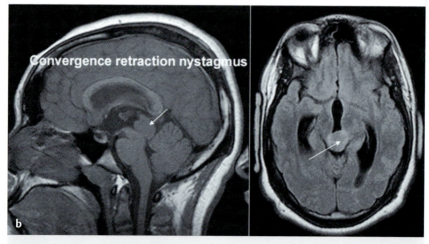

Fig. 16.16 (a) Convergence–retraction nystagmus (*blue arrows*) with attempted upgaze (*black arrow*). (b) Lesion (*arrows*) with mass effect on the posterior commissure.

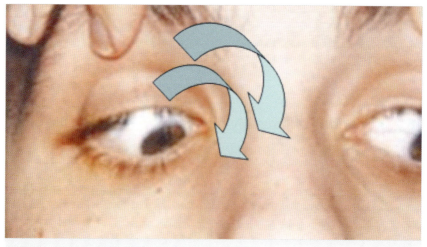

Fig. 16.17 Right superior oblique myokymia (*blue arrows*).

Treatment includes carbamazepine, baclofen, or propanolol. Surgical weakening of the superior oblique muscle may be performed in refractory cases.

16.2.3 Ocular Bobbing

Ocular bobbing is characterized by conjugate eye movements beginning with a fast downward movement, followed by a slow drift back to the midline (similar to a fish bob in the water). It is commonly found in comatose patients with a massive pontine lesion or metabolic encephalopathy.

16.3 Saccadic Intrusions

Saccadic intrusions are often mistaken for nystagmus. In contrast to nystagmus, in which there is always a slow-phase eye movement, saccadic oscillations are saccades (rapid refixational eye movements) without any slow phases.

16.3.1 Ocular Flutter

Ocular flutter (▶ Fig. 16.18) is characterized by intermittent bursts of back-to-back horizontal saccades without any interval between saccades. There is no vertical component. Bursts of ocular flutter typically last for seconds at a time. The strictly horizontal direction distinguishes ocular flutter from opsoclonus, and the lack of interval between the saccades distinguishes ocular flutter from square-wave jerks.

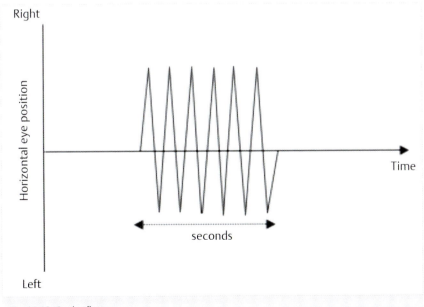

Fig. 16.18 Ocular flutter.

16.3.2 Opsoclonus

Opsoclonus is back-to-back saccades in multiple directions, including horizontal, vertical, and torsional (sometimes referred to as saccadomania). These movements are higher amplitude and last longer than typical ocular flutter. Eye movements are often associated with blinking, facial twitching, myoclonus, and ataxia ("dancing eyes and dancing feet").

Causes of Ocular Flutter and Opsoclonus

Causes of ocular flutter and opsoclonus include the following:
- Paraneoplastic:
  - Neuroblastoma in children: 50% of children with opsoclonus harbor a neuroblastoma; 2% of children with neuroblastoma have opsoclonus.
  - Small cell carcinomas and other cancers associated with anti-Ri antibodies in adults
- Encephalitis, cerebellitis
- Intracranial tumor, hydrocephalus, thalamic hemorrhage, multiple sclerosis, nonketotic hyperosmolar coma, drug toxicity (lithium, phenytoin, and cocaine)

16.3.3 Square-Wave Jerks and Macrosquare-Wave Jerks

Horizontal to-and-fro saccades that interrupt fixation are referred to as squarewave jerks (▶ Fig. 16.19). Unlike ocular flutter, square-wave jerks have intersaccadic intervals. They are termed macrosquare-wave jerks when the amplitude is > 5 degrees.

Common causes include cerebellar diseases, Parkinson disease, and progressive supranuclear palsy.

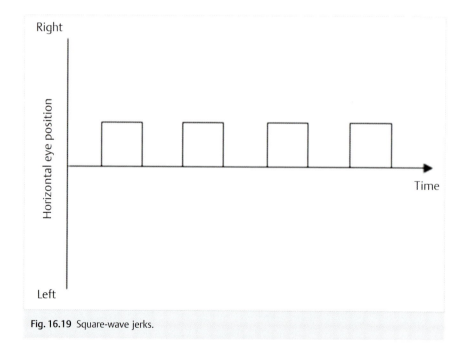

Fig. 16.19 Square-wave jerks.

16.3.4 Ocular Dysmetria

In ocular dysmetria, the eye overshoots (saccadic hypermetria) or undershoots (saccadic hypometria) the target upon refixation. It then saccades back or forward to the intended fixation point (back-up or catch-up saccade).

It is a sign of cerebellar dysfunction similar to limb dysmetria.

16.3.5 Voluntary Nystagmus

Some normal subjects can induce ocular oscillations (often with convergence and subtle movements of the eyelids such as squinting) mimicking ocular flutter accompanied by convergence effort.

16.4 Summary of the Evaluation of the Patient with Ocular Oscillations (▶ Fig. 16.20)

The diagram below summarizes the steps necessary for the characterization of ocular oscillations.

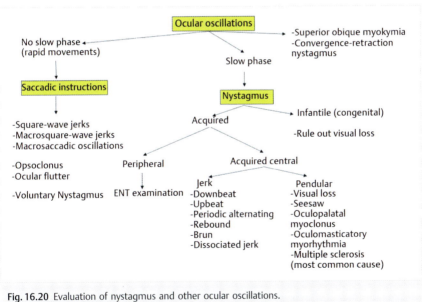

Fig. 16.20 Evaluation of nystagmus and other ocular oscillations. ENT, ear, nose, and throat.

17 Disorders of the Eyelid

The eyelid protects the eye and helps maintain the corneal tear film. Eyelid disorders compromise vision by covering the eye (and covering the visual axis) or by exposing the cornea (resulting in abnormal tear film and blurry vision and complications from corneal exposure).

Abnormalities of the eyelid commonly encountered in neuro-ophthalmology include ptosis (drooping of the eyelid), retraction (abnormal elevation of the eyelid), facial weakness (incomplete eyelid closure), and abnormal blinking (decreased or increased).

17.1 Anatomy and Examination of the Eyelid

Eyelid closure (▶ Fig. 17.1, ▶ Fig. 17.2, ▶ Fig. 17.3) involves the orbicularis oculi muscle (innervated by branches of the facial nerve: cranial nerve [CN] VII).

Eyelid opening involves the frontalis muscle (facial nerve), the levator palpebrae (oculomotor nerve: CN III), the Müller muscle and inferior tarsal muscles (sympathetic innervation), and the aponeurosis of the levator muscle attached to the superior tarsal plate.

Eyelid position depends on the resting tone of the levator muscle, which varies with the patient's state of arousal. Eyelid movements are coordinated with vertical eye movements: the eyelids move up and down with the eyes.

Examination of the eyelid includes evaluation of the position of the eyelids (looking for possible ptosis and retraction) and lid function, and inspection of the eyelid for any swelling or mass. It includes measurements of the palpebral fissure (9–12 mm), the margin reflex distance (4–5 mm), and the levator function, or the difference of position of the lid margin when the patient looks down, then up (> 12 mm) (▶ Fig. 17.4 and ▶ Fig. 17.5).

Palpation and inversion of the eyelids should be performed in all patients with ptosis.

When the eyelids are abnormal, the examiner should look for the presence of an orbital syndrome, diplopia with abnormal extraocular movements, and pupillary abnormalities, and should determine whether the findings are unilateral or bilateral.

17.2 Ptosis

Ptosis can be either congenital or acquired.

17.2.1 Congenital Ptosis

Congenital ptosis is present at birth or early childhood. It can be isolated or accompanied by an elevation deficit of the eye (elevator palsy). There is also incomplete lowering of the eyelid in downgaze, resulting in lid lag. The abnormal eyelid does not stretch well in downgaze (▶ Fig. 17.6) because there is congenital maldevelopment of the levator palpebrae or its tendon.

Causes of lid droop at birth include the following:
- Congenital ptosis
- Marcus Gunn jaw winking
- Congenital fibrosis

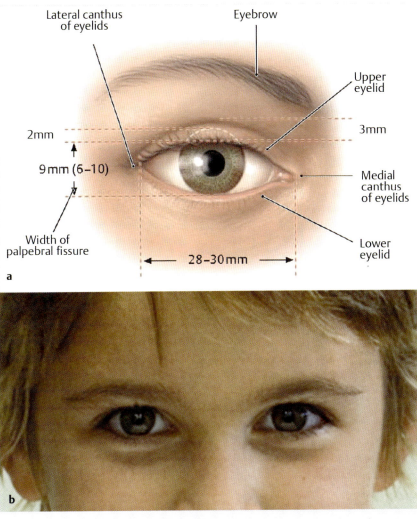

Fig. 17.1 (a) External appearance of the eyelid. (From Schuenke M, Schulte E, Schumacher U, Ross LM, Lamperti ED, Voll M. THIEME Atlas of Anatomy, Head and Neuroanatomy. Stuttgart, Germany: Thieme; 2007. Illustration by Markus Voll.) (b) Normal eyelids. In normal individuals, the upper lid covers the superior 1 to 2 mm of the iris, and the lower lid just reaches the inferior aspect of the iris.

- Blepharophimosis syndrome (bilateral ptosis, telecanthus, epicanthus inversus)
- Congenital (neonatal) myasthenia
- Congenital third nerve palsy
- Birth trauma (third nerve palsy, Horner syndrome)
- Lid or orbital tumors (neurofibroma, hemangioma, dermoid)

Marcus Gunn jaw winking is a form of congenital ptosis associated with trigemino-oculomotor synkinesis (▶ Fig. 17.7)

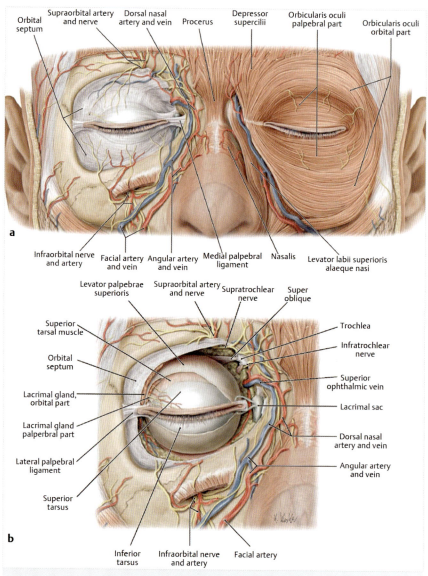

Fig. 17.2 Anatomy of the eyelid showing the superficial (a) and deep (b) layers. (From Schuenke M, Schulte E, Schumacher U, Ross LM, Lamperti ED, Voll M. THIEME Atlas of Anatomy, Head and Neuroanatomy. Stuttgart, Germany: Thieme; 2007. Illustration by Karl Wesker.)

- Ptotic eyelid that retracts during contraction of the external pterygoid muscle (e.g., while sucking, opening the mouth, or moving the jaw)
- Aberrant connection between the motor branches of the trigeminal nerve (CN V3) innervating the external pterygoid muscle and the fibers of the superior division of the oculomotor nerve (CN III) that innervate the levator superioris muscle of the upper eyelid (trigemino-oculomotor synkinesis)

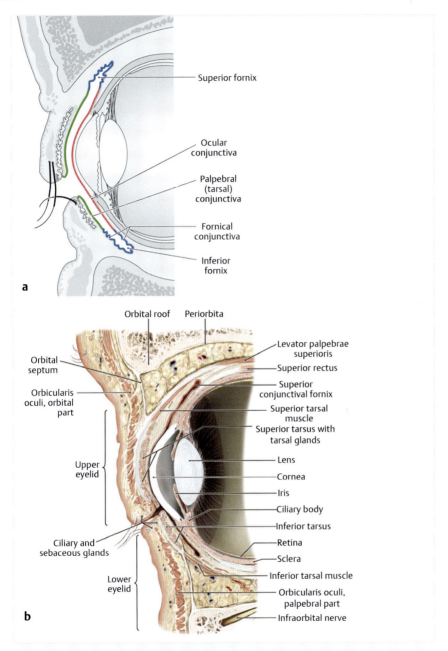

Fig. 17.3 **(a)** Sagittal view through the eyelid. (From Schuenke M, Schulte E, Schumacher U, Ross LM, Lamperti ED, Voll M. THIEME Atlas of Anatomy, Head and Neuroanatomy. Stuttgart, Germany: Thieme; 2007. Illustration by Markus Voll.) **(b)** Sagittal view through the eyelid. (From Schuenke M, Schulte E, Schumacher U, Ross LM, Lamperti ED, Voll M. THIEME Atlas of Anatomy, Head and Neuroanatomy. Stuttgart, Germany: Thieme; 2007. Illustration by Karl Wesker.)

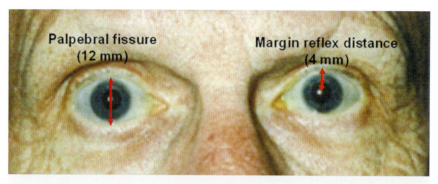

Fig. 17.4 Measurement of the palpebral fissure and margin reflex distance. The palpebral fissure is the distance between the upper and lower eyelid in vertical alignment with the center of the pupil (normal 9–12 mm). The margin (or marginal) reflex distance (normal 4–5 mm) can be measured for the upper and the lower eyelids:
— Marginal reflex distance-1 (MRD-1): distance between the center of the pupillary light reflex and the upper eyelid margin with the eye in primary gaze
— Marginal reflex distance-2 (MRD-2): distance between the center of the pupillary light reflex and the lower eyelid margin with the eye in primary gaze

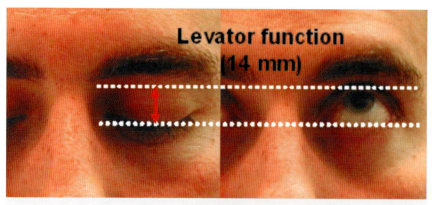

Fig. 17.5 Measurement of levator function. The levator function is the distance the eyelid travels from downgaze to upgaze while the frontalis muscle is held inactive at the brow. A measurement of > 10 mm is considered excellent, whereas 0 to 5 mm is considered poor.

17.2.2 Acquired Ptosis

Causes of acquired unilateral or bilateral ptosis include the following:
• Mechanical ptosis
  ○ Aponeurotic defect (levator dehiscence)
    – Aging
    – Trauma, surgery (ocular with use of speculum, orbital)
    – Contact lens use

- ○ Dermatochalasis
- ○ Cicatricial
- ○ Eyelid or orbital tumor
- ○ Inflammation
  - – Edema
  - – Allergy
  - – Chalazion
  - – Blepharitis
  - – Blepharochalasis
- Myogenic ptosis
  - ○ Chronic progressive external ophthalmoplegia (CPEO)
  - ○ Myotonic dystrophy
  - ○ Oculopharyngeal dystrophy
  - ○ Chronic use of topical ocular steroid drops

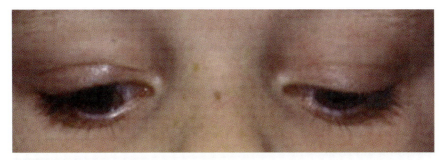

Fig. 17.6 Congenital right ptosis. Note that the right eyelid remains elevated when the patient looks down.

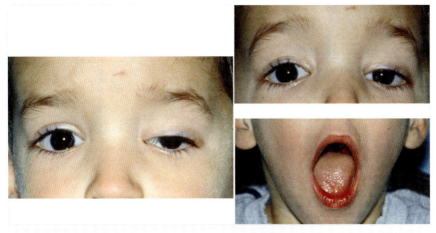

Fig. 17.7 Left Marcus Gunn jaw-winking sign. Note the left ptosis, which improves with mouth opening.

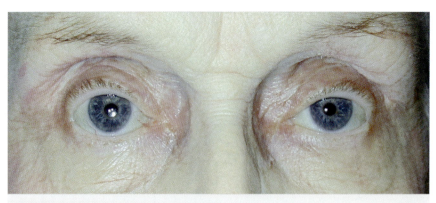

Fig. 17.8 Aponeurotic defect from senile ptosis.

- Disorder of neuromuscular transmission
  - Myasthenia gravis
  - Botulism
- Neurogenic ptosis
  - Horner syndrome (oculosympathetic paresis)
  - Third nerve palsy
  - Apraxia of lid opening

Mechanical Ptosis

Aponeurotic ptosis (▶ Fig. 17.8) is usually bilateral. The upper eyelid crease is high or indistinct, and levator function is relatively preserved.

In elderly patients, an aponeurotic defect may be associated with dermatochalasis. The aponeurosis of the levator muscle dehisces or disinserts from the tarsal plate of the upper lid (usually bilateral). It is also common after ocular surgery requiring a speculum (usually unilateral). In younger patients, it is usually secondary to contact lens wear.

Pearls

Aponeurotic defect is the most common cause of acquired ptosis in adults.

Lesions of the eyelid (e.g., tumor, chalazion, and vascular malformations) can produce a mechanical ptosis (▶ Fig. 17.9 and ▶ Fig. 17.10).

Pearls

Palpation and inversion of the eyelids should be performed in all patients with ptosis.

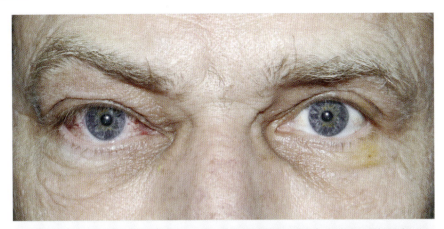

Fig. 17.9 Vascular malformation of the anterior right orbit responsible for redness of the right eye and right ptosis. (There is a dilated vein in the right upper eyelid.)

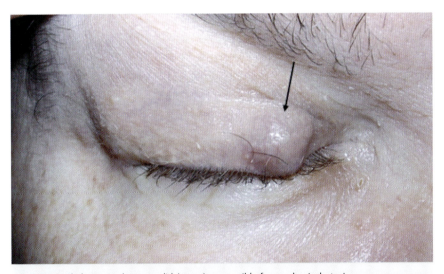

Fig. 17.10 Chalazion in the upper lid (*arrow*) responsible for mechanical ptosis.

Myogenic Ptosis

Myogenic ptosis (▶ Fig. 17.11 and ▶ Fig. 17.12) is usually bilateral and progressive. It is commonly associated with impaired eye movements. There may not be diplopia if the eyes are straight in primary position and if the ophthalmoplegia is complete. The pupils are always normal. Chronic progressive external ophthalmoplegia (mitochondrial disorder) is a classic cause.

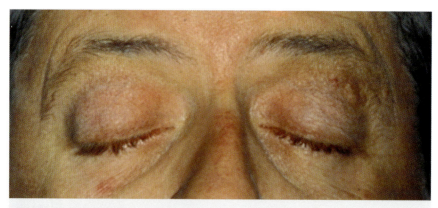

Fig. 17.11 Bilateral complete ptosis in chronic progressive external ophthalmoplegia. The patient also had complete bilateral ophthalmoplegia.

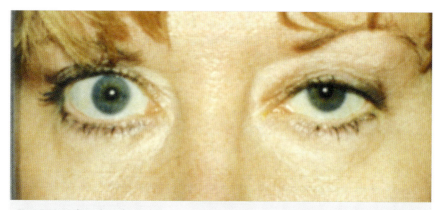

Fig. 17.12 Unilateral moderate left ptosis in chronic progressive external ophthalmoplegia. The patient had diffusely reduced eye movements in both eyes. The pupils were normal.

Pearls

It is essential to rule out myasthenia gravis in all patients with presumed myogenic ptosis.

Ptosis Resulting from a Neuromuscular Transmission Disorder

Myasthenia gravis is a classic cause of unilateral or bilateral ptosis (▶ Fig. 17.13). Myasthenic ptosis may be isolated, or it may be associated with oculomotor paresis. The pupils are always normal. The hallmark of myasthenic ptosis is fluctuation. The ptosis usually reverses with a Tensilon test (see Chapter 13).

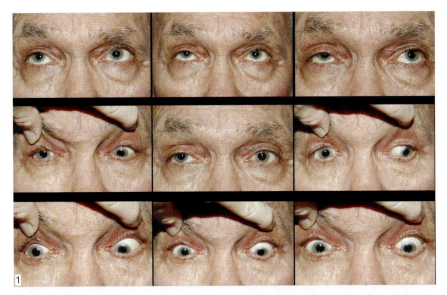

Fig. 17.13 Bilateral ptosis (right worse than left) with diffuse bilateral ophthalmoplegia (right worse than left) from myasthenia gravis.

Neurogenic Ptosis

Lesions of the Oculosympathetic Pathways

Lesions of the oculosympathetic pathways produce an ipsilateral Horner syndrome, which consists of mild ptosis (reduced palpebral fissure) and impaired dilation of the pupil, with anisocoria worse in the dark and dilation lag (▶ Fig. 17.14 and ▶ Fig. 17.15a). The ptosis results from denervation of the Müller muscle and inferior tarsal muscle of the lower lid. It is usually mild and usually 1 to 2 mm, although 3 or 4 mm of ptosis can sometimes be observed. The ptosis from Horner syndrome resolves after administration of topical apraclonidine 0.5% or 1.0%. Apraclonidine drops are useful for the diagnosis of Horner syndrome (it reverses the anisocoria). It can also be used to improve the ptosis (▶ Fig. 17.15b).

Lesions of the Third Nerve

Lesions of the third cranial nerve produce an ipsilateral ptosis. The ptosis results from weakness of the levator palpebrae muscle and may be complete or mild. It is never isolated: the eye movements are abnormal, and the pupil may be dilated. When the ptosis is complete, diplopia may not be noticed by the patient (▶ Fig. 17.16). A lesion of the third nerve nucleus in the midbrain produces bilateral ptosis.

Apraxia of Eyelid Opening

Apraxia of eyelid opening is the inability to open the eyelid not explained by levator dysfunction. It is believed to be a supranuclear disorder. Patients can often open their

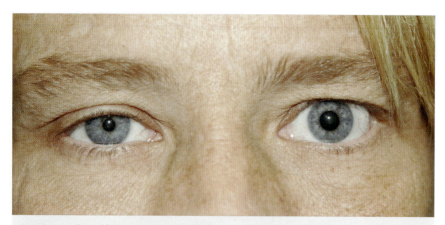

Fig. 17.14 Right mild ptosis with anisocoria from a right Horner syndrome.

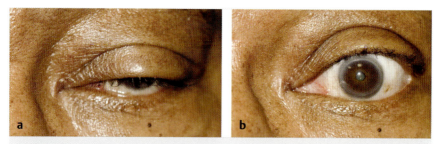

Fig. 17.15 (a) Unusually severe left ptosis with miosis from a left Horner syndrome. (b) After apraclonidine, the ptosis has dramatically improved.

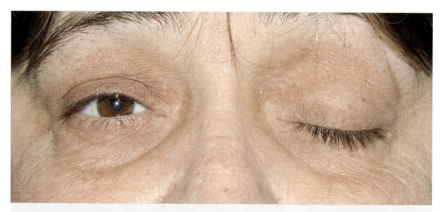

Fig. 17.16 Complete left ptosis from a left third nerve palsy.

eyelids after touching the orbital rim or after sudden command. Apraxia occurs in association with essential blepharospasm, Parkinson syndromes, Huntington disease, and cerebral lesions.

Cerebral Ptosis

Very rarely, a unilateral hemispheric lesion can cause unilateral or bilateral ptosis without third nerve palsy. It is called cerebral ptosis, and it is believed to be a supranuclear disorder.

17.2.3 Pseudoptosis

In all cases of ptosis, pseudoptosis needs to be ruled out (▶ Fig. 17.17 and ▶ Fig. 17.18).
  Causes of pseudoptosis include the following:
- Dermatochalasis
- Contralateral lid retraction
- Contralateral peripheral facial palsy
- Duane syndrome

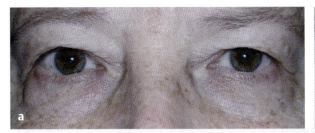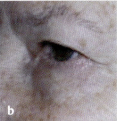

Fig. 17.17 (a) Dermatochalasis with pseudoptosis. Note the excess skinfolds over the eyelids. The levator function and the eyelid position are normal when the excess skin is pulled up. (b) Dermatochalasis. Note the redundant fold of skin over the eyelid.

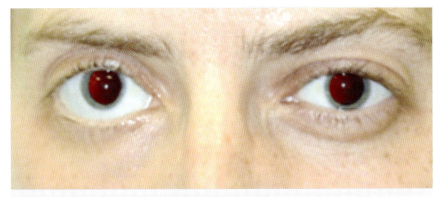

Fig. 17.18 Pseudoptosis on the left. There is abnormal widening of the right palpebral fissure (lagophthalmos) from right peripheral facial palsy.

- Microphthalmos
- Enophthalmos
- Voluntary ptosis (see ▸ Fig. 18.11)
- Blepharospasm

17.3 Eyelid Retraction

Eyelid retraction is diagnosed when sclera is seen between the lower edge of the upper eyelid and the limbus (edge of the iris).

Causes of lid retraction can be mechanical, myogenic, or neurogenic. The three most common causes of lid retraction are thyroid eye disease, dorsal midbrain syndrome (Collier sign), and contralateral ptosis.

Causes of lid retraction include the following:

- Mechanical
  - Proptosis
  - High myopia (pseudoproptosis)
  - Ocular or orbital surgery
  - Eyelid scarring
  - Contralateral ptosis
- Myogenic
  - Thyroid eye disease
  - Congenital
- Neurogenic
  - Dorsal midbrain syndrome (Collier sign)
  - Marcus Gun jaw winking
  - Aberrant regeneration of the third nerve
  - Third nerve palsy with cyclic spasms
  - Neuromyotonia involving the third nerve
  - Facial nerve paresis

Lid retraction from thyroid eye disease is usually bilateral and is often associated with lid lag in downgaze (▸ Fig. 17.19, ▸ Fig. 17.20, ▸ Fig. 17.21).

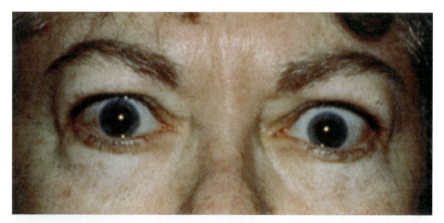

Fig. 17.19 Bilateral lid retraction with proptosis and ocular misalignment in thyroid eye disease.

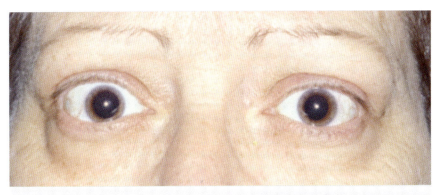

Fig. 17.20 Bilateral lid retraction with only mild proptosis in thyroid eye disease.

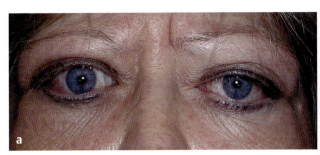

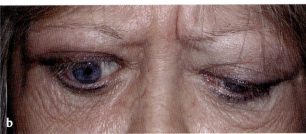

Fig. 17.21 **(a)** Mild right lid retraction from thyroid eye disease. Note the conjunctival hyperemia. **(b)** When the patient looks down, the right upper lid remains elevated (lid lag).

Pretectal eyelid retraction (Collier sign) is observed in the dorsal midbrain (Parinaud) syndrome (▶ Fig. 17.22). It is usually accompanied by upgaze paresis and convergence–retraction nystagmus.

Patients with unilateral ptosis tend to raise their eyebrows to compensate for their ptosis (they use their frontalis muscles more). This may result in lid retraction in the normal fellow eye (▶ Fig. 17.23). The examiner should raise the ptotic lid to observe spontaneous resolution of the lid retraction.

17.4 Peripheral Facial Weakness

Peripheral facial weakness results in decreased closure of the eyelid and a larger palpebral fissure. When the Bell phenomenon is preserved, the cornea is still partially

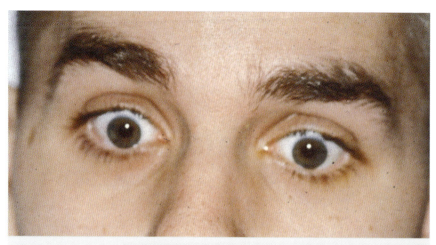

Fig. 17.22 Collier sign in dorsal midbrain syndrome.

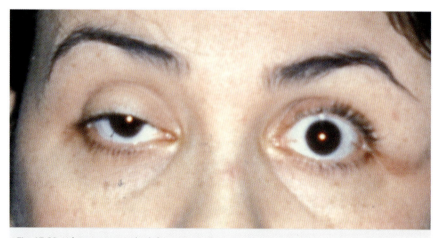

Fig. 17.23 Lid retraction in the left eye secondary to right upper lid ptosis in a patient with myasthenia.

protected during sleep (▶ Fig. 17.24). When there is complete facial palsy and no Bell phenomenon, the cornea is exposed (▶ Fig. 17.25).

Complications of incomplete eye closure include ocular surface irritation (pain, redness, and visual loss), corneal exposure, and risk of corneal infection and perforation (▶ Fig. 17.26).

These patients need to be evaluated by an ophthalmologist. Artificial tears and lubricant ointment need to be applied to the cornea every few hours. If the eye closure is incomplete, then the eyelid may be temporarily closed by placing tape horizontally on the upper lid (▶ Fig. 17.27).

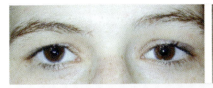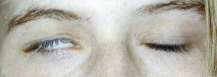

Fig. 17.24 Right peripheral facial weakness with good Bell phenomenon during eye closure (right).

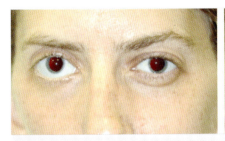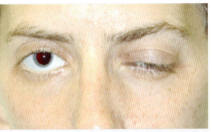

Fig. 17.25 Right complete peripheral facial paresis with poor Bell phenomenon during eye closure (right) resulting in permanent exposure of the cornea. Note the larger palpebral fissure with lagophthalmos (inability to completely close the eye) in the right eye.

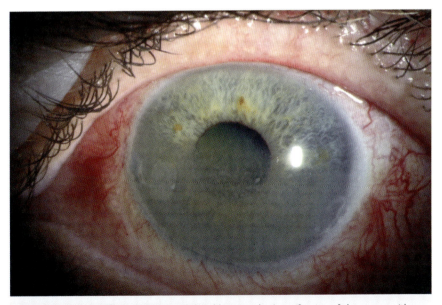

Fig. 17.26 Chronic corneal exposure with band keratopathy (opacification of the cornea with deposits in the exposed cornea).

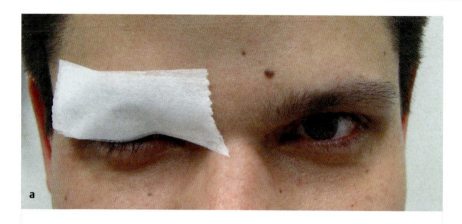

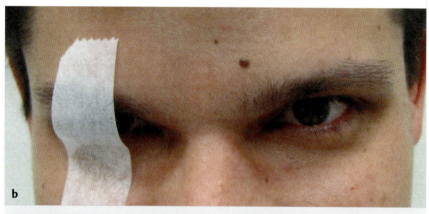

Fig. 17.27 (a) Layers of tape appropriately placed horizontally on the upper eyelid, keeping the upper eyelid down. The tape cannot rub on the cornea, and it is still possible to apply topical drops and ointment. (b) Tape inappropriately placed vertically on the eyelid. When the patient sweats, the eyelid opens, and the tape may rub on the cornea.

When the cornea is exposed, the upper and lower eyelids can be sewn together to keep the eye closed and the cornea protected. This procedure is called a tarsorrhaphy, which can be performed at bedside (▶ Fig. 17.28). If the facial weakness does not improve, various procedures can be performed later to improve eye closure (▶ Fig. 17.29).

Patients with a peripheral facial palsy may ultimately develop hemifacial spasm (involuntary contraction of the hemiface, often predominating around the eye). This occurs more commonly when there is a compressive lesion of the facial nerve.

Pearls

All patients with hemifacial spasm need magnetic resonance imaging (MRI) of the brain, with contrast, looking for a lesion compressing the facial nerve.

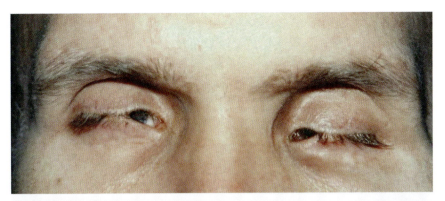

Fig. 17.28 Temporary tarsorrhaphy performed to protect both corneas in a patient with Guillain-Barré syndrome and bilateral facial weakness. Note that only the central part of each eyelid is closed, allowing the patient to see to the sides.

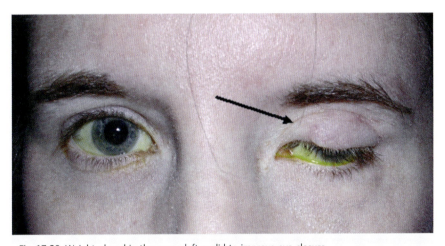

Fig. 17.29 Weight placed in the upper left eyelid to improve eye closure.

17.5 Abnormal Blinking

Regular blinking, which is defined as 20 to 30 blinks per minute, keeps the eye from drying out by evenly distributing the lacrimal fluid and glandular secretions.

17.5.1 Decreased Blinking

Decreased spontaneous blinking is common in patients with Parkinson syndromes.

Patients with facial weakness also have decreased (and often incomplete) blinking.

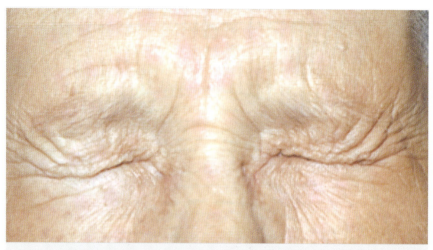

Fig. 17.30 Essential blepharospasm with sustained spasm of the orbicularis oculi.

17.5.2 Blepharospasm

Blepharospasm, or involuntary intermittent bilateral eyelid closure, ranges from an increased blink rate to severe, sustained spasms of the orbicularis oculi. Spasms are worse with wind, sun, light, and stress.

Causes of blepharospasm include the following:

• Ocular surface irritation (severe dry eye syndrome)
• Essential blepharospasm (idiopathic dystonia)
• Parkinson syndrome
• Pontine lesions

Blepharospasm accompanied by dystonic movements of the lower face or neck (oromandibular dystonia) is called Meige syndrome.

Severe spontaneous eyelid closure from blepharospasm can result in functional blindness and severe disability. Some patients cannot keep their eyes open long enough to cross a street. They cannot read and cannot drive. Pain is common (described as cramps of the involved muscles) (▶ Fig. 17.30).

The treatment of choice in patients with blepharospasm or hemifacial spasm is local subcutaneous injections of botulinum toxin. Botulinum toxin is injected subcutaneously in the muscles responsible for the spasms (in the orbicularis oculi and other facial muscles if necessary). Botulinum toxin blocks the release of acetylcholine at the neuromuscular junction, thereby rendering the muscle unable to contract for a period of approximately 3 months. The effect on pain is immediate. The effect on the spasms is usually delayed by a few days and lasts several weeks. The injections are repeated every few months. Ocular lubrication is also important.

18 Nonorganic Neuro-ophthalmic Symptoms and Signs

Nonorganic visual symptoms and signs—patients' visual complaints that are not supported by clinical examination—are common in neuro-ophthalmology. Classic nonorganic symptoms and signs include unilateral or bilateral visual loss, which ranges from blurred vision to complete blindness; peripheral visual field loss, which is usually visual field constriction; monocular diplopia; spasm of the near reflex; voluntary nystagmus; pharmacologic dilation of one or both pupils; disturbance of accommodation; and voluntary ptosis and blepharospasm.

This chapter discusses warning signs that visual symptoms and signs are nonorganic and offers examination strategies to confirm their nonorganic nature.

18.1 Types of Visual Symptoms and Signs

The neuro-ophthalmologist is often in the position of showing that the visual system is actually normal and that these symptoms and signs are associated with various psychiatric disorders that present with nonorganic (functional or psychogenic) neuro-ophthalmic symptoms and signs.

Most patients in these cases are found to have the following:

- Nonspecific visual symptoms that are part of a depressive or anxiety disorder (e.g., chronic eye pain, photosensitivity, or asthenopia)
- Visual symptoms and signs that are part of a conversion disorder, hypochondriasis, or somatization disorder syndrome (in these cases, the patient may not be aware of the nonorganic nature of the symptoms)
- Visual symptoms and signs that are part of a factitious disorder (Munchausen syndrome)
- Visual symptoms and signs that are being feigned to seek compensation or disability (malingering)
- Visual symptoms and signs that are being used to seek medical help and escape from a difficult situation (if abuse is suspected, patients should be admitted for further evaluation)

Psychiatric evaluation should be suggested when an underlying psychiatric disorder is suspected.

18.2 Examination Strategies to Confirm That Symptoms and Signs Are Nonorganic

The only way to confirm that the symptoms and signs are nonorganic is to prove that visual function is normal during the examination. Specific examination strategies can be used, but only if the visual symptoms and signs are suspected to be nonorganic prior to the examination.

Nonorganic visual symptoms and signs are usually suspected early during the interaction with the patient. A discrepancy between the patient's complaints and the patient's activities in the waiting room should raise a red flag. Another tipoff is that patients claiming nonorganic visual loss often wear sunglasses, even in the examination room.

Patients with true visual loss tend to look at the examiner during the interview and examination, whereas patients with nonorganic visual loss tend to look in other directions and often pretend to have difficulty following instructions during the examination.

Pearls

The diagnosis of nonorganic visual loss should be made cautiously and only when the examiner is able to prove normal vision. It is common to see patients with true organic disease but superimposed nonorganic symptoms (e.g., a patient with true visual loss from brain injury may worsen his complaints to avoid having to return to work, or the same patient may have secondary depression and somatization).

18.2.1 When the Complaint Is Visual Loss

1. Observe the patient walking without help from the waiting room into the examination room.
2. Visual acuity testing:
   - *Start at the very bottom of the Snellen chart* (at the 20/10 line) and encourage the patient to see the letters, emphasizing that the size of the letters doubles at each line. Most patients read the letters by the time you reach the 20/30 or 20/40 line.
   - *Attempt a fake refraction* (by placing neutral lenses in front of the tested eye); it often improves vision, particularly in children.
   - *"Magic drop" test:* emphasize that the drops you are placing in the eyes (artificial tears) are going to improve the vision temporarily and help you understand the mechanism of vision loss (this is particularly helpful in children).

When the Complaint Is Substantial Visual Loss in One Eye Only

If the patient has clear ocular media, no major refractive error determined by retinoscopy, and no history of amblyopia, try the following:
1. *Check for normal pupillary responses* (absence of relative afferent pupillary defect), which suggest that unilateral visual loss is not related to an optic neuropathy or severe retinopathy.
2. *Test stereovision* to objectively measure visual acuity in both eyes (equal vision in both eyes is required for stereopsis) (▶ Fig. 18.1; ▶ Table 18.1).
3. *Fog the good eye* with plus lenses while measuring visual acuity with both eyes open so that only the "bad eye" sees (the patient is usually not aware of which eye is being tested).
4. *Perform a prism shift test.* A normal prism shift test requires binocular vision. Ask the patient to look at the Snellen chart showing small letters (smaller than what the patient claims to be able to see in the bad eye). Place a 4-diopter prism (base in) in front of the alleged bad eye. If the patient truly sees the letters with both eyes, then a compensatory movement of both eyes toward the apex of the prism is followed by a convergence movement of the good eye as the patient tries to suppress diplopia. If vision is organically reduced in the bad eye, there will be no compensatory eye movement.

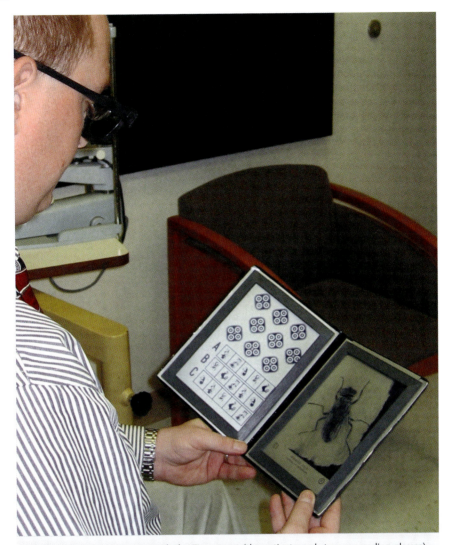

Fig. 18.1 Stereovision testing with the Titmus test (the patient needs to wear reading glasses).

Table 18.1 Relationship of visual acuity to stereopsis

Visual acuity in each eye is at least	Stereopsis (arc seconds)[a]
20/20	40
20/25	43
20/30	52
20/40	61
20/50	89
20/70	94
20/100	124
20/200	160

[a]The Titmus test gives results in seconds of arc.

When the Complaint Is No Light Perception or Hand Motion Vision in Both Eyes

1. *Surprise the patient:* Unexpected actions from the examiner can elicit a surprise response from the patient.
2. *Test proprioception:* Truly blind patients have no difficulty performing tests that appear to require vision but are actually proprioception tasks (e.g., "Look at your hand," "Bring the tips of your index fingers together," and "Sign your name") (► Fig. 18.2).
3. *Test for optokinetic nystagmus:* A positive response indicates vision of at least 20/400 vision in the tested eye (► Fig. 18.3).
4. *Perform the mirror test:* The mirror test is helpful in patients with "no light perception" or "light perception" vision. Patients with nonorganic visual loss will be unable to avoid eye movements following their own image in a mirror that is held close to their face and rocked back and forth and up and down (► Fig. 18.4).
   The optokinetic test and the mirror test can be performed with both eyes open if the patient claims complete bilateral blindness. It should be performed with the good eye patched if the patient claims blindness in only one eye.
5. *Use visual evoked potentials:* Normal visual evoked responses indicate intact visual pathways for central vision. Abnormal visual evoked responses do not prove organic visual loss (they can be abnormal from defocusing, poor fixation, and poor effort).

18.2.2 When the Complaint Is Constriction of Visual Fields

Constricted visual fields are seen with automated and Goldmann visual fields.

There is generalized constriction, and on Goldmann visual fields, the size of the visual field does not vary with the size of the stimulus, or isopters may be overlapping, reversed, or spiraled (► Fig. 18.5).

1. *Test the confrontation visual field:* Ask the patient to mime what you are doing in the peripheral vision of one or both eyes (► Fig. 18.6).
   - Tell the patient that you are testing coordination, not vision.
   - Next, quickly tell the patient to "hold up your hands," "show me two fingers," then "do this" (and do something with your hands—wave or make fists—without saying aloud what you are doing).
   - Often, a patient will follow along even though the patient says he or she cannot see your hands (this is a sort of "Simon Says" game).
2. *Test tangent screen visual field:* With nonorganic constricted visual field, the size of the visual field does not physiologically increase when the distance at which the visual field is tested increases (tubular visual field) (► Fig. 18.7, ► Fig. 18.8).

18.2.3 When the Complaint Is Monocular Diplopia

Patients with ocular misalignment have binocular diplopia (diplopia resolves with closing either eye).

When diplopia does not resolve when closing either eye, the diplopia is monocular.

In most cases, there is no true diplopia, but rather ghosting or distortion of images, which improves or resolves by looking through a pinhole (monocular diplopia of optical origin).

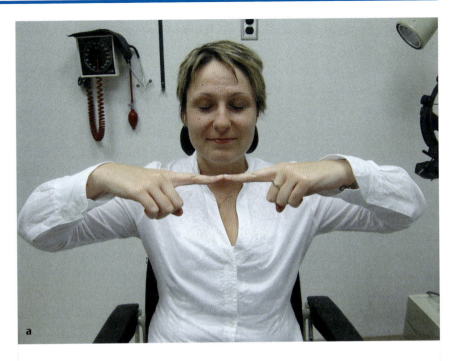

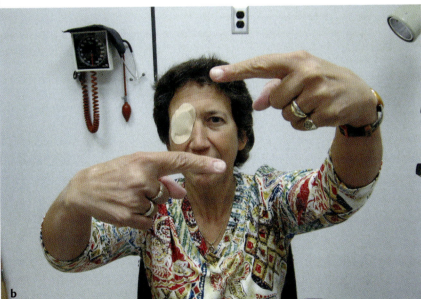

Fig. 18.2 (a) A person who is truly blind can touch the tips of the fingers properly. (b) A person with nonorganic visual loss is often "unable" to touch the tips of the fingers properly.

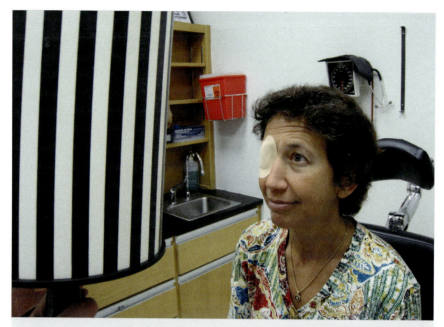

Fig. 18.3 Positive optokinetic nystagmus indicates vision of at least 20/400. It is tested one eye at a time with the other eye completely occluded.

Have the patient draw what he or she sees: True monocular diplopia (when two separate and equal images of an object are seen by one eye only) is almost always nonorganic.

18.2.4 When the Complaint Is Binocular Diplopia

In these cases, spasm of the near triad is very common and is characterized by episodes of intermittent convergence, accommodation, and miosis (▶ Fig. 18.8). When ductions are tested with one eye covered, eye movements are normal, and the miosis resolves.

18.2.5 When the Complaint Is Nystagmus

Voluntary nystagmus is characterized by rapid movements of the eyes that are purposely initiated. These rapid alternating saccades can usually be sustained for only a few seconds. Fluttering of eyelids during episodes, often with convergence, can be seen.

18.2.6 When the Complaint Is Pupillary Dilation

Pharmacologic pupillary dilation results in widely dilated pupils. It can be unilateral or bilateral. The dilated pupil does not constrict in response to light or near stimulation. There is no constriction with dilute pilocarpine (unlike tonic pupil), and there is no or incomplete constriction with pilocarpine 1% (▶ Fig. 18.9).

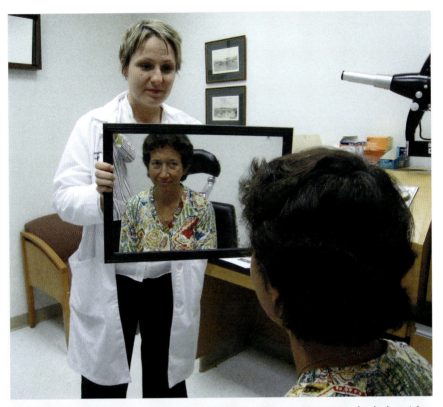

Fig. 18.4 Use of a mirror to detect nonorganic blindness. The patient is instructed to look straight ahead at the mirror. The mirror is then rotated from side to side. Eye movements indicate that the patient can see his or her own image in the mirror.

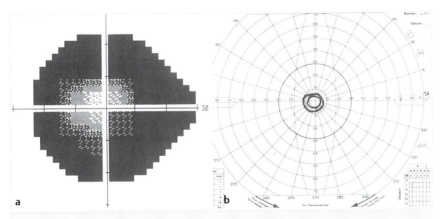

Fig. 18.5 (a) Nonorganic constricted visual field of the left eye on automated perimetry. (b) Nonorganic constricted visual field of the left eye on Goldmann perimetry. Often, constricted visual fields result from unreliable testing and not from "nonorganic" disease.

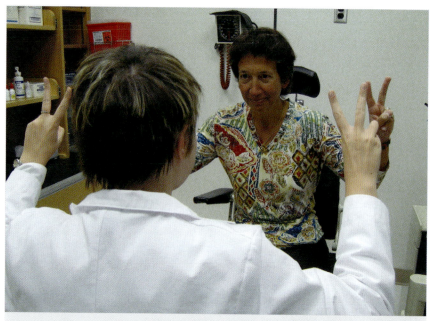

Fig. 18.6 Demonstration of a full visual field by confrontation.

When evaluating a patient with suspected pharmacologic mydriasis, dilute pilocarpine should be used first. If there is no pupillary constriction after 45 minutes, then 1% pilocarpine can be used.

> **Pearls**
>
> Mydriasis from a third nerve palsy will fully constrict with pilocarpine 1%.

18.2.7 When the Complaint Is Accommodation Paralysis

Patients with nonorganic weakness or paralysis of accommodation are unable to read at near, even with a plus lens. Some patients improve only partially with a corrective plus lens (all patients with organic accommodation paralysis should be able to read at near with the appropriate plus lens correction).

18.2.8 When the Complaint Is Ptosis

Nonorganic unilateral or bilateral ptosis is rare. These patients voluntarily close the eye and lower the ipsilateral brow (unlike patients with true ptosis, who elevate the ipsilateral brow) (▶ Fig. 18.10 and ▶ Fig. 18.11).

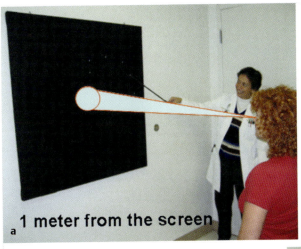

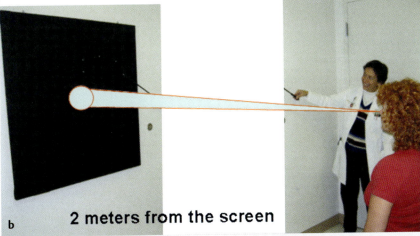

Fig. 18.7 (a) Nonorganic constriction of visual field on tangent screen test. (b) The size of the visual field does not increase when the patient is moved farther away from the screen.

18.2.9 When the Complaint Is Blepharospasm

Although blepharospasm is most often organic and involuntary, repeated eyelid closure may be nonorganic. In both cases, treatment with botulinum toxin may be highly effective.

> **Pearls**
>
> Because nonorganic visual symptoms and signs often result from anxiety and depression, reassurance that there is no underlying lesion and that visual symptoms should spontaneously resolve often results in improvement. Once normal visual function is proven, there is no need to pursue further testing.

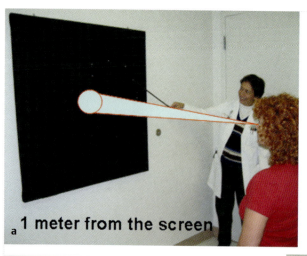

a **1 meter from the screen**

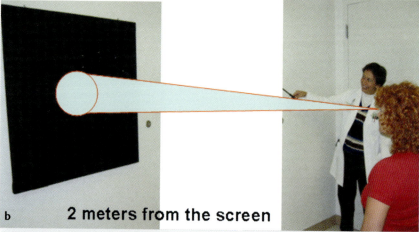

b **2 meters from the screen**

Fig. 18.8 (a) Organic constriction of visual field on tangent screen test. (b) The size of the visual field increases when the patient is moved farther away from the screen.

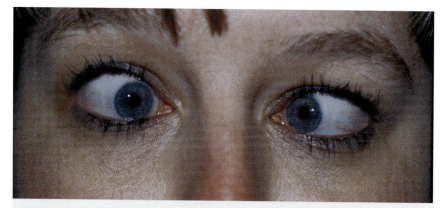

Fig. 18.9 Spasm of the near triad (convergence spasm). With voluntary convergence, there is esotropia, accommodation, and miosis.

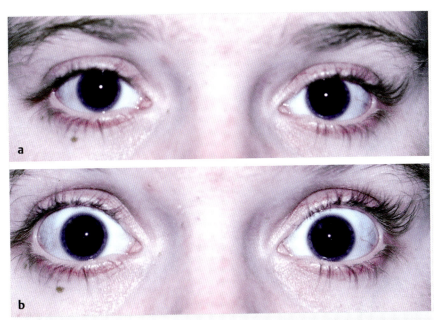

Fig. 18.10 (a) Bilateral pharmacologic mydriasis. The pupils do not react to light or with near stimulation. (b) The size of the pupils does not change after placing pilocarpine 1% in both eyes.

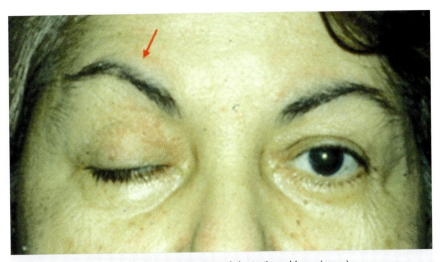

Fig. 18.11 True right ptosis. Note the elevation of the ipsilateral brow (*arrow*).

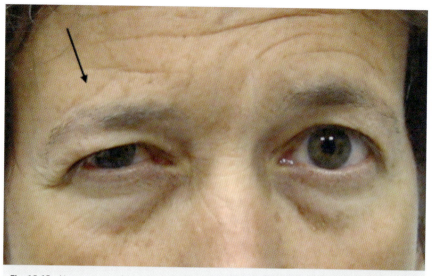

Fig. 18.12 Nonorganic right ptosis. Note the lowering of the ipsilateral eyebrow (*arrow*).

19 Diagnosis of Headache and Facial Pain

Headache and facial pain accompany or reveal many neuro-ophthalmic disorders. The diagnosis of the cause of headache and facial pain is based on clinical history. In particular, the mode of onset of pain and its temporal profile are of great importance. These characteristics are the key indicators of whether the pain is due to a benign headache, a facial pain syndrome, or a neuro-ophthalmic disorder.

19.1 Clinical Diagnosis of Headache and Facial Pain

The clinical diagnosis of headache and facial pain depends on characterization of the *mode of onset of pain* (▶ Fig. 19.1). For example, an *acute, recent onset* is usually related to an emergency, whereas *episodic pain, with pain-free intervals between attacks*, is usually related to a benign, primary headache or facial pain disorder. *Progressive, permanent pain over a few days or a few weeks* is usually related to an intracranial space-occupying lesion. *A long-standing, chronic headache* is usually related to a benign process.

19.1.1 Other Characteristics of the Pain

The following characteristics of the pain guide further evaluation:
- Location of pain (diffuse, hemicrania, periorbital, occipital, or cervical)
- Side of pain (unilateral, alternating, or bilateral)
- Type of pain (dull, constant, or throbbing)

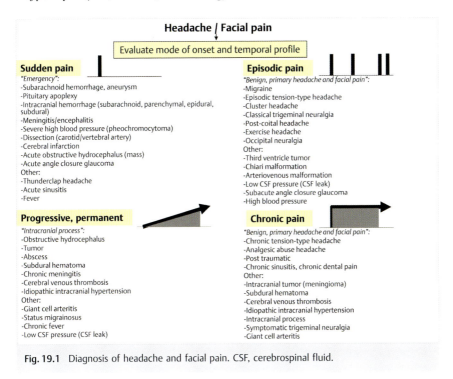

Fig. 19.1 Diagnosis of headache and facial pain. CSF, cerebrospinal fluid.

- Duration of pain (without treatment)
- Severity of pain (using a scale from 1 to 10, particularly considering its impact on activities)
- Frequency of episodes (per day, week, or month)
- Temporal profile (age of onset, recent worsening, and progressive)
- Precipitating factors
- Prodromes (i.e., early symptoms preceding onset)
- Associated symptoms and signs (nausea, vomiting, photophobia, tearing, ocular redness, visual loss, Horner syndrome, diplopia, and sleep apnea)
- Treatments tried and their efficacy

19.2 Clinical Evaluation of the Patient with Headache/Facial Pain

Clinical evaluation should include a detailed neurologic examination, including cranial nerve examination; a funduscopic examination looking for disc edema, which would reveal papilledema from raised intracranial pressure, and spontaneous venous pulsations, which would suggest normal intracranial pressure; palpation of the temporal arteries (for patients > age 50); blood pressure and temperature; and a general physical examination.

In most cases, the cause of headache or facial pain is identified at this point. The International Headache Society (IHS) has proposed a classification of headaches according to their underlying mechanisms. It is important to recognize the primary headaches or facial pain (usually benign disorders) and differentiate them from the secondary headaches and facial pain, which reveal an underlying disease. Further investigations are obtained when a secondary cause of pain is suspected (▶ Fig. 19.2).

Pearls

- Blood pressure should be checked in all headache patients (acute or chronic).
- Examination of the ocular fundus is required in all patients presenting with chronic or new-onset headaches.
- The presence of optic nerve head edema suggests raised intracranial pressure.
- Giant cell arteritis should be considered in all patients > age 50 who present with any type of headache or facial pain.
- Intraocular pressure and detailed ocular examination need to be performed in patients with recurrent, unilateral pain localized around the eye.

19.3 Classification of Headache and Facial Pain

The following classification is adapted from the Headache Classification Subcommittee of the International Headache Society. International Classification of Headache Disorders, 3rd ed. (ICHD-III). Cephalalgia 2013;33(9):629–808. In each subgroup, we have detailed only disorders that may present with neuro-ophthalmic symptoms and signs.
a) Primary headaches
  - Migraine
    - Migraine with visual aura
  - Tension-type headache and new daily persistent headache

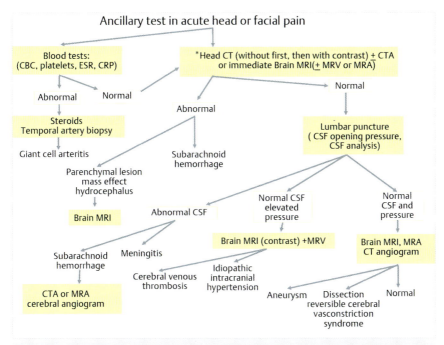

Fig. 19.2 Evaluation of the patient with acute head or facial pain. All patients with headaches need an examination of the ocular fundus to look for disc edema (this is part of the clinical examination and is not included in the ancillary tests). *The type of brain imaging obtained urgently varies based on local resources and protocols. CBC, complete blood count; CRP, C-reactive protein; CSF, cerebrospinal fluid; CT, computed tomography; CTA, computed tomographic angiography; ESR, erythrocyte sedimentation rate; MRA, magnetic resonance angiography; MRI, magnetic resonance imaging; MRV, magnetic resonance venography.

- Cluster headache and other trigeminal autonomic cephalalgias
  - Cluster headache (episodic and chronic)
  - Paroxysmal hemicrania (episodic and chronic)
  - Short-lasting unilateral neuralgiform headache with conjunctival injection and tearing (SUNCT)
- Other primary headaches
  - Hemicrania continua
b) Secondary headaches
  - Headaches attributed to head and/or neck trauma
  - Headaches attributed to cranial or cervical vascular disorders
    - Ischemic and hemorrhagic strokes
    - Unruptured and ruptured vascular malformations (aneurysm, arteriovenous malformation, dural arteriovenous fistula, cavernous angioma, Sturge–Weber syndrome)
    - Giant cell arteritis
    - Central nervous system vasculitis
    - Carotid or vertebral artery dissection
    - Reversible vasoconstriction syndrome
    - Cerebral venous thrombosis

- Cerebral autosomal dominant arteriopathy with subcortical infarcts and leukoencephalopathy (CADASIL)
- Mitochondrial myopathy, encephalopathy, lactic acidosis, and stroke-like episodes (MELAS)
- Pituitary apoplexy
- Headaches attributed to nonvascular intracranial disorders
  - High cerebrospinal fluid (CSF) pressure
  - Low CSF pressure
  - Meningeal processes
  - Intracranial neoplasms
  - Chiari malformation
- Headaches attributed to a substance or its withdrawal
- Headaches attributed to infection
  - Meningitis, encephalitis, intracranial abscess
- Headaches attributed to disorders of homeostasis
  - Hypoxia
  - High altitude
  - Sleep apnea
  - Dialysis
  - Arterial hypertension
  - Hypoglycemia
- Headaches or facial pain attributed to disorders of the cranium, neck, eyes, ears, nose, sinuses, teeth, mouth, or other facial or cranial structures
  - Acute glaucoma
  - Refractive errors
  - Heterophoria or heterotropia
  - Ocular inflammatory disorders (uveitis, scleritis, orbital inflammation, optic neuritis)
- Headaches attributed to psychiatric disorder

c) Cranial neuralgias, central and primary facial pain, other headaches
- Cranial neuralgias and central causes of facial pain
  - Trigeminal neuralgia (classic, symptomatic)
  - Nasociliary neuralgia
  - Supraorbital neuralgia
  - Optic neuritis
  - Herpes zoster
- Other headaches, cranial neuralgia, central or primary facial pain

Pearls

Thunderclap headache is a high-intensity headache of abrupt onset mimicking that of a ruptured cerebral aneurysm. The search for an underlying cause should be immediate (and performed in an emergency department) and exhaustive. Thunderclap headache is frequently associated with serious vascular intracranial disorders, particularly subarachnoid hemorrhage, intracerebral hemorrhage, cerebral venous thrombosis, unruptured vascular malformation (mostly aneurysm), arterial dissection (intra- and extracranial), central nervous system vasculitis, reversible vasoconstriction syndrome, pituitary apoplexy, colloid cyst of the third ventricle, CSF hypotension, and acute sinusitis (particularly with barotrauma).

Primary thunderclap headache should be the diagnosis only when all organic causes have been excluded.

19.3.1 Diagnostic Criteria for Migraine without Aura

The following information is based on ICHD-III Diagnostic Criteria for Migraine.

Description

Migraine is defined as a recurrent headache disorder with attacks lasting 4 to 72 hours. Typical characteristics of the headache are unilateral location, pulsating quality, moderate or severe intensity, aggravation by routine physical activity, and association with nausea and/or photophobia.

Diagnostic Criteria

a) At least five attacks fulfilling criteria B to D
b) Headache attacks lasting 4 to 72 hours (untreated or unsuccessfully treated)
c) Headache has at least two of the following characteristics:
  • Unilateral location
  • Pulsating quality
  • Moderate or severe intensity
  • Aggravation by or causing avoidance of routine physical activity (e.g., walking or climbing stairs)
d) During headache, at least one of the following:
  • Nausea and/or vomiting
  • Photophobia and phonophobia
e) Not attributable to another disorder

19.3.2 Diagnostic Criteria for Migraine with Aura

The following information is based on ICHD-II Diagnostic Criteria for Migraine with Aura.

Description

Migraine with aura is defined as a recurrent headache disorder with attacks of reversible neurologic symptoms, usually developing gradually over 5 to 20 minutes and lasting for < 60 minutes. Headaches with the features of migraine without aura usually follow the migraine with aura symptoms. Less commonly, headaches without the features of migraines or no headaches follow.

Diagnostic Criteria

a) At least two attacks fulfilling criteria B and C of migraine headache
b) Migraine fulfilling criteria for typical aura
c) Not attributed to another disorder

A typical aura consists of visual and/or sensory and/or speech symptoms. Gradual development, duration no longer than 1 hour, a mix of positive and negative features, and complete reversibility characterize the aura.

Visual aura is the most common type, often presenting as a fortification spectrum (zigzag figure near the point of fixation that may gradually spread right or left and assuming a laterally convex shape with an angulated scintillating edge leaving variable degrees of absolute or relative scotoma in its wake). A progressively enlarging scotoma without positive phenomena may occur (▸ Fig. 6.1, ▸ Fig. 11.2).

Pearls

Some of the treatments used to abort migrainous headaches are vasoconstrictors and should not be used during the aura. The patients should be instructed to wait until the aura has resolved to take such medications (e.g., ergotamine and triptans).

19.4 Differential Diagnosis of Facial Pain

▸ Table 19.1 outlines the characteristics of various facial pain syndromes: classic trigeminal neuralgia, symptomatic trigeminal neuralgia, cluster headache, episodic or chronic paroxysmal hemicrania, SUNCT syndrome, and hemicrania continua.

In most cases with new-onset facial pain or hemicrania, a workup is required to rule out underlying lesions (e.g., dissections, aneurysms, or cavernous sinus or skull base lesions).

19.5 Evaluation of the Patient with Suspected Secondary Headache or Facial Pain

The type of workup depends primarily on the mode of onset of the pain and available resources (▸ Fig. 19.1 and ▸ Fig. 19.2). All patients with acute headache or facial pain, or rapidly progressive pain, require an urgent evaluation. Patients with abnormal clinical examination, with optic nerve head edema (▸ Fig. 19.3), or with associated neuro-ophthalmic symptoms or signs also need to be further evaluated. In most cases of long-standing episodic pain suggesting a primary headache or pain disorder with a normal examination (including normal funduscopic evaluation), no further investigation is necessary.

In cases with acute or subacute headache, ancillary investigations are usually obtained in the following order:
1. *Blood tests* in patients > age 50 (complete blood count, platelet count, erythrocyte sedimentation rate, and C-reactive protein)
2. *Head computed tomography* (CT) without contrast first to rule out a subarachnoid hemorrhage and screen for hydrocephalus, followed by contrast to screen for mass lesions and meningeal processes or brain magnetic resonance imaging (MRI) with contrast. Depending on the type of headache, computed tomographic angiography (CTA) with contrast may be obtained immediately after the initial head CT without contrast
3. *Lumbar puncture* with CSF opening pressure and CSF analysis
4. *Brain MRI with contrast* if the above investigations are normal.
5. *Brain and neck magnetic resonance angiography (MRA) or magnetic resonance venography (MRV)* may also be needed, depending on associated symptoms and signs. Dedicated orbital views are necessary if there is an orbital syndrome or if there is unilateral visual loss.

Table 19.1 Diagnosis of facial pain

Characteristics	Classic trigeminal neuralgia	Symptomatic trigeminal neuralgia	Cluster headache	Episodic or chronic paroxysmal hemicrania	SUNCT syndrome	Hemicrania continua
Age/gender ratio	50-year-old M:W: 1:4	Any W = M	Young M:W 9:1	Any M:W 1:3	Any M:W 8:1	Any W > M
Side of pain Location of pain	Unilateral V2/V3 > V1	May be bilateral V1, V2, or V3	Unilateral Periorbital	Unilateral Periorbital	Unilateral Periorbital	Unilateral Hemicrania
Type of pain	Stabbing	Dull, persistent	Boring, very severe	Very severe	Very severe	Sharp pain
Duration of pain	<1 s	Chronic	15–180 min	2–30 min	5–240 s	<1 min
Temporal profile	Few to many per day for a few weeks or months Pain-free between attacks	Fluctuations but no remission	1–8/d Attack phase: 4–16 wk Remission: 6 mon–2 y>	5/d	Numerous in a day Sometimes dull pain between attacks Remissions with irregular pattern	Associated with continuous headache Fluctuating intensity
Associated signs	None Look for trigger	Hypoesthesia V Dysesthesia V Motor deficit V Other cranial nerve palsies	Horner Eye redness Tearing, rhinorrhea	Horner Eye redness Tearing rhinorrhea	Eye redness Tearing	Nausea, vomiting, photophobia ± Horner
Interictal examination	Normal	Hypoesthesia V Motor deficit V	Normal ± permanent Horner	Normal ± permanent Horner	Normal	Normal
Specific treatment	Carbamazepine	Variable response	Acute: oxygen, injectable triptans, and DHE Chronic: lithium steroids, calcium channel inhibitors	Indomethacin stops pain	None Variable response	Indomethacin

Abbreviations: DHE, dihydroergotamine mesylate; SUNCT, short-lasting unilateral neuralgiform headache with conjunctival injection and tearing; V, trigeminal nerve; M, men; W, women.

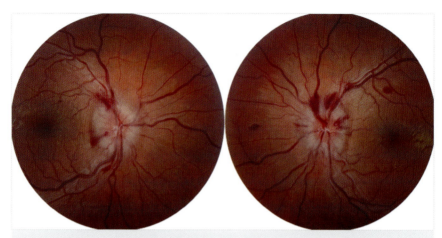

Fig. 19.3 Bilateral papilledema seen on fundus photographs obtained in a patient with new-onset headaches. The optic nerves are elevated, and there are a few hemorrhages at the edge of the optic discs. This patient presented to an emergency department with a 2 week history of new-onset headaches. Ocular fundus photographs were obtained with a nonmydriatic camera as part of the systematic evaluation of headache patients.

Depending on its availability and on the clinical suspicion, the MRI may replace the head CT, and vascular imaging (with MRA/MRV or CTA) may be obtained initially. The only cause of headache that could be seen on a CT scan and missed by MRI is a subarachnoid hemorrhage, especially during the first week.

6. *Cerebral angiography* is indicated only in patients with subarachnoid hemorrhage. Arterial dissections, cerebral venous thrombosis, and most aneurysms can usually be diagnosed noninvasively with MRI, MRA, MRV, computed tomographic angiography, or computed tomographic venography.

20 Disorders Commonly Encountered in Neuro-ophthalmology

Some neurologic or systemic disorders are commonly encountered in neuro-ophthalmology. Patients with common neurologic disorders such as multiple sclerosis, strokes, traumatic brain injuries, or brain tumors may have visual loss or diplopia. However, it is important to realize that these patients often can also have routine ocular disorders (such as refractive errors, corneal surface disease, or cataracts) that can be easily treated. In addition, even patients with neurologic disorders can have urgent acute ocular disorders such as retinal detachment, retinal vascular occlusions, or intraocular hypertension.

> **Pearls**
>
> Neurologists evaluating a known neurologic patient with new-onset visual loss should not automatically assume that visual loss is related to the neurologic disease. They should obtain an ophthalmic consultation prior to making management and therapeutic decisions.

Some disorders, such as pituitary tumors, occipital lesions, intracranial aneurysms, and raised intracranial pressure, commonly affect the visual pathways. Systematic neuro-ophthalmologic follow-up with careful examination of visual function (including repeat visual fields) can document worsening of the intracranial process.

A few diseases have pathognomonic ocular findings that facilitate early diagnosis. These patients are often sent to neuro-ophthalmology for "screening." This is often the case when the diagnoses of Wilson disease, Whipple disease, or neurofibromatosis type 1 are being considered, or when it is necessary to determine if an incidental finding (such as Chiari malformation or an intracranial aneurysm) is symptomatic and, therefore, should be treated.

20.1 Cerebrovascular Disease

The term *stroke* includes cerebral ischemia (transient ischemic attacks and cerebral infarctions) and cerebral hemorrhage. A stroke is suspected when a patient presents with *acute* neurologic symptoms and signs (*acute* usually means that the mechanism is vascular). Stroke patients often have neuro-ophthalmic complaints, including visual loss, visual field defects, and diplopia. Retinal vascular disorders are equivalent to strokes involving various ocular vascular territories.

Once the diagnosis of stroke is suspected, the first step is to determine whether the vascular event is ischemic or hemorrhagic. In the eye, this can be done by looking at the fundus; for the brain, it requires neuroimaging, usually a head computed tomographic (CT) scan without contrast (▶ Fig. 20.1 and ▶ Fig. 20.2)

Questions to be answered in patients with suspected cerebrovascular disease (and retinal vascular diseases) include the following:

1. Is it a vascular event?
2. Where in the brain or the eye has the vascular event occurred (parenchymal and vascular topography)?
3. What type of vascular event is it (pathology)?

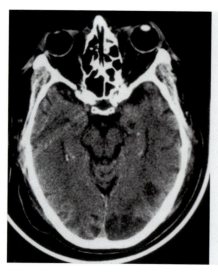

Fig. 20.1 Computed tomographic scan of the brain without contrast showing hypodensities at the level of both occipital lobes consistent with bilateral occipital infarctions.

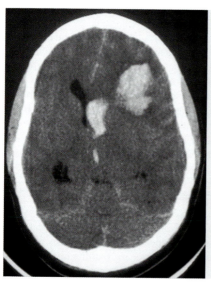

Fig. 20.2 Computed tomographic scan of the brain without contrast showing hyperdensities in the left frontal lobe and ventricles, consistent with intraparenchymal hemorrhages with ventricular extension.

4. What has caused the vascular event (mechanism)?
5. What are the consequences of the vascular event (impairments, disabilities, and handicap)?
6. What other medical problems coexist?

20.1.1 Cerebral Infarctions

Once a stroke is confirmed and the mechanism (ischemic vs. hemorrhagic) is determined, the cause should be clarified to offer the best secondary prevention to the patient (▶ Fig. 20.3).

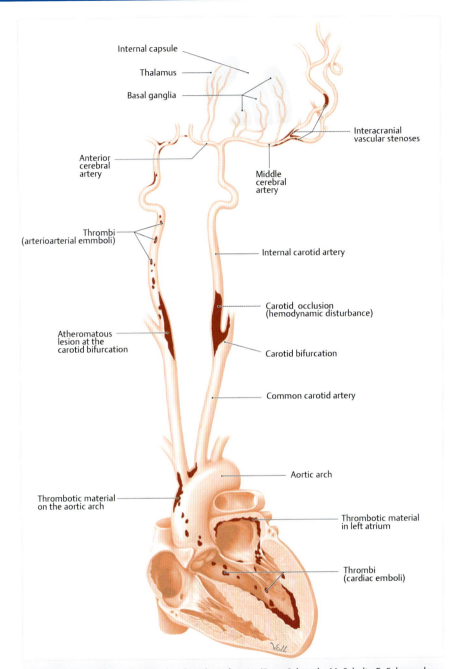

Fig. 20.3 Mechanisms of cerebral and ocular ischemia. (From Schuenke M, Schulte E, Schumacher U, Ross LM, Lamperti ED, Voll M. THIEME Atlas of Anatomy; Head and Neuroanatomy. Stuttgart, Germany: Thieme; 2007. Illustration by Markus Voll.)

Causes of Cerebral Infarction (see ▶ Fig. 20.3)

Four main mechanisms can result in cerebral ischemia.
- Thrombosis of a vessel
  - Large-vessel or macrovascular (arterial) disease
  - Small-vessel or microvascular (arterial) disease
- Emboli
  - Cardiac source of emboli
  - Artery to artery
- Hypoperfusion
- Venous thrombosis

Ocular Manifestations of Carotid Disease

Carotid disease (mostly interval carotid artery) often presents with ocular symptoms and signs.
- Asymptomatic retinal emboli
- Transient monocular visual loss
- Central or branch retinal artery occlusion
- Ophthalmic artery occlusion
- Episcleral artery dilation
- Venous stasis retinopathy
- Ocular ischemic syndrome
- Ischemic optic neuropathy (rare)
- Optic nerve compression (rare)
- Horner syndrome
- Ocular motor nerve paresis (rare)
- Referred pain

Differential Diagnosis of Carotid Artery Disease

The carotid artery can be affected by the following diseases:
- Arterial wall
  - Atheroma
  - Dissection
  - Fibromuscular dysplasia
  - Arteritis
    - Infectious
    - Noninfectious (Takayasu, giant cell arteritis)
  - Trauma
  - External radiation
  - Tumors (carotid glomus)
- External compression
  - Tumors
  - Trauma
- Blood flow
  - Coagulation disorders
  - Emboli (heart, artery to artery)

Cervical Artery Dissections

Dissections of the internal carotid artery commonly present with an ipsilateral acute Horner syndrome associated with orbital, face, or head pain. These patients are at risk for a cerebral infarction and should be evaluated and treated emergently (▶ Fig. 20.4 and ▶ Fig. 20.5)

Dissections involve the extracranial carotid or vertebral arteries more often than the intracranial arteries. They may occur spontaneously or after cervical trauma

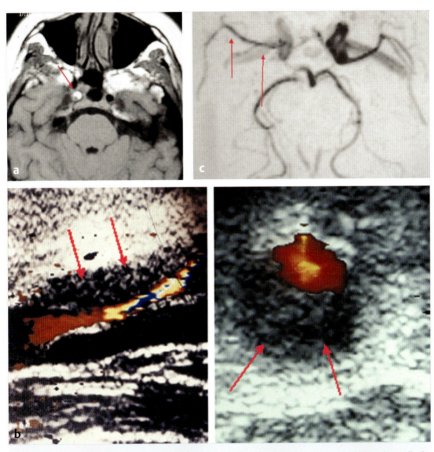

Fig. 20.4 (a) Axial T1-weighted magnetic resonance imaging showing a hypersignal in the wall of the dissected right internal carotid artery (*arrow*). Note the normal black signal (flow void) of the normal left internal carotid artery. (b) Carotid ultrasound (sagittal view on the left and axial cut on the right) showing the residual normal flow in the dissected artery (in color) and the hematoma in the wall of the artery (*arrows*). (c) Magnetic resonance angiography of the head demonstrating decreased signal in the middle cerebral artery (*arrows*) ipsilateral to the dissected carotid artery. This finding suggests that the patient is at risk for hemodynamic cerebral infarction. This patient should be admitted to the hospital and maintained on strict bed rest until normal blood flow is restored (this is best seen with transcranial Doppler).

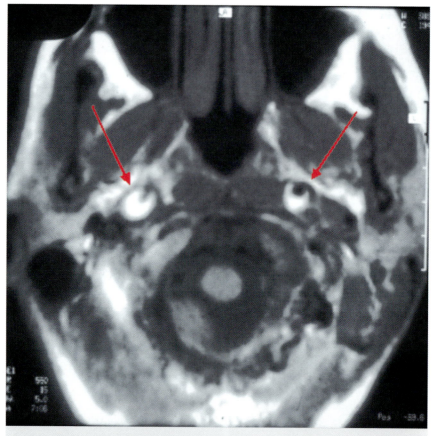

Fig. 20.5 Axial T1-weighted magnetic resonance imaging showing hypersignals in the wall of the dissected internal carotid arteries (*arrows*). This patient presented with bilateral painful acute Horner syndrome.

(car accident, strangulation, chiropractic manipulation). There is often a symptom-free interval of a few days between the trauma and the first sign of the dissection. Pain is often present immediately after the trauma.

Cardiac Sources of Embolism and Embolic Risk

The risk of cerebral emboli in cardiac disease is classically defined as "high" (needing urgent treatment) and "low or uncertain" (often not directly responsible for the cerebral infection)

High Risk

- Atrial
  - Atrial fibrillation
  - Sustained atrial flutter
  - Sick sinus syndrome

- Left atrial thrombus
- Left atrial appendage thrombus
- Left atrial myxoma
- Valvular disease
  - Mitral stenosis
  - Prosthetic valves
    - Mechanical
    - Bioprosthetic
  - Endocarditis
    - Infective
    - Noninfective
      a. Marantic
      b. Liebman Sachs (systemic lupus erythematosus; antiphospholipid antibodies)
  - Ventricular
    - Recent anterior myocardial infarction
    - Left ventricular thrombus
    - Left ventricular myxoma
    - Dilated cardiomyopathy
  - Iatrogenic
    - Cardiac catheterization
    - Cardiac surgery

Low or Uncertain Risk

- Atrial
  - Patent foramen ovale
  - Atrial septal aneurysm
  - Spontaneous echo contrast on transesophageal echocardiogram (TEE)
- Valvular disease
  - Mitral annulus calcification
  - Mitral valve prolapse
  - Calcified aortic stenosis
  - Fibroelastoma
  - Giant Lambl excrescences
- Ventricular
  - Akinetic/dyskinetic ventricular wall segment
  - Subaortic hypertrophic cardiomyopathy
  - Congestive heart failure

Classification of Small Vessel Disease

Cerebral infarctions can be related to occlusion of a large intracranial vessel (such as posterior cerebral artery or middle cerebral artery), or can be related to diseases affecting small intracranial vessels. Small vessel diseases include abnormalities in the vessel content and vessel wall abnormalities.

20.1.2 Abnormalities in the Vessel Content

- Hypercoagulable states

20.1.3 Vessel Wall Abnormalities (Veins and Arteries)

- Acute
  - Vasculitis
  - Noninflammatory vasculopathies
- Chronic
  - Arteriolar sclerosis ("lacuna" due to hypertension)
  - Cerebral amyloid angiopathy
  - Cerebral autosomal dominant arteriopathy with subcortical infarcts and leukoencephalopathy (CADASIL)
  - Mitochondrial encephalopathy with lactic acidosis and stroke-like episodes (MELAS)

Risk Factors for Ischemic Stroke

Vascular risk factors should be evaluated in all patients with cerebral or ocular ischemia. Aggressive treatment of modifiable risk factors is essential in secondary prevention.

Risk factors for ischemic stroke include the following:

- Nonmodifiable
  - Age
  - Gender (men > women)
  - Ethnicity (African Americans and Hispanics > Caucasians)
  - Heredity
  - Migraine
- Modifiable
  - Elevated blood pressure
  - Cardiovascular disease
  - Diabetes
  - Hyperlipidemia
  - Cigarette smoking
  - Alcohol abuse
  - Obesity
  - Sedentary lifestyle
  - Obstructive sleep apnea
  - Asymptomatic carotid stenosis
  - Hyperhomocysteinemia
  - Chronic infection
  - Oral contraceptives

Laboratory and Diagnostic Tests Recommended for Patients with Suspected Stroke

Some tests are systematically obtained in the emergency department in patients with suspected strokes. Other tests are obtained based on the patient's characteristics and risk factors.

These tests include the following (* tests are indicated only for certain patients, depending on stroke type and clinical setting):

- Laboratory
  - Complete blood count
  - Platelet count
  - Blood glucose level

- ○ Serum electrolytes, including magnesium and calcium
- ○ Serum creatinine level
- ○ Prothrombin time and activated partial prothrombin time, international normalized ratio
- ○ Urinalysis (may detect occult blood indicating embolic events in the kidney)
- ○ Hepatic function tests*
- ○ Toxicology screen*
- ○ Blood alcohol determination*
- ○ Pregnancy test*
- • Other tests
  - ○ Electrocardiogram (or cardiac monitoring)
  - ○ Chest X-ray (helpful in assessing cardiac disease and aspiration pneumonia)
  - ○ Brain CT or magnetic resonance imaging (MRI)—often with computed tomographic angiography (CTA) or magnetic resonance angiography (MRA) of head and neck
  - ○ Carotid duplex ultrasound* (in anterior circulation infarctions when CTA or MRA are not performed immediately)
  - ○ Holter monitor*
  - ○ Transthoracic or transesophageal echocardiogram*
  - ○ Lumbar puncture*

Hypercoagulable States

Hypercoagulable states can produce a cerebral or retinal infarction by occluding an artery. Many of these factors are congenital (thrombophilia), and the thrombotic episode is triggered by an acquired factor. For example, a woman born with congenital activated protein C resistance may have a normal childhood and may develop a cerebral venous thrombosis only when she starts an oral contraceptive pill or when she is pregnant.

Hypercoagulable states are only rarely responsible for cerebral or ocular arterial ischemia. The workup should be obtained only in specific situations, such as the following:
- • Younger patients
- • No obvious risk factor for cerebral or ocular ischemia
- • Family history of thrombophilia, or recurrent thrombosis
- • Prior history of thrombosis
- • Recurrent, unexplained episodes of thrombosis
- • Venous thrombosis at unusual sites (e.g., cerebral venous thrombosis)

Risk Factors for Thrombosis

- • Congenital factors
  - ○ Protein C defect/deficiency
  - ○ Protein S defect/deficiency
  - ○ Antithrombin III deficiency
  - ○ Activated protein C resistance (factor V Leiden)
  - ○ Prothrombin gene (factor II 20210A) mutation
  - ○ Heparin cofactor II deficiency
  - ○ Dysfibrinogenemia
  - ○ Plasminogen activator inhibitor (PAI-1) gene polymorphism
  - ○ Congenital plasminogen deficiency
  - ○ Thrombomodulin gene mutation

- ○ Sickle cell disease
- ○ Platelet defects
- Acquired factors
  - ○ Antiphospholipid syndrome
  - ○ Myeloproliferative disorder
  - ○ Paroxysmal nocturnal hemoglobinuria
  - ○ Thrombotic thrombocytopenic purpura
  - ○ Disseminated intravascular coagulation
  - ○ Malignancy
  - ○ Sepsis
  - ○ Hyperviscosity syndrome
  - ○ Trauma
  - ○ Immobilization
  - ○ Surgery
  - ○ Pregnancy
  - ○ Oral contraceptives
  - ○ Heparin-induced thrombocytopenia
- Combined risk (both acquired and genetic factors)
  - ○ Hyperhomocysteinemia
  - ○ Elevated factor VIII levels
  - ○ Elevated fibrinogen levels

Pearls

Multiple congenital thrombophilia often coexist in the same patient; therefore, all patients at risk should be screened for all types of thrombophilia.

Angiopathies of the Central Nervous System Associated with Ocular Manifestations

▶ Table 20.1 lists angiopathies of the central nervous system associated with ocular manifestations.

20.1.4 Cerebral Venous Thrombosis

Because a large part of the cerebrospinal fluid (CSF) drains into the venous sinuses and the internal jugular veins (▶ Fig. 20.6 and ▶ Fig. 20.7), thrombosis of an intracranial venous sinus usually results in raised intracranial pressure with headaches and papilledema. Ultimately, the thrombus may extend to the deep cerebral veins and the cortical veins, resulting in acute cerebral venous infarctions and hemorrhages.

The cortical veins empty into the dural venous sinuses, which have an anteroposterior drainage into the transverse sinuses and the jugular veins. Occlusion of a sinus usually results in reversal of the flow in some veins, producing specific clinical manifestations based on the anatomical location of the thrombosed sinus (e.g., when the cavernous sinus is thrombosed, the orbital veins drain anteriorly instead of posteriorly, and there is orbital congestion with proptosis). In most cases, the CSF drainage is compromised, and there are symptoms and signs of raised intracranial pressure.

Table 20.1 Angiopathies of the central nervous system associated with ocular manifestations

Mechanism of ocular disease	Angiopathy	Transmission	Manifestations
Homocystinuria and homocysteinemia	Premature athero-sclerotic occlusion of carotid arteries and large cerebral arteries	Autosomal recessive	Retinal ischemia
Fabry disease (angio-keratoma corporis diffusum)	Glycosphingolipid deposit in endothelial cells, cerebral aneur-ysms	X-linked recessive	Lens subluxation, whorl-like corneal opacification
Neurofibromatosis 1	Arterial dissections, aneurysms, fistulae, moyamoya disease, ganglioneuromas, neurofibromas	Autosomal dominant	Tortuosity of vessels, neurofibromas, Lisch nodules, optic nerve gliomas, retinal hamartomas
MELAS (mitochondrial myopathy, encephal-opathy, lactic acidosis, strokelike episodes) syndrome	Proliferation of mitochondria in smooth muscle cells of cerebral vessels	Maternally inherited (point mutation in mitochondrial DNA)	Optic atrophy, pig-mentary retinopathy, chronic progressive external ophthalmo-plegia
von Hippel–Lindau disease	Cerebellar, brainstem, and spinal cord hemangioblastoma	Autosomal dominant	Retinal angiomas
Tuberous sclerosis (Bourneville disease)	Intracranial aneur-ysms, moyamoya disease	Autosomal dominant	Retinal hamartomas
Rendu–Osler–Weber syndrome (hereditary hemorrhagic telangi-ectasia)	Arteriovenous malfor-mations, venous angiomas, aneurysms, meningeal telangiectasia	Autosomal dominant	Retinal telangiectasia
Ataxia-telangiectasia (Louis-Bar syndrome)	Telangiectasia	Autosomal recessive	Oculocutaneous telangiectasia
CADASIL (cerebral autosomal arteriopa-thy with subcortical infarcts and leukoen-cephalopathy)	Nonatherosclerotic, nonamyloidotic angi-opathy of leptome-ningeal and small penetrating arteries	Autosomal dominant	Mild vascular retinopathy
HERNS (Hereditary endotheliopathy with retinopathy, nephrop-athy, and stroke)	Nonatherosclerotic arteriopathy of retina, small penetrating cerebral arteries, and kidneys	Autosomal dominant	Vascular retinopathy
Menkes syndrome (kinky hair disease)	Tortuosity, elongation, and occlusion of cere-bral arteries	X-linked recessive	Ocular ischemia
Marfan syndrome	Aneurysms, aortic dissection	Autosomal dominant	Lens subluxation, retinal detachment
Hereditary cerebral amyloid angiopathy	Hereditary cerebral hemorrhage with	Autosomal dominant	None

Table 20.1 (continued)

Mechanism of ocular disease	Angiopathy	Transmission	Manifestations
	amyloidosis (HCHWA)–Dutch type (beta-amyloid) HCHWA–Iceland type (cystatin C)		
Fibromuscular dysplasia	Arterial stenosis, arterial dissections, aneurysms, carotid cavernous fistulae	May be autosomal dominant; mostly sporadic	Retinal emboli
Ehler–Danlos syndrome (type IV)	Aneurysms, carotid cavernous fistulae, carotid or vertebral artery dissection	Heterogeneous	Ocular ischemia, angioid streaks
Pseudoxanthoma elasticum (Grönblad–Strandberg syndrome)	Premature atherosclerosis, aneurysms, carotid cavernous fistulae		Angioid streaks, peau d'orange fundus
Moyamoya disease	Noninflammatory occlusive intracranial vasculopathy	May be associated with other hereditary disorders	Morning glory disc, ocular ischemia
Sturge–Weber syndrome (encephalofacial angiomatosis)	Leptomeningeal venous angioma, arteriovenous malformations, venous and dural sinus abnormalities	Possibly autosomal dominant; mostly sporadic	Skin, conjunctiva, episclera, uveal angiomas, glaucoma
Wyburn-Mason syndrome	Cerebral arteriovenous malformations (usually brainstem)	Sporadic	Retinal arteriovenous (racemose angioma) malformations

Dilation and thrombosis of the cortical veins produce catastrophic venous infarctions that are often hemorrhagic.

There are multiple veins draining the cerebellum and the brainstem (▶ Fig. 20.8). Thrombosis of some veins may result in dilation of these veins and compression or ischemia of the adjacent cranial nerves. This explains why petrosal sinus thrombosis can produce multiple cranial nerve palsies such as sixth, fifth, seventh, and third nerve palsies. Isolated diplopia with pain may rarely be the first sign of cerebral venous thrombosis.

Classic clinical presentations of cerebral venous thrombosis include the following:
• Raised intracranial pressure (headache, papilledema, sixth nerve palsy)
• Seizures
• Altered mental status
• Neurologic deficit (hemiparesis, aphasia based on the location of cerebral infarctions)
• Deficits on alternating sides or occurring bilaterally (unlike in cerebral arterial ischemia)

Urgent treatment is necessary to prevent multiple cerebral venous infarctions and death.

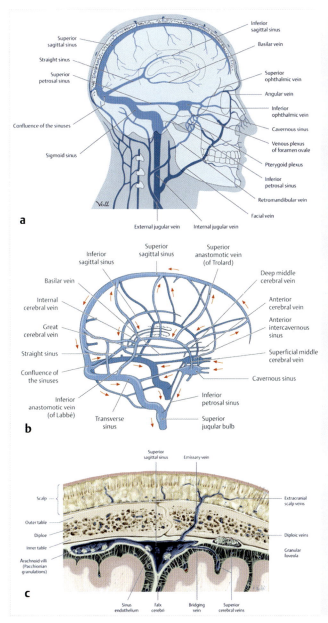

Fig. 20.6 (a) Sagittal view of the intracranial venous system. (b) Anteroposterior drainage of the intracranial venous blood. ([a, b] From Schuenke M, Schulte E, Schumacher U, Ross LM, Lamperti ED, Voll M. THIEME Atlas of Anatomy; Head and Neuroanatomy. Stuttgart, Germany: Thieme. 2007. Illustrations by Markus Voll.) (c) Drainage of the CSF into the superior sagittal sinus. ([c] From Schuenke M, Schulte E, Schumacher U, Ross LM, Lamperti ED, Voll M. THIEME Atlas of Anatomy; Head and Neuroanatomy. Stuttgart, Germany: Thieme; 2007. Illustration by Karl Wesker.)

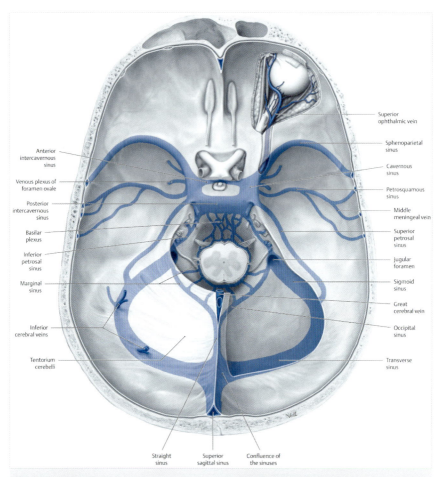

Fig. 20.7 Intracranial venous sinuses. View from above. (From Schuenke M, Schulte E, Schumacher U, Ross LM, Lamperti ED, Voll M. THIEME Atlas of Anatomy; Head and Neuroanatomy. Stuttgart, Germany: Thieme; 2007:255, Fig. 8.5c).

Pearls

Permanent visual loss from papilledema is a classic complication of cerebral venous thrombosis. Early treatment of intracranial hypertension is necessary. When possible, a lumbar puncture should be performed *prior* to anticoagulation to reduce the intracranial pressure and help preserve vision.

Diagnosis of Cerebral Venous Thrombosis

MRI and magnetic resonance venography (MRV) usually allow very good noninvasive visualization of the intracranial venous sinuses (▶ Fig. 20.9 and ▶ Fig. 20.10). Artifacts

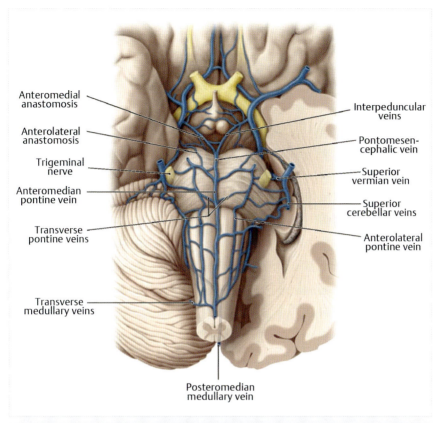

Fig. 20.8 Veins of the brainstem (anterior view). (From Schuenke M, Schulte E, Schumacher U, Ross LM, Lamperti ED, Voll M. THIEME Atlas of Anatomy; Head and Neuroanatomy. Stuttgart, Germany: Thieme; 2007. Illustration by Markus Voll).

are common, and CT venography often complements these tests. A catheter cerebral venogram is only rarely required.

20.1.5 Intracranial Hemorrhage

Intracranial hemorrhages are classified as follows (▸ Fig. 20.11):
- *Epidural hemorrhage* (between the skull and meninges): Usually results from skull fracture (temporal bone with rupture of the middle meningeal artery). There can be rapid expansion of the hematoma with uncal herniation, ipsilateral third nerve palsy, and death if the hematoma is not drained emergently.
- *Subdural hemorrhage* (between the dura and the subarachnoid space): Usually results from mild head trauma or may be spontaneous (rupture of the bridging veins). Particularly common in the elderly. There is relatively slow expansion of the hematoma with headaches and mass effect on the adjacent cerebral hemisphere. Visual field defects are common. Subdural hematoma can be subacute (over days) or chronic (over months).

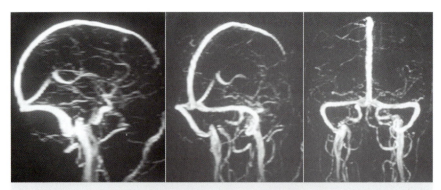

Fig. 20.9 Magnetic resonance venogram (sagittal, three quarter posterior view, and posterior view) showing the normal cerebral venous sinuses.

- *Subarachnoid hemorrhage* (in the subarachnoid space): Usually results from aneurysmal rupture, or may be spontaneous or from head trauma. The blood in the subarachnoid space can produce arterial spasm with cerebral ischemia, or it may block CSF passage and cause obstructive hydrocephalus.
- *Intraparenchymal hemorrhage* (▶ Fig. 20.12 and ▶ Fig. 20.13): Intraparenchymal hemorrhages usually result from bleeding of the small perforating arteries and most often involve the basal ganglia. Superficial intracerebral hemorrhages are often associated with subarachnoid hemorrhage from aneurysmal or arteriovenous malformation rupture.

Risk Factors for Intraparenchymal Hemorrhage

Cerebral hemorrhages may result from the following:
- Arterial hypertension
- Vascular malformations
  - Arteriovenous malformations
  - Cavernous hemangiomas
  - Aneurysms
- Cerebral amyloid angiopathy
- Brain tumor/metastases
- Bleeding disorders
  - Coagulopathies
  - Thrombocytopenia
  - Anticoagulants
  - Thrombolytic treatment
- Head trauma
- Vasculitis
- Endocarditis
- Cerebral venous thrombosis
- Drugs (sympathomimetic agents)
- Alcohol use
- Low cholesterol

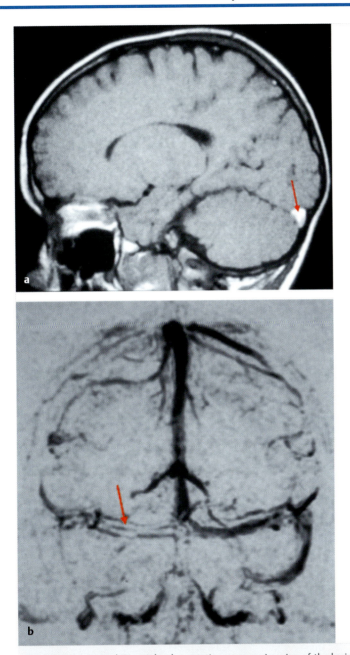

Fig. 20.10 (a) Sagittal T1-weighted magnetic resonance imaging of the brain showing a hyperintense signal in the right transverse sinus (*arrow*) in a patient with headaches and papilledema. This is suggestive of subacute thrombosis of the transverse sinus. (b) Magnetic resonance venogram (posterior view) showing the absence of signal in the thrombosed right transverse sinus (*arrow*).

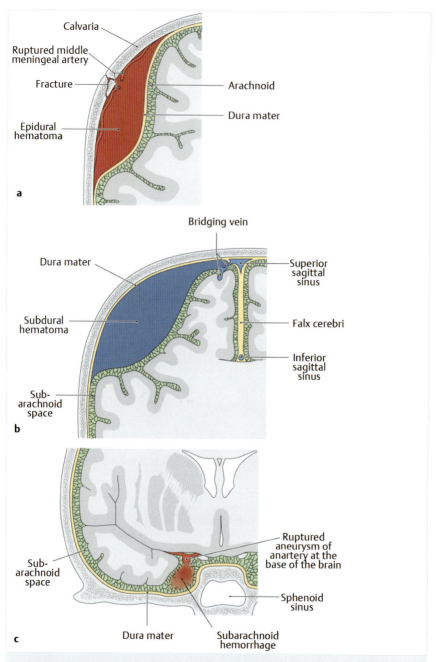

Fig. 20.11 Classification of intracranial hemorrhages. (**a**) Epidural hematoma, (**b**) subdural hematoma, (**c**) subarachnoid hemorrhage (From Schuenke M, Schulte E, Schumacher U, Ross LM, Lamperti ED, Voll M. THIEME Atlas of Anatomy, Head and Neuroanatomy. Stuttgart, Germany: Thieme; 2007. Illustration by Markus Voll.)

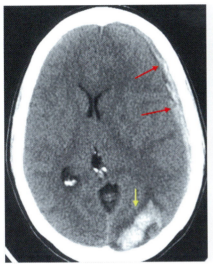

Fig. 20.12 Axial computed tomographic scan of the brain without contrast showing a left occipital intraparenchymal hemorrhage (*yellow arrow*) and left subdural hematoma (*red arrows*) in a patient with bacterial endocarditis and multiple mycotic aneurysms.

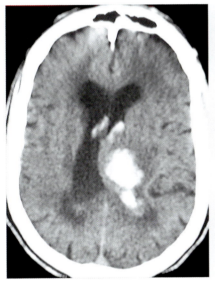

Fig. 20.13 Axial computed tomographic scan of the brain without contrast showing a left intraparenchymal hemorrhage in a patient with uncontrolled arterial hypertension.

When evaluating a patient with an acute intraparenchymal hemorrhage, it is important to determine the source of the hemorrhage. It is sometimes impossible acutely because the hemorrhage may hide an underlying lesion. Repeat brain imaging a few weeks later (once the blood has partially resolved) sometimes allows visualization of a cavernous hemangioma or a mass (► Fig. 20.14 and ► Fig. 20.15).

Funduscopic examination is sometimes useful by revealing retinal vascular malformations (► Fig. 20.16 and ► Fig. 20.17).

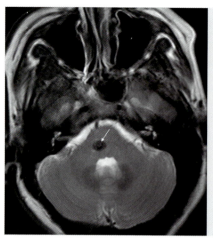

Fig. 20.14 Axial T2-weighted brain magnetic resonance imaging showing bleeding of a cavernous hemangioma in the right pons (*arrow*). This patient had an acute right sixth nerve palsy.

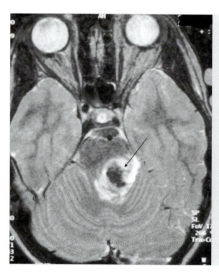

Fig. 20.15 Axial T2-weighted brain magnetic resonance imaging showing bleeding of a cavernous hemangioma of the left midbrain (*arrow*) producing a right fourth nerve palsy.

Subarachnoid Hemorrhage

Bleeding in the subarachnoid space (▶ Fig. 20.18) is usually revealed by an acute, explosive headache. There may be a third nerve palsy if the subarachnoid hemorrhage is related to rupture of an aneurysm of the posterior communicating artery (▶ Fig. 20.19).

The prognosis of subarachnoid hemorrhage is poor. Immediate diagnosis and treatment are essential. Subarachnoid hemorrhage should be suspected in all patients presenting with a very severe headache. Other neurologic symptoms and signs depend on the cause of the subarachnoid hemorrhage and the location of the aneurysm (if related to an aneurysmal rupture). The most common complications are vasospasm with cerebral infarction and obstructive hydrocephalus.

Visual fields often reveal a contralateral homonymous defect when the vascular malformation involves the retrochiasmal visual pathways (▶ Fig. 20.20).

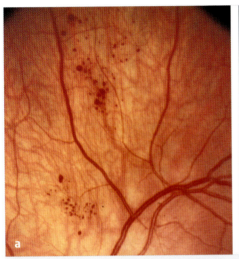 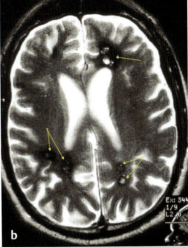

Fig. 20.16 (a) Retinal cavernous hemangioma (grapelike hemangiomas) in a patient with familial cerebral and retinal cavernous hemangiomas. (b) Axial T2-weighted brain magnetic resonance imaging showing multiple cavernous hemangiomas (*arrows*).

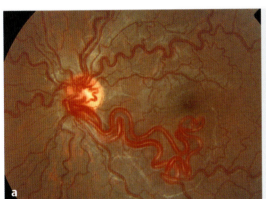

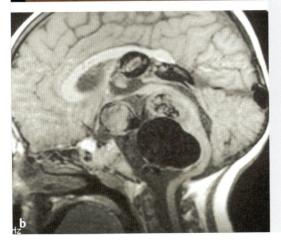

Fig. 20.17 (a) Retinal vascular malformation (a true arteriovenous malformation) in the setting of Wyburn-Mason syndrome. Note additionally the diffusely tortuous vessels. (b) Sagittal T1-weighted magnetic resonance imaging of the brain without contrast showing a large intracranial vascular malformation (the areas in black correspond to dilated vascular flow voids).

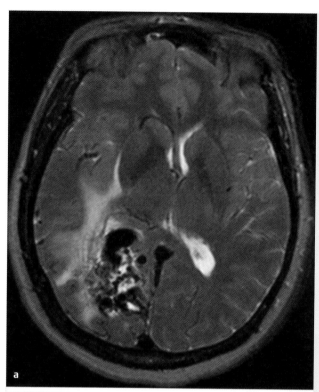

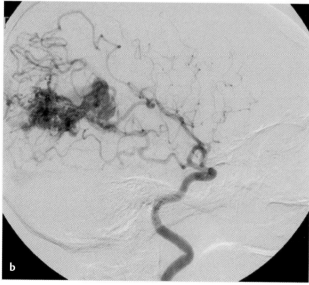

Fig. 20.18 (a) Axial T2-weighted magnetic resonance imaging of the brain in a patient with a left homonymous hemianopia, showing a large arteriovenous malformation in the right occipital lobe. (b) Sagittal catheter angiogram with selective catheterization of a vertebral artery showing the occipital arteriovenous malformation.

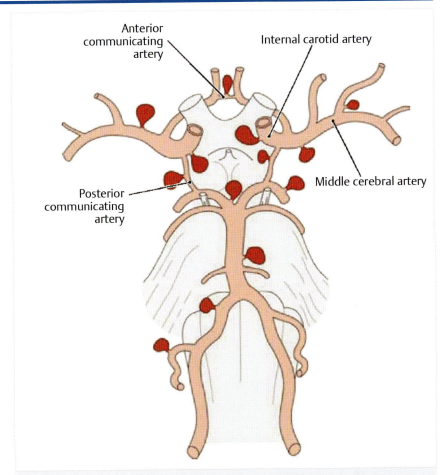

Fig. 20.19 Most common sites of intracranial aneurysms. (From Schuenke M, Schulte E, Schumacher U, Ross LM, Lamperti ED, Voll M. THIEME Atlas of Anatomy, Head and Neuroanatomy. Stuttgart, Germany: Thieme; 2007. Illustration by Markus Voll).

Etiologies of Subarachnoid Hemorrhage

- Aneurysm rupture
- Vascular malformation bleeding
- Bleeding diathesis
- Trauma
- Drug (cocaine, methamphetamine)
- Amyloid angiopathy
- Hypertension
- Brain tumors
- Spinal lesions
  - Aneurysms
  - Arteriovenous malformations
  - Tumors

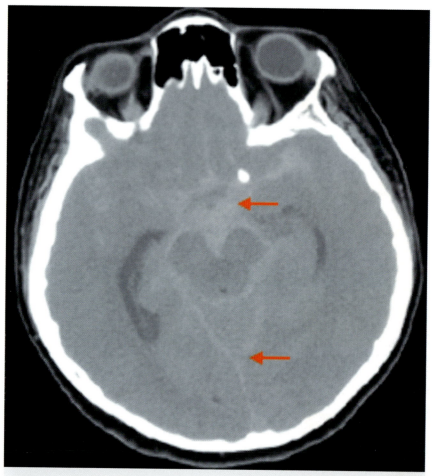

Fig. 20.20 Axial computed tomographic scan of the brain without contrast showing a subarachnoid hemorrhage. Note the hyperdensities filling the subarachnoid space (*arrows*).

Terson Syndrome

Subarachnoid hemorrhage produces a very acute increase in intracranial pressure, sometimes associated with Terson syndrome (retinal and vitreous hemorrhages) (▶ Fig. 20.21 and ▶ Fig. 20.22). Terson syndrome is a classic cause of unilateral or bilateral visual loss in patients with subarachnoid hemorrhage. Because these patients are often unconscious, the diagnosis of Terson syndrome is typically delayed unless funduscopic examination is systematically performed.

Classic findings include the following:

- Optic nerve head edema, often with hemorrhages
- Retinal hemorrhages
- Subhyaloid hemorrhages
- Vitreous hemorrhages

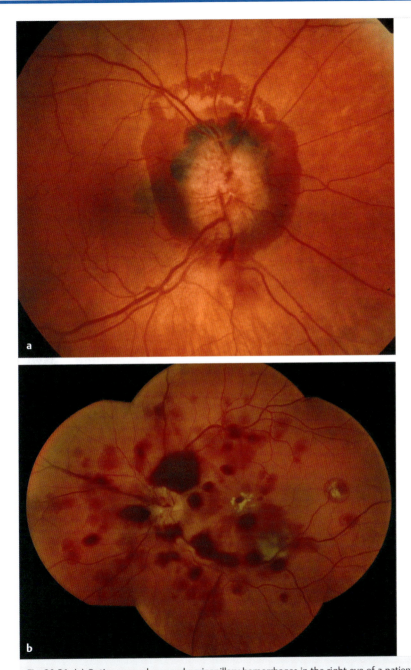

Fig. 20.21 (a) Optic nerve edema and peripapillary hemorrhages in the right eye of a patient with aneurysmal rupture and subarachnoid hemorrhage, suggesting Terson syndrome. (b) There are multiple subhyaloid hemorrhages (dark hemorrhages) as well as intraretinal hemorrhages and disc edema in the left eye.

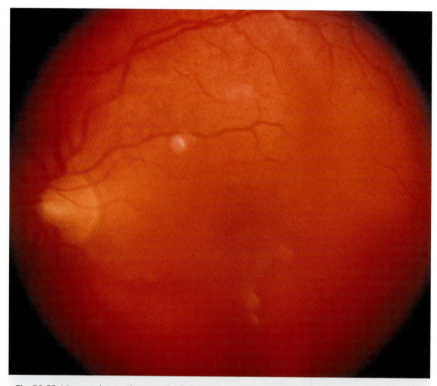

Fig. 20.22 Vitreous hemorrhage in the left eye in a patient with aneurysmal rupture and subarachnoid hemorrhage (Terson syndrome). Note that the view of the fundus is blocked by the intravitreal blood.

The intraocular hemorrhages likely result from acute venous pressure secondary to the subarachnoid hemorrhages; they do *not* result from diffusion of the blood from the subarachnoid space into the eye.

In many cases, the hemorrhages resolve spontaneously over a few weeks or months. Macular hemorrhages may result in permanent visual loss. Persistent vitreous hemorrhage may require a vitrectomy for removal of the blood. Traction retinal detachment may develop.

Intracranial Aneurysms

Intracranial aneurysms represent the most common cause of subarachnoid hemorrhage. This is why catheter angiography is always performed immediately when a subarachnoid hemorrhage is diagnosed: early treatment of the ruptured aneurysm allows prevention of complications and rebleeding. All intracranial vessels are examined because about 20% of patients have more than one intracranial aneurysm.

Intracranial aneurysms (▶ Table 20.2, ▶ Fig. 20.23) may manifest in various ways:
- May be asymptomatic, found on imaging performed for another reason
- Compression of adjacent structures (mass effect of the aneurysm)
- Distal emboli from the sac of the aneurysm
- Rupture with devastating subarachnoid hemorrhage

Table 20.2 Clinical manifestations of intracranial aneurysms according to their anatomical location on the circle of Willis

Location of aneurysm	Frequency %	Neuro-ophthalmic manifestations
Carotid-ophthalmic aneurysms Ophthalmic artery Superior hypophyseal artery	5	Compression, ischemia, hemorrhage of anterior visual pathways: • Optic nerve (monocular visual loss, junctional scotoma) • Chiasm (bitemporal hemianopia) • Optic tract (homonymous hemianopia) Orbital pain
Anterior communicating artery aneurysm	30	Compression, ischemia, hemorrhage of anterior visual pathways: • Optic nerve (monocular visual loss, junctional scotoma) • Chiasm (bitemporal hemianopia) Orbital pain, headache
Internal carotid artery bifurcation aneurysm	4	Compression, ischemia, hemorrhage of visual pathways: • Optic nerve (monocular visual loss, junctional scotoma) • Chiasm (bitemporal hemianopia) • Optic tract (contralateral homonymous hemianopia) Orbital pain, headache
Cavernous sinus aneurysm	2	Sixth nerve palsy Horner syndrome Third, fourth, and fifth (V1 and V2) nerve palsies Compression of anterior visual pathways: • Optic nerve (monocular visual loss) • Chiasm (bitemporal hemianopia) Orbital pain
Middle cerebral artery aneurysm	20	Compression, ischemia, hemorrhage of retrochiasmal visual pathways: • Optic radiations (contralateral homonymous hemianopia) Headache
Posterior communicating artery aneurysm	35	Ipsilateral third nerve palsy Orbital pain, headache
Basilar artery aneurysm	3–5	Ipsilateral third nerve palsy: uni- or bilateral Compression of the adjacent midbrain or pons: • Horizontal gaze palsy, skew deviation, internuclear ophthalmoplegia, lid retraction nystagmus, sixth nerve palsy Occipital headache
Posterior cerebral artery aneurysm	<3	Ipsilateral third nerve palsy Compression of the retrochiasmal visual pathways: • Optic radiations (contralateral homonymous hemianopsia) Occipital headache
Superior cerebellar artery aneurysm	<3	Ipsilateral third nerve palsy Occipital headache

Table 20.2 (*continued*)

Location of aneurysm	Frequency %	Neuro-ophthalmic manifestations
Anterior inferior cerebellar artery (AICA) aneurysm	<3	Ipsilateral sixth nerve palsy Occipital headache
Posterior inferior cerebellar artery (PICA) aneurysm	<3	Ipsilateral sixth nerve palsy Occipital headache
Vertebral artery aneurysm	<3	Ipsilateral sixth nerve palsy Occipital headache
Rupture of the aneurysm (subarachnoid hemorrhage)		Papilledema (raised intracranial pressure) Sudden headache Terson syndrome Sixth Nerve Palsy

20.2 Vasculitis (Angiitis)

Cerebral vasculitis may occur primarily (without any systemic manifestations) or may be secondary to systemic vasculitis. The terms *vasculitis* and *angiitis* imply that there is inflammation in or around the blood vessels. It is a pathological term and the diagnosis of cerebral angiitis or vasculitis should be made only after it is confirmed by cerebral and leptomeningeal biopsy. All other cases should be called cerebral vasculopathy.

20.2.1 Patient Evaluation

Classic clinical presentations include the following:
- Headaches
- Seizures
- Focal neurological symptoms and signs (transient ischemic attacks, cerebral infarctions, or cerebral hemorrhages)
- Altered mental status
- Retinal vasculitis (rare and usually suggests a systemic vasculitis)

The patient's condition often worsens rapidly. Workup and treatment often need to be performed emergently.
Confirmation of the diagnosis involves the following steps:
- Brain MRI with contrast and diffusion-weighted imaging (▶ Fig. 20.24a)
  - Increased T2 signals involving the white and gray matter (often small and multiple)
  - Cerebral infarction, cerebral hemorrhage, or diffuse white matter changes
- Electroencephalogram: often abnormal
- Lumbar puncture: often abnormal (lymphocytic meningitis)
- Vascular imaging demonstrates irregularity of the intracranial arteries
  - MRA and CTA are poorly sensitive because most cerebral angiitis involves the small intracranial vessels, which are not well visualized on MRA and CTA.
  - Catheter angiography is necessary in most cases (▶ Fig. 20.24b).
- Cerebral and leptomeningeal biopsy confirms the diagnosis.

The diagnosis of cerebral angiitis should be made only after it is confirmed by cerebral and leptomeningeal biopsy

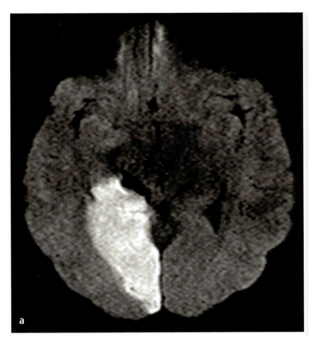

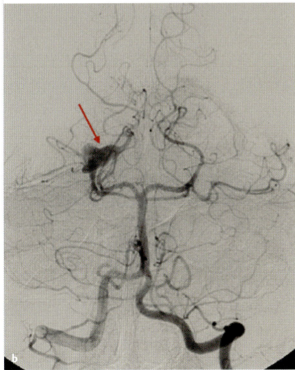

Fig. 20.23 (a) Axial brain magnetic resonance imaging (diffusion-weighted) showing a right occipital infarction (as hyperintense) from an occlusion of the right posterior cerebral artery due to an embolus from the sac of a proximal aneurysm on the posterior cerebral artery. (b) Catheter angiogram (frontal view) showing a large aneurysm on the right posterior cerebral artery (*arrow*).

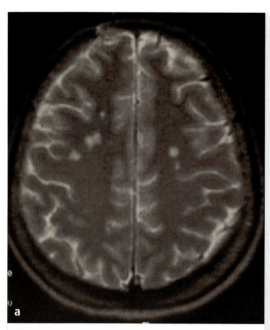

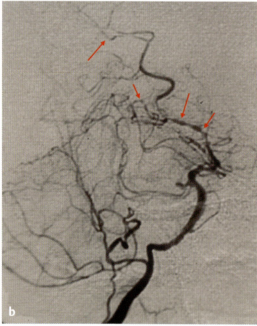

Fig. 20.24 (a) Axial T2-weighted magnetic resonance imaging of the brain showing multiple small hypersignals in the white matter in a patient with primary central nervous system vasculitis. (b) Catheter angiogram (lateral view, posterior circulation) showing irregular intracranial vessels with dilation and stenosis suggestive of vasculitis (*arrows*).

20.2.2 Classification

Central nervous system angiitis is classified as follows:
- Cerebral angiitis associated with systemic diseases
  - Systemic vasculitides
  - Connective tissue diseases
- Cerebral angiitis associated with infections
  - Bacterial
    - Bacterial meningitis
    - Bacterial endocarditis
    - Lyme disease
    - *Chlamydia pneumoniae*
    - *Mycoplasma pneumoniae*
    - Tuberculosis
    - Syphilis
    - Cat scratch disease (Bartonella henselae)
  - Viral
    - Herpes zoster and herpes simplex
    - Cytomegalovirus
    - Human immunodeficiency virus (HIV)
  - Parasitic
    - Toxoplasmosis
    - Cysticercosis
  - Fungal
    - Aspergillosis
    - Coccidioidomycosis
    - Histoplasmosis
    - Cryptococcosis
    - Mucormycosis
- Cerebral angiitis associated with neoplasm
  - Carcinomatous meningitis
  - Lymphoma
- Primary angiitis
  - Primary granulomatous angiitis
  - Benign cerebral angiitis
  - Postpartum benign cerebral angiitis

Certain conditions mimic cerebral angiitis:
- Noninflammatory vasculopathies
  - Benign cerebral angiopathy
  - Reversible cerebral vasoconstriction syndrome
  - Cholesterol emboli
  - Susac syndrome
  - Cerebral autosomal dominant arteriopathy with subcortical infarcts and leukoencephalopathy (CADASIL)
  - Hereditary endotheliopathy with retinopathy, nephropathy, and stroke (HERNS)
  - Vasospasm (subarachnoid hemorrhage, pheochromocytoma, malignant systemic hypertension, ergotism, amphetamines, nasal spray vasoconstrictors)

- ○ Intracranial dissection
- ○ Fibromuscular dysplasia
- ○ Moyamoya disease
- ○ Sneddon syndrome
- Vasculopathies associated with drugs
  - ○ Vasoconstrictors
  - ○ Amphetamines
  - ○ Cocaine
- Coagulopathies
  - ○ Antiphospholipid antibody syndrome
  - ○ Disseminated intravascular coagulation
  - ○ Thrombotic thrombocytopenic purpura
  - ○ Sickle cell disease
  - ○ Hyperviscosity syndrome
- Cardiac emboli
- Severe infections
  - ○ Meningococcemia
  - ○ Hemorrhagic fever
  - ○ Malaria
  - ○ Leptospirosis
- Neoplasia
  - ○ Central nervous system lymphoma
  - ○ Endovascular lymphoma
- Metabolic diseases
  - ○ Fabry disease
  - ○ Cerebrotendinous xanthomatosis
  - ○ MELAS

20.3 Giant Cell Arteritis

Giant cell arteritis (temporal arteritis, cranial arteritis, or Horton disease) is an inflammatory vasculopathy of the medium and large arteries, with a propensity to affect the aorta and its extracranial branches. It is the most common primary vasculitis in adults, occurring almost exclusively in individuals older than 50 years and being much more common in patients older than 70. It is more prevalent in whites, relatively uncommon in blacks, and rare in Hispanics.

20.3.1 Patient Evaluation

Patients with giant cell arteritis present clinically as follows:
- Systemic symptoms (polymyalgia rheumatica)
- Ocular symptoms with permanent, devastating visual loss
  (usually follow the systemic symptoms, but can be isolated in 25% of cases)

Pearls

- The diagnosis of giant cell arteritis must be made prior to visual loss. Immediate treatment with steroids prevents visual loss.
- Headaches or visual loss in a patient older than 50 should raise the possibility of giant cell arteritis.
- Anterior ischemic optic neuropathy (AION) is the most common ophthalmic manifestation of giant cell arteritis (▶ Fig. 20.25 and ▶ Fig. 20.26). Posterior ischemic optic neuropathy (PION) may also occur in giant cell arteritis, but caution is advised when making this diagnosis because ophthalmic artery aneurysms, pituitary apoplexy, and tumor infiltration are also classic causes of acute or subacute retrobulbar optic neuropathy in this age group.
- Always consider giant cell arteritis in the differential diagnosis of older patients with diplopia. The diplopia associated with giant cell arteritis may be transient, particularly when the cause is extraocular muscle ischemia.

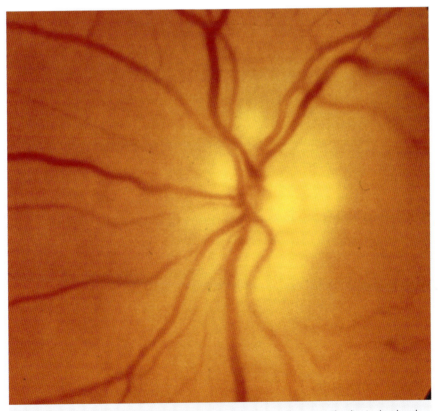

Fig. 20.25 Acute anterior ischemic optic neuropathy from giant cell arteritis. The disc is already pale.

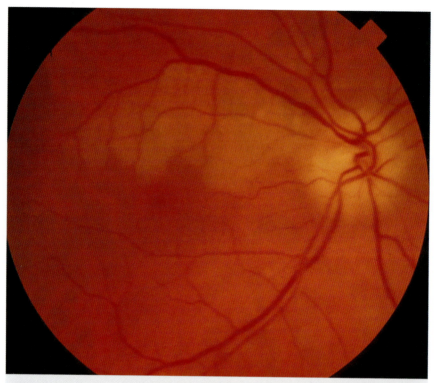

Fig. 20.26 Acute anterior ischemic optic neuropathy and branch retinal artery occlusion from giant cell arteritis. The optic nerve head is swollen and there is retinal whitening (retinal edema) around the superior vascular arcade.

Non-neuro-ophthalmic Manifestations of Giant Cell Arteritis

Systemic symptoms are very common and include the following:
- Headache (most common)
- Temporal artery abnormalities (prominence, tenderness, pulselessness)
- Systemic symptoms and signs of vasculitis (polymyalgia rheumatica):
  - Fever
  - Asthenia
  - Arthralgias, peripheral synovitis
  - Myalgias
  - Weight loss/Anorexia
  - Cough
- Ischemic complications
  - Jaw claudication
  - Scalp necrosis
  - Tongue necrosis
  - Sore throat
  - Hoarseness
  - Cerebral infarction or transient ischemic attack

- ○ Angina, myocardial infarction
- ○ Upper extremity ischemia (pain, claudication)
- Mental status changes
  - ○ Depression
  - ○ Delusions
  - ○ Memory impairment/dementia

Neuro-ophthalmic Manifestations of Giant Cell Arteritis

25% of patients with giant cell arteritis develop visual symptoms without systemic symptoms. They include the following:
- Permanent visual loss occurs in 15 to 20% of patients with giant cell arteritis.
- Visual loss associated with giant cell arteritis usually results from one or more of the following:
  - ○ Optic nerve ischemia (vasculitic involvement of the short posterior ciliary arteries)
  - ○ Choroidal ischemia (also vascularized by posterior ciliary arteries)
  - ○ Retinal infarction (less common; vasculitic involvement of the central retinal artery)
  - ○ Bilateral occipital infarction (exceedingly rare in giant cell arteritis)
- Diplopia occurs in up to 15% of patients with giant cell arteritis.
  - ○ Results most often from ischemia of the extraocular muscles (orbital ischemia), although cranial nerve involvement or brainstem ischemia may also occur in giant cell arteritis

Pearls

Visual loss in arteritic ischemic optic neuropathy is usually severe (hand motion to no light perception vision) and usually permanent. It may be preceded by recurrent episodes of transient monocular visual loss or transient diplopia (premonitory visual symptoms occur in about 65% of patients, usually within the week preceding permanent visual loss)

Summary of the Neuro-ophthalmic Manifestations of Giant Cell Arteritis

- Optic neuropathy
  - ○ Anterior ischemic optic neuropathy
  - ○ Posterior ischemic optic neuropathy
- Retinal ischemia
  - ○ Central retinal artery occlusion
  - ○ Branch retinal artery occlusion
  - ○ Diffuse or focal retinal ischemia
  - ○ Cotton wool spots
  - ○ Retinal hemorrhages
- Choroidal ischemia
- Ocular ischemic syndrome
  - ○ Corneal edema
  - ○ Anterior uveitis
  - ○ Cataract

- Increased intraocular pressure (neovascular glaucoma)
- Ocular hypotony
- Retinal hemorrhages (venous stasis retinopathy)
- Retinal neovascularization
- Orbital ischemia
  - Orbital pain
  - Diplopia (ischemia of the extraocular muscles)
  - Proptosis
- Cranial nerve ischemia
  - Diplopia (third, fourth, and sixth nerve ischemia)
- Cerebral ischemia
  - Brainstem ischemia (diplopia)
  - Occipital lobe infarction (cerebral blindness)
  - Visual hallucinations
- Pupillary abnormalities
  - Tonic pupil
  - Horner syndrome

Fluorescein angiography shows choroidal ischemia (delayed and patchy choroidal filling) in many patients with giant cell arteritis (▶ Fig. 20.27). Although nonspecific, this feature is very suggestive of giant cell arteritis in elderly patients with visual loss and normal carotid arteries.

The fluorescein angiogram normalizes within 2 weeks of steroid treatment.

Pearls

Ischemic optic neuropathy in giant cell arteritis is often bilaterally sequential and may be associated with a concurrent choroidal or retinal infarction. The combination of an ischemic optic neuropathy and retinal infarction or choroidal ischemia should strongly suggest the diagnosis of giant cell arteritis.

Ophthalmic Signs Suggesting a High Risk for Giant Cell Arteritis

the following ophthalmic signs are very suggestive of giant cell arteritis and should prompt immediate evaluation and treatment:
- AION with one or more of the following:
  - Severe visual loss
  - A large cup-to-disc ratio (no disc-at-risk for nonarteritic AION)
  - Pale/milky/chalky white optic disc edema acutely
  - Cotton wool spots suggesting associated retinal ischemia
  - Choroidal ischemia
  - Transient visual loss preceding the AION
  - Transient diplopia preceding the AION
  - Headache, orbital or ocular pain
- PION in the absence of prior surgery, severe blood loss, or hypotension—manifests acutely as vision loss with an ipsilateral relative afferent pupillary defect and normal-appearing optic nerve

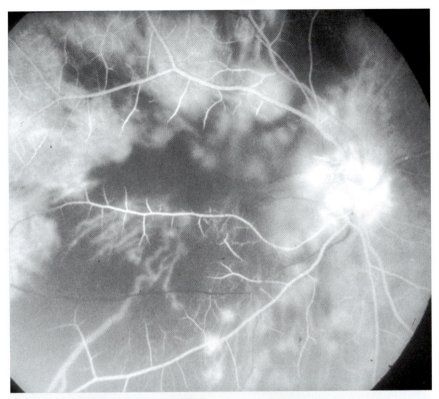

Fig. 20.27 Fluorescein angiogram in a patient with giant cell arteritis and visual loss. There is patchy choroidal filling (there is poor blood flow to the dark areas).

- Any combination of ophthalmic vascular events in close temporal proximity, especially those affecting separate vascular territories (i.e., posterior ciliary and retinal arteries) or affecting both eyes simultaneously or sequentially (▶ Fig. 20.28)
- Cilioretinal artery occlusion (especially with AION)

Pearls

In the elderly, the association of very severe visual loss with ocular ischemia and pallid optic nerve head edema acutely is essentially diagnostic of giant cell arteritis. Steroids must be started immediately to prevent visual loss in the fellow eye (intravenous methylprednisolone is started immediately in the emergency room prior to admitting the patient for workup and further treatment).

20.3.2 Diagnosis of Giant Cell Arteritis

- Clinical suspicion (age, clinical manifestations)
  - Ocular manifestations isolated in up to 25% of cases

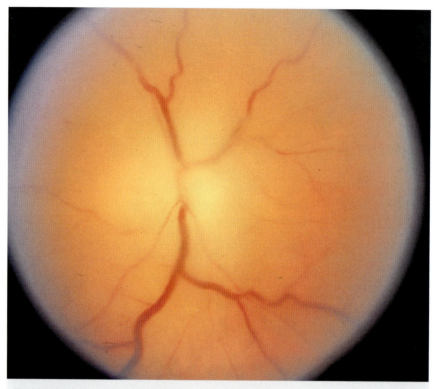

Fig. 20.28 Acute severe ocular ischemia in giant cell arteritis. The patient has no light perception vision. There is a central retinal artery occlusion with pale optic nerve edema and very attenuated arteries, suggesting very severe ocular ischemia.

- Demonstration of biological inflammatory syndrome
  - Erythrocyte sedimentation rate (ESR) elevated—may be normal in up to 20% of cases
  - C-reactive protein (CRP) elevated
  - Low hematocrit
  - Platelet count elevated
  - Fibrinogen elevated
- Temporal artery biopsy (▶ Fig. 20.29 and ▶ Fig. 20.30)
  - Only definite confirmation of the diagnosis
  - Must always be performed
  - False-negative in about 4 to 5% of cases
- Fluorescein angiogram
  - Delayed choroidal filling
  - Useful when diagnosis is uncertain
- Imaging of the aorta and its branches
  - Useful when the diagnosis is uncertain

Superficial temporal artery biopsy (see ▶ Fig. 20.29 and ▶ Fig. 20.30) is performed under local anesthesia and is a relatively benign procedure. The artery is identified

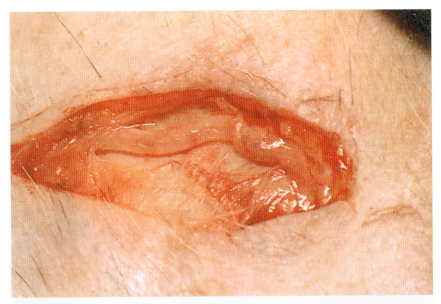

Fig. 20.29 Biopsy of the superficial temporal artery. The skin is open, exposing the artery.

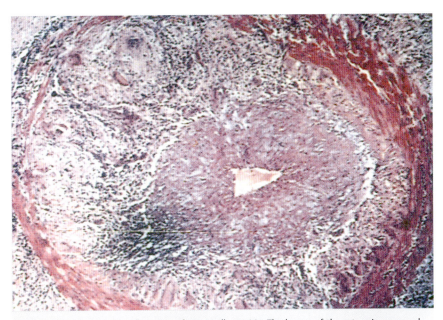

Fig. 20.30 Pathological confirmation of giant cell arteritis. The lumen of the artery is narrowed, and there is an inflammatory infiltrate in the wall of the artery. There are giant cells and interruption of the internal elastic lamina.

under the skin by either palpation or Doppler ultrasonography. A superficial incision is made along the course of the artery. Blunt dissection allows visualization of an arterial segment long enough to remove at least 2 to 3 cm for pathological examination. The artery is either ligated or cauterized at the proximal and distal ends of the specimen, and the skin is closed. Stitches are removed a week later. Complications are rare and include injury to the frontal branch of the facial nerve (paralysis of the ipsilateral forehead), infection, bleeding, and skin necrosis.

Rheumatologic Criteria for the Diagnosis of Giant Cell Arteritis

The diagnosis of giant cell arteritis requires at least three of these five criteria to be present:
1. Age at disease onset 50 years or older
2. New onset or new type of headache
3. Temporal artery tenderness to palpation or decreased pulsation, unrelated to arteriosclerosis of cervical arteries
4. Elevated sedimentation rate (≥ 50 mm/h) by the Westergren method
5. Abnormal artery biopsy showing vasculitis characterized by a predominance of mononuclear cell infiltration or granulomatous inflammation, usually with multinucleated giant cells.

20.3.3 Treatment

The treatment of giant cell arteritis is urgent and the temporal artery biopsy is often performed after treatment is initiated. Laboratory testing should be done prior to initiating any treatment.

Treatment with steroids cures the arteritis, and the typical pathological signs of giant cell arteritis resolve within a few weeks. Ideally the temporal artery biopsy should be performed within 2 weeks of treatment with steroids.

Giant cell arteritis is exquisitely responsive to steroids. Steroids must be started as soon as the diagnosis is suspected to prevent visual loss (the temporal artery biopsy is done a few days later to confirm the diagnosis). Dose and route depend on the clinical manifestations. These patients need to be treated with steroids until there is no evidence of disease activity (no clinical symptoms and no biological inflammatory syndrome)—the total duration of treatment is at least 1 to 2 years, during which the steroids are slowly tapered. In all cases, careful follow-up with monitoring and treatment of complications of steroid treatment is mandatory.

Systemic forms of giant cell arteritis (polymyalgia rheumatica) usually require only low doses of oral prednisone. Ischemic complications of giant cell arteritis (visual loss) usually require high doses of steroids (1 mg prednisone/kg/d). Intravenous (IV) treatment with methylprednisolone (1 g/d for 3 days) followed by oral prednisone (1 mg/kg/d) is often chosen in patients with acute visual loss when there is no contraindication.

As a general rule, the taper should be slow (~ 10 mg/mon) so that patients reach 20 mg of prednisone/d after 6 months, and 10 mg of prednisone/d after 1 year. Patients are seen monthly while tapering the prednisone (for neuro-ophthalmic examination, evaluation of side effects, biological markers). Any clinical or biological indication of activity of the disease should result in an increase of the steroids and a slower taper.

20.4 Multiple Sclerosis

Multiple sclerosis (MS) is a demyelinating disease affecting the white matter of the central nervous system (brain, optic nerves, and spinal cord). Young women are more commonly affected. The disease is more common in Caucasians than in other races.

20.4.1 Patient Evaluation

MS present with relapsing - remitting neurological and visual symptoms and signs.

Common Symptoms and Signs of Multiple Sclerosis

Themost common symptoms and signs of MS include the following:
- Optic neuritis (often with Uhthoff phenomenon)
- Vertigo
- Trigeminal neuralgia
- Diplopia
- Sensory disturbances
- Cerebellar syndrome with ataxia
- Lhermitte sign (electric shock–like sensation down the back when flexing the neck)
- Spasticity and weakness
- Urinary incontinence

Symptoms are often multiple, and they come and go over days to weeks.

There are no systemic manifestations of MS (no other organ than the central nervous system is affected). Headaches are uncommon as are seizures (only the white matter is typically affected). Altered mental status is uncommon.

> **Pearls**
>
> The association of neurologic signs with other organ failure, headaches, altered mental status, or seizures, should suggest a diagnosis other than MS, such as vasculitis.

Neuro-ophthalmic Manifestations of Multiple Sclerosis

Visual symptoms and signs are very common and include the following:
- Optic neuritis is very common
  - Posterior (retrobulbar) in 65%
  - Anterior (with disc edema) in 35%
- Uveitis (most often pars planitis) is rare
- Retinal periphlebitis (asymptomatic)
- Visual field defects (optic tract lesion)
- Cranial nerve palsies (sixth, third, or fourth nerve palsy)
- Vertigo is very common
- Nystagmus is very common
- Internuclear ophthalmoplegia (bilateral > unilateral) is very common
- Skew deviation

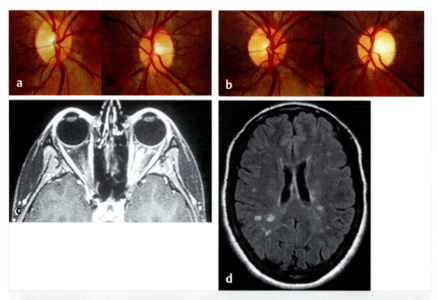

Fig. 20.31 a–e (a) Left acute optic neuritis. Both optic nerves are normal. (b) A few weeks later, the left optic nerve is pale temporally. (c) Axial T1-weighted magnetic resonance imaging (MRI) of the orbits with contrast and fat suppression showing diffuse enhancement of the left optic nerve. (d) Axial fluid-attenuated inversion recovery MRI of the brain showing multiple hypersignals in the white matter, ovoid, and periventricular, highly suggestive of multiple sclerosis. (*continued*)

Pearls

Optic neuritis is often the first sign of multiple sclerosis. Almost all patients with multiple sclerosis develop optic nerve involvement during the course of the disease (▶ Fig. 20.31). Optical coherence tomography (OCT) is routinely used to follow patients with MS and is particularly useful in clinical trials (▶ Fig. 20.31 **e**).

Peripheral venous sheathing and pars planitis are usually asymptomatic and found only when a careful dilated funduscopic examination is performed (▶ Fig. 20.32 and ▶ Fig. 20.33). They are not specific to MS, and they are often found in isolation or in patients with sarcoidosis.

20.4.2 Diagnosis

The diagnosis of MS is made when there is evidence of dissemination of the lesions in space (more than one type of deficit or more than one radiologic lesion) and time (relapse of events).

The diagnosis is suspected clinically and is confirmed by brain MRI. When patients present initially with a clinically isolated syndrome (such as optic neuritis), the clinical diagnosis of MS cannot be confirmed until a second clinical event occurs (clinically definite MS). ▶ Table 20.3 presents the 2010 revised McDonald criteria for the diagnosis of MS.

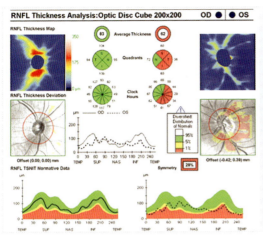

Fig. 20.31 (*continued*) (**e**) Optical coherence tomography (OCT) of the peripapillary retinal nerve fiber layer (RNFL) obtained 3 months after the episode of left optic neuritis. The right eye has a normal RNFL thickness measured at 83 µm; the left eye (affected) has thinning of the RNFL measured at 62 µm and worse temporally.

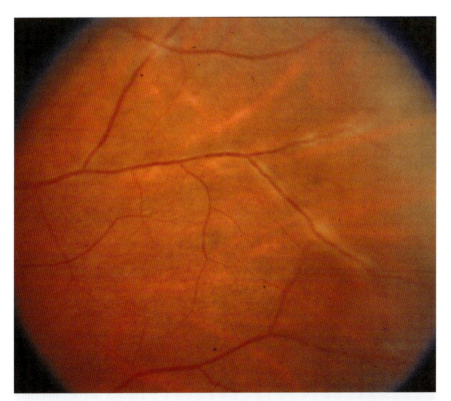

Fig. 20.32 Retinal vascular sheathing (periphlebitis) in the peripheral retina.

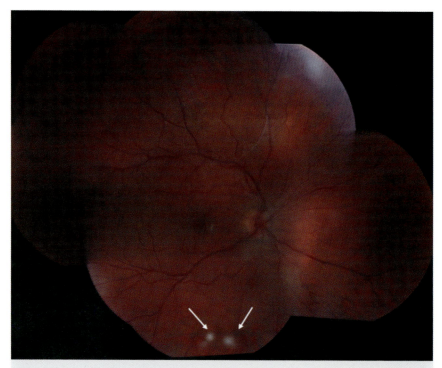

Fig. 20.33 Pars planitis in a patient with multiple sclerosis (note the small white dots in the vitreous at the periphery of the retina inferiorly) (*arrows*).

20.4.3 Course of the Disease

A relapsing and remitting course is typical: the neurologic symptoms and signs of MS tend to improve spontaneously within a few weeks. They may resolve completely or improve only partially. Each relapse may be associated with a different type of deficit and may leave a residual deficit (neurologic deficit or visual loss) (relapsing-remitting form of MS).

In the later course of the disease, the deficits (particularly weakness and spasticity) tend to progress slowly, without remission (secondary progressive form of MS). In a minority of cases, the deficit is slowly progressive from the beginning (primary progressive form of MS).

20.4.4 Treatment of Multiple Sclerosis–Related Neuro-ophthalmic Symptoms

Most MS patients develop visual symptoms at some point during the course of the disease. Monocular or binocular visual loss secondary to recurrent episodes of optic neuritis is common, and numerous patients experience binocular diplopia, often with oscillopsia related to nystagmus. The treatment of these neuro-ophthalmic manifestations of MS is similar to the one recommended for any neurologic flare of MS and is

Table 20.3 2010 Revised McDonald criteria for the diagnosis of multiple sclerosis

Clinical presentation	Additional data needed for the diagnosis of MS
Two or more attacks (relapses) Two or more objective clinical lesions	None Clinical evidence sufficient
Two or more attacks with objective evidence of one lesion	Dissemination in space demonstrated by MRI[a] or Two or more lesions characteristic of MS on MRI *with* positive CSF (oligoclonal bands or raised IgG index)
One attack with objective clinical evidence of two or more lesions	Dissemination in time demonstrated by MRI[b] or second clinical attack
One attack with objective clinical evidence of one lesion (clinically isolated syndrome)	Dissemination in space demonstrated by one or more T2 lesions in at least two of four MS-typical regions of the CNS (periventricular, juxtacortical, infratentorial, or spinal cord) *or* second clinical attack implicating a different CNS site Dissemination in time demonstrated by simultaneous presence of asymptomatic gado-linium-enhancing and nonenhancing lesions at any time *or* a new T2 and/or gadolinium-enhancing lesion(s) on follow-up MRI, irrespective of its timing with reference to a baseline scan *or* second clinical attack.
Insidious neurological progression suggestive of MS (primary progressive MS)	One year of disease progression and two or three of the following: Positive CSF Dissemination in space in the brain demonstrated by MRI Dissemination in space in the brain demonstrated by MRI

Abbreviations: CNS, central nervous system; CSF, cerebrospinal fluid; IgG, immunoglobulin G; MRI, magnetic resonance imaging; MS, multiple sclerosis.
Adapted from: Polman CH, Reinglod SC, Banwell, et al. Diagnostic criteria for multiple sclerosis: 2010 revisions to the McDonald criteria. Ann Neurol 2010;69(2):292–302.
[a]MRI lesions disseminated in space = at least three of the following:
Dissemination in space can be demonstrated by the presence of one or more T2 lesions in at least two of four of the following areas of the CNS: periventricular, juxtacortical, infratentorial, or spinal cord.
[b]Dissemination in time, demonstrated by simultaneous presence of asymptomatic gadolinium-enhancing and nonenhancing lesions at any time; or a new T2 and/or gadolinium-enhancing lesion(s) on follow-up MRI, irrespective of its timing with reference to a baseline scan (no longer a need to have separate MRI scans run).

usually administered by the treating neurologist. Symptomatic treatment of persistent visual loss and diplopia is essential and requires a close collaboration with ophthalmologists (see Chapter 21). The treatment of pendular nystagmus is often challenging. It is important for MS patients to be followed by an ophthalmologist who will be able to confirm a diagnosis of optic neuritis when visual loss occurs (and will rule out other causes of visual loss).

20.5 Sarcoidosis

Sarcoidosis is a granulomatous inflammation that can affect every organ, particularly the lungs, the lymph nodes, the skin, and the eyes.

20.5.1 Patient Evaluation

Sarcoidosis may present with numerous systemic, neurologic, and neuroophthalmic symptoms and signs.

Most Common Presenting Symptoms of Sarcoidosis

- Respiratory symptoms in 50%
- Generalized symptoms (fatigue, fever, weight loss) in 20%
- Extrathoracic symptoms in 5 to 10%
- Asymptomatic (abnormal chest X-ray, abnormal liver function tests, hypercalcemia) in 20%

Clinical Manifestations of Sarcoidosis

- Pulmonary involvement in 90%
- Generalized symptoms (fatigue, fever, weight loss) in 20%
- Peripheral lymphadenopathy in 75%
- Cutaneous manifestations
- Liver involvement
- Neurologic manifestations in 5%
- Musculoskeletal manifestations in 5%
- Ocular involvement in 20%
- Cardiac dysfunction
- Renal manifestations
- Heerfordt syndrome (uveoparotid fever)
  - Uveitis
  - Parotid enlargement
  - Fever
  - Sometimes with seventh nerve palsy

Neurologic manifestations of sarcoidosis (neurosarcoidosis), organized from the most common to the least common manifestation (▶ Fig. 20.34, ▶ Fig. 20.35, ▶ Fig. 20.36), include the following:
- Cranial neuropathy
  - Seventh nerve palsy (facial weakness)
  - Eighth nerve palsy (deafness)
  - Ocular motor nerve (diplopia)
  - Optic neuropathy (optic neuritis)
- Aseptic lymphocytic meningitis
- Meningeal thickening (pachymeningitis)
- Hypothalamic dysfunction
- Intracranial mass (granuloma)
- Intraspinal mass (granuloma)
- Seizures
- Encephalopathy
- Peripheral neuropathy

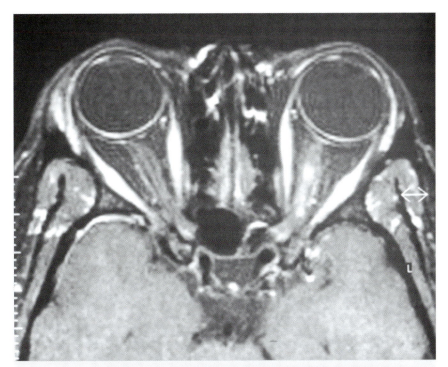

Fig. 20.34 Axial T1-weighted magnetic resonance imaging of the orbits with contrast and fat suppression showing diffuse enhancement of the left optic nerve in a patient with sarcoidosis.

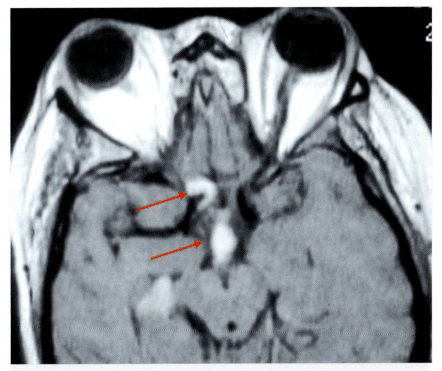

Fig. 20.35 Axial T1-weighted magnetic resonance imaging of the orbits with contrast showing enhancement in the hypothalamic region in a patient with sarcoidosis (*arrows*).

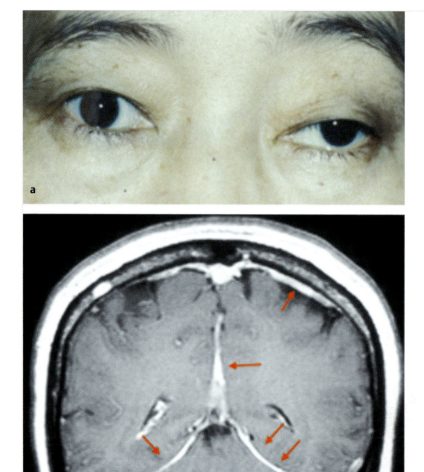

Fig. 20.36 (a) Left third nerve palsy in a patient with sarcoidosis. The patient also has a left optic neuropathy. (b) T1-weighted coronal magnetic resonance imaging with contrast showing diffuse leptomeningeal enhancement (*arrows*).

Neuro-ophthalmic manifestations of systemic sarcoidosis are common, and systemic sarcoidosis may present with isolated ocular or neuro-ophthalmic manifestations (▶ Fig. 20.37, ▶ Fig. 20.38, ▶ Fig. 20.39).

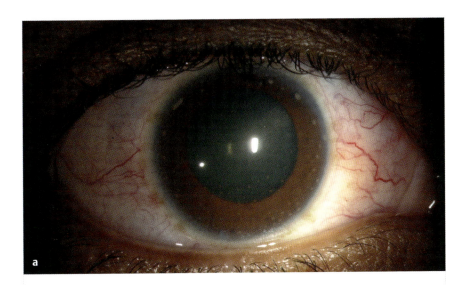

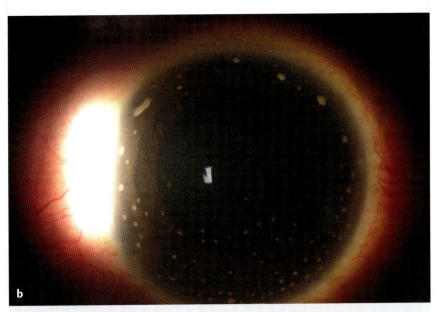

Fig. 20.37 (a) Unilateral (right eye) anterior granulomatous uveitis in sarcoidosis. The eye is red, and the view of the anterior chamber is hazy. (b) Slit-lamp view of the same patient, showing "mutton fat" granulomatous keratic precipitates.

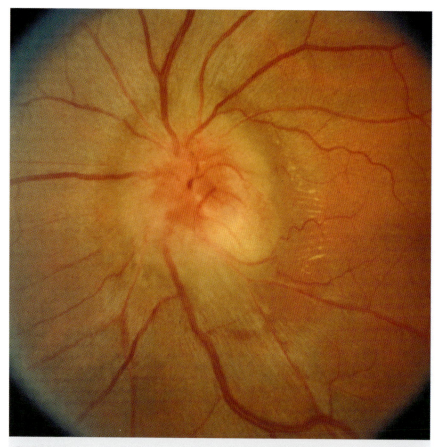

Fig. 20.38 Optic nerve granuloma from sarcoidosis. Note the elevation of the left optic nerve by a whitish mass.

Ocular and neuro-ophthalmic manifestations of sarcoidosis, organized anatomically, include the following:

- Enlargement of the lacrimal gland
  - Pseudoptosis
  - Dry eye syndrome
- Anterior granulomatous uveitis
  - Visual loss
  - Intraocular hypertension
  - Posterior synechiae
  - Cataract
- Pars planitis (intermediate uveitis)
- Posterior uveitis
- Retinal vasculitis
- Retinal infiltrates (granuloma)
- Optic nerve granuloma

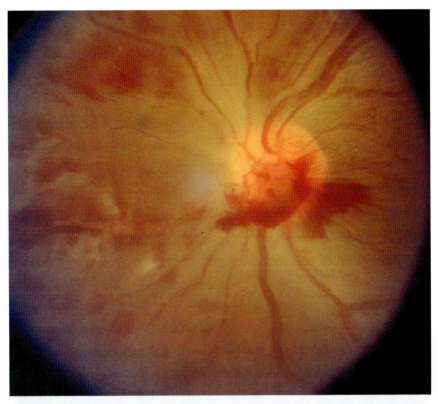

Fig. 20.39 Retinal vasculitis with retinal ischemia and neovascularization responsible for subhyaloid hemorrhages over the optic nerve in a patient with sarcoidosis.

- Optic neuritis
- Chiasmal neuritis
- Papilledema (from raised intracranial pressure)

20.5.2 Diagnosis

Confirmation of the diagnosis of sarcoidosis may be difficult and is mostly aimed at identifying abnormal inflammatory tissue that can be biopsied.
- The gold standard is the histologic confirmation of sarcoid granulomas.
- Chest X-ray is the most useful screening and diagnostic test for sarcoidosis (▶ Fig. 20.40).
  - Bilateral hilar adenopathy
  - Parenchymal infiltrates
- Chest CT
  - Early fibrosis
  - Hilar adenopathy
- Gallium scanning (▶ Fig. 20.41)
  - Increased metabolic activity in the lungs; mediastinum; and lacrimal, parotid, and submandibular glands

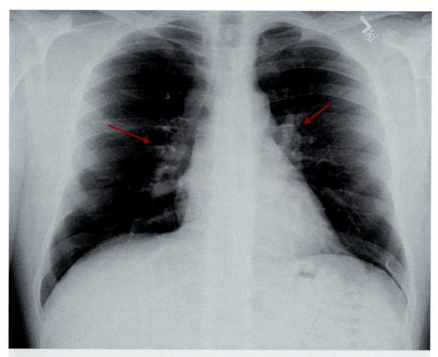

Fig. 20.40 Chest X-ray showing bilateral hilar lymphadenopathy (*arrows*).

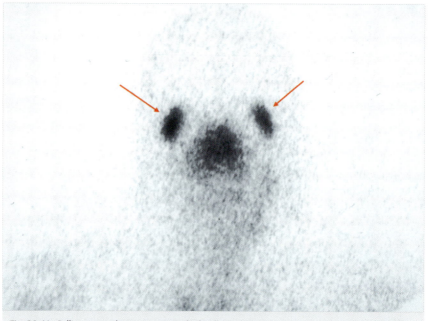

Fig. 20.41 Gallium scan showing increased of gallium update by the lacrimal glands (*arrows*).

- Whole body positron-emission tomography (PET) scan with fluorodeoxyglucose (FDG) is often used instead of a gallium scan
- Angiotensin-converting enzyme (ACE) in the blood
  - Often elevated in sarcoidosis (not specific)
- Hypercalcemia, hypercalciuria
- Cutaneous anergy to skin tests
- Bronchoalveolar lavage
  - Lymphocytosis in the bronchoalveolar lavage fluid

20.5.3 Treatment

- Sarcoidosis is classically very sensitive to steroids.
- In addition to local steroid treatment given for ocular complications of sarcoidosis (treatment of uveitis), systemic steroids are necessary. The dose, route, and duration of treatment depend on the severity of the manifestations.
- Neurosarcoidosis is usually treated more aggressively; other immunosuppressive treatments are usually necessary.

20.6 Infectious Diseases

Systemic infections can produce various neuro-ophthalmic manifestations. Infections can invade the intracranial space, the orbit, and the eye and can produce visual loss, visual field defects, and diplopia.

All infections (bacterial, viral, fungal, and parasitic) may invade the central nervous system and the eye, although some have a particular tropism for these organs. For example, cryptococcal infection (fungus) is a classic cause of acute meningitis in immunodeficient patients; secondary and tertiary syphilis (spirochete) are classic causes of meningitis, uveitis, and optic neuritis; zoster virus infection produces ocular signs and often ophthalmoplegia when involving the first branch of the trigeminal nerve; cat scratch disease (*Bartonella henselae* infection) is a classic cause of neuroretinitis.

The neurologic and ocular complications of systemic infections include the following:
- Intracranial infection
  - Cerebral abscess
  - Cerebral empyema (▶ Fig. 20.12)
  - Infectious meningitis
  - Optic neuritis
  - Encephalitis
  - Ventriculitis
  - Vasculitis
    - Cerebral infarction
    - Cerebral hemorrhages
  - Cavernous sinus abscess or thrombosis
- Orbital cellulitis
- Ocular infection
  - Endophthalmitis
  - Retinitis
  - Choroiditis

- Endocarditis
  - Cerebral infarction
  - Mycotic intracranial aneurysm
  - Retinal emboli (Roth spots)
- Cerebral venous thrombosis
  - Raised intracranial pressure (papilledema)
  - Venous infarction

> **Pearls**
>
> Infectious meningitis often produces an increase in intracranial pressure and severe papilledema. Visual loss from unrecognized papilledema is a common cause of nonreversible visual loss in meningitis. Repeat lumbar punctures and treatment of intracranial hypertension are crucial in this setting. Acute bacterial meningitis, tuberculous meningitis, and cryptococcal meningitis are particularly frequently associated with severe papilledema and visual loss.

20.6.1 Syphilis

Neuro-ophthalmic complications of syphilis (▶ Fig. 20.42 and ▶ Fig. 20.43) include the following:
- Uveitis (all types)
- Retinitis
- Choroiditis
- Optic neuritis
- Lymphocytic meningitis
  - Papilledema
  - Basilar meningitis with cranial nerve palsies
  - Vasculitis
    - Cerebral infarction
- Intracranial mass (gumma)

20.6.2 Acquired Immunodeficiency Syndrome

Posterior segment manifestations of acquired immunodeficiency syndrome (AIDS) include the following (▶ Fig. 20.43, ▶ Fig. 20.44, ▶ Fig. 20.45, ▶ Fig. 20.46):
- Infectious
  - Herpes zoster ophthalmicus and optic neuritis
  - Herpes simplex optic neuritis
  - Progressive outer retinal necrosis (PORN)
  - Cytomegalovirus retinitis and optic neuritis
  - Toxoplasmosis chorioretinitis and optic neuritis
  - Syphilis retinitis and optic neuritis
  - *Pneumocystis jiroveci* (formerly *P. carinii*) choroiditis
  - Fungal choroiditis
  - Papilledema from meningitis (cryptococcal meningitis most common)

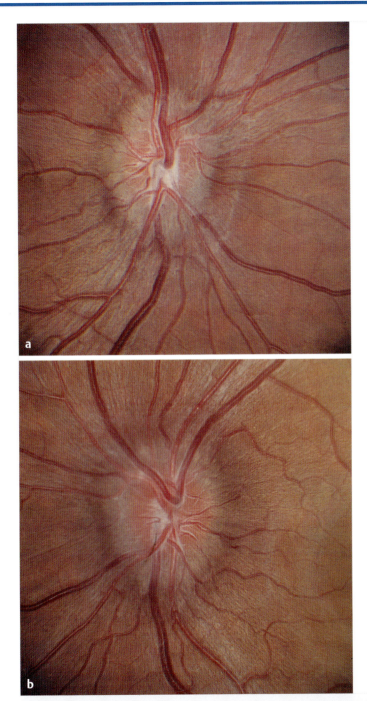

Fig. 20.42 a,b Bilateral papilledema in a patient with secondary syphilis and chronic lymphocytic meningitis. This patient was found to be positive for human immunodeficiency virus.

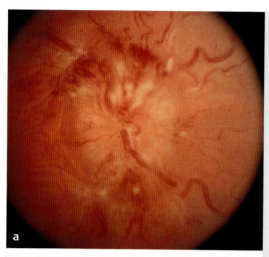

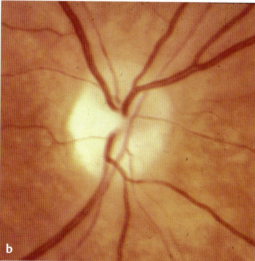

Fig. 20.43 (a) Severe optic nerve head edema in a patient with cryptococcal meningitis. (b) Optic atrophy and severe visual loss after treatment of cryptococcal meningitis.

- Noninfectious
  - Retinal microvasculopathy
  - Retinal cotton wool spots
  - Ocular lymphoma
  - HIV optic neuritis

20.6.3 Cat Scratch Disease (*Bartonella Henselae* Infection)

Bartonella henselae infection produces various ocular manifestations, including anterior segment inflammation, retinitis, and optic neuritis (▶ Fig. 20.47 and ▶ Fig. 20.48). Retinal vascular occlusions are also common.

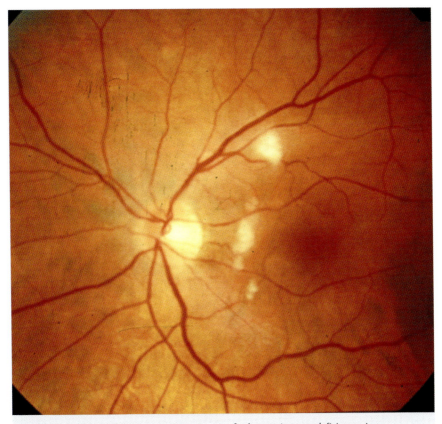

Fig. 20.44 Cotton wool spots in a patient positive for human immunodeficiency virus.

20.6.4 Whipple Disease

This rare disorder is often discussed in neuro-ophthalmology because it is frequently associated with eye movement abnormalities. It is caused by a gram-positive bacillus (*Tropheryma whipplei)*, which mostly resides in the gut.

Clinical Presentation

- Weight loss, fever
- Diarrhea, abdominal pain
- Arthralgias
- Lymphadenopathy
- Neurologic manifestations (may be isolated):
  - Slowly progressive memory loss with cognitive impairment
  - Oculomasticatory movements (myorhythmia)
  - Supranuclear vertical (more than horizontal) gaze palsy

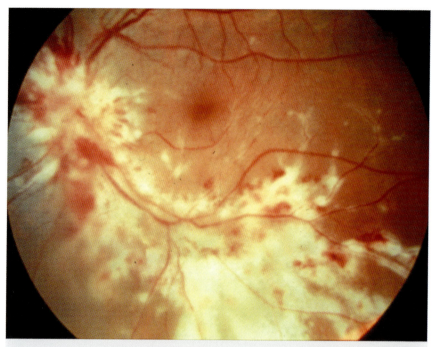

Fig. 20.45 Cytomegalovirus retinitis in a patient with acquired immunodeficiency syndrome. The disc is swollen and hemorrhagic. There is involvement of the inferior half of the retina.

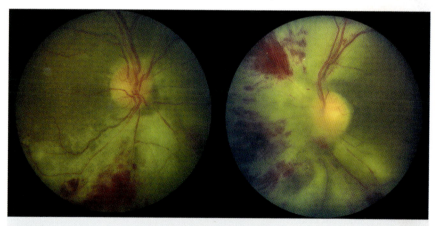

Fig. 20.46 Progressive outer retinal necrosis is a necrotizing acute retinopathy most often secondary to infection by herpes zoster (also possible with herpes simplex and cytomegalovirus) in immunodeficient patients. The entire retina is necrotic (yellow) with hemorrhages and very attenuated arteries. It progresses rapidly over a few days, beginning at the periphery of the retina.

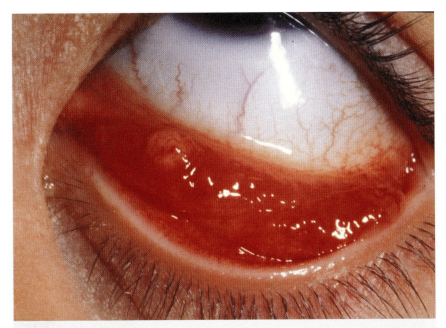

Fig. 20.47 Conjunctival granuloma from cat scratch disease.

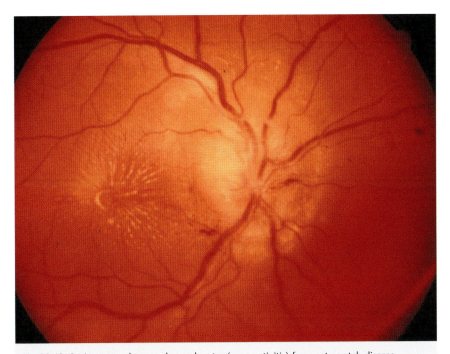

Fig. 20.48 Optic nerve edema and macular star (neuroretinitis) from cat scratch disease.

Diagnosis

- Positive polymerase chain reaction (PCR) for *Tropheryma whipplei* in the CSF
- Biopsy of jejunal mucosa with periodic acid-Schiff stain (PAS-positive organisms)
- Positive PCR for *Tropheryma whipplei* in the jejunal biopsy

Treatment

Treatment consists of long-term antibiotics.

Tumors

Intracranial tumors (all types) often produce neuro-ophthalmic symptoms and signs.

20.6.5 Mechanisms

The mechanisms by which brain tumors produce neuroophthalmic symptoms and signs include the following.
- Raised intracranial pressure (from the mass or from obstructive hydrocephalus)
  - Papilledema
  - Diplopia (from sixth nerve palsy)
- Mass effect or infiltration
  - Choroidal metastasis
  - Intracranial optic nerve (optic neuropathy)
  - Chiasm (bitemporal hemianopia)
  - Retrochiasmal visual pathways (homonymous hemianopia)
  - Ocular motor cranial nerve (diplopia)
- Carcinomatous meningitis
  - Raised intracranial pressure
  - Multiple cranial nerve palsies
- Paraneoplastic syndrome from a cancer
  - Retinopathy
  - Optic neuropathy
  - Nystagmus, opsoclonus, brainstem syndromes
- Toxicity of treatment
  - Postsurgical complication
  - Radiation
    - Radiation necrosis of the brain
    - Radiation optic neuropathy (see Chapter 8)
    - Radiation retinopathy
  - Chemotherapy
    - Optic nerve toxicity

Cancer patients who develop neuro-ophthalmic symptoms or signs (such as optic neuropathy, papilledema, visual field defect, diplopia, or nystagmus) need immediate neuroimaging (MRI of the brain, often with the orbits, and *with contrast).* If the imaging is normal, then a lumbar puncture with CSF opening pressure, cytology, and flow cytometry needs to be performed.

20.6.6 Carcinomatous Meningitis

Carcinomatous meningitis must be ruled out in all patients with raised intracranial pressure and a known history of cancer. Imaging is often normal or may show leptomeningeal enhancement. A lumbar puncture with CSF opening pressure and CSF analysis, including cytology and flow cytometry, is mandatory. If normal, the lumbar puncture should be repeated for repeat cytologic examination. Sometimes, it is necessary to perform at least three lumbar punctures to make a diagnosis of carcinomatous meningitis.

The most common sites or types of cancer in patients with carcinomatous meningitis are as follows:
- Breast
- Lung
- Lymphoma
- Melanoma
- Adenocarcinoma of unknown origin

> **Pearls**
>
> The three classic causes of raised intracranial pressure in patients with known cancer are (1) metastasis, (2) carcinomatous meningitis, (3) cerebral venous thrombosis (from cancer-induced hypercoagulable state).

20.6.7 Paraneoplastic Syndromes

Paraneoplastic syndromes represent rare nonmetastatic complications of cancer, which can affect multiple levels of the nervous system. Autoantibodies are usually found in the CSF or serum. Paraneoplastic syndromes may complicate a known cancer or may be the first sign of a very localized cancer.

Neuro-ophthalmic symptoms and signs are relatively common and include the following:
- Abnormal eye movements
  - Opsoclonus (Ri antibodies)
  - Ocular flutter (Ri antibodies)
  - Cerebellar degeneration (Yo antibodies)
  - Nystagmus
  - Slow saccades, limited vertical movements (Hu, Ma/Ta antibodies)
- Neuromuscular junction disorder (Lambert–Eaton syndrome or myasthenic syndrome)
  - Voltage-gated calcium channel antibodies
- Visual loss
  - Retinal degeneration
    - Cancer-associated retinopathy (CAR) antibodies
    - Melanoma-associated retinopathy (MAR) antibodies
  - Optic neuropathy with disc edema and intraocular inflammation
    - CRMP-5 antibodies

20.7 Traumatic Brain Injury

Neuro-ophthalmic manifestations of traumatic brain injury include the following:
- Visual loss
  - Monocular
    - Trauma to the eye
    - Orbital trauma
    - Optic nerve injury (direct/indirect)
  - Binocular
    - Trauma to both eyes or both optic nerves
    - Traumatic chiasmopathy (bitemporal hemianopia)
    - Trauma to the retrochiasmal visual pathways (homonymous hemianopia)
  - Higher cortical function impairment from brain injury
- Diplopia
  - Orbital trauma (entrapment, fibrosis of extraocular muscles)
  - Cranial nerve palsies (fourth, sixth, and third)
  - Intracranial lesions

Causes of posttraumatic acute visual loss include the following:
- Refractive error
  - Glasses or contact lenses are lost or damaged at the time of trauma (may be overlooked in patients with difficulty communicating)
- Ocular injury
  - Ruptured globe (anterior with corneal laceration or posterior with scleral laceration)
  - Intraocular foreign body
  - Exposure keratopathy (secondary to proptosis, lid laceration, or seventh nerve dysfunction)
  - Corneal edema (from airbag injury)
  - Corneal abrasion
  - Hyphema (blood in anterior chamber)
  - Traumatic iritis (often delayed by about 24 hours)
  - Traumatic mydriasis (and decreased accommodation)
  - Lens subluxation or luxation
  - Vitreous hemorrhage
  - Commotio retinae
  - Retinal detachment
  - Retinal ischemia from carotid dissection
  - Retinal fat emboli
  - Choroidal rupture
- Optic nerve
  - Direct traumatic optic neuropathy
  - Indirect traumatic optic neuropathy
  - Intrasheath hematoma
  - Avulsion of the optic nerve head
  - Penetrating injuries of the orbit with direct optic nerve injury
  - Intraorbital foreign body
  - Optic nerve ischemia from carotid dissection
- Orbit
  - Orbital fracture (direct optic nerve damage)
  - Orbital hemorrhage (optic nerve ischemia)

- Orbital emphysema (optic nerve ischemia)
- Carotid cavernous fistula (increased intraocular pressure)
- Subperiosteal hemorrhage (direct optic nerve damage or optic nerve ischemia)
- Intracranial optic pathways
  - Chiasmal or retrochiasmal direct injury
  - Chiasmal or retrochiasmal indirect injury
  - Hemorrhage or hematoma compressing the chiasm
  - Cerebral diffuse axonal injury with homonymous hemianopia
  - Intraparenchymal hemorrhage with homonymous hemianopia
  - Cerebral infarction (posterior cerebral artery) secondary to increased intracranial pressure/herniation with homonymous hemianopia or cerebral blindness
  - Cerebral infarction secondary to cervical artery dissection with homonymous hemianopia

20.8 Visual Loss during Ocular or Cranial Surgery

Damage to the intracranial visual pathways or to the optic nerves may occur during surgery. Visual loss is particularly common during ocular and intracranial surgery, but it may occur as a complication of any surgical procedure. The first step when evaluating a patient with postoperative visual loss is to localize the lesion by an ophthalmic examination.

Visual loss during ocular surgery can result from the following:
- Optic neuropathy
  - Direct damage to the retrobulbar optic nerve from retrobulbar anesthesia, orbital surgery, orbital hemorrhage after blepharoplasty
  - Fluctuation in intraocular pressure during ocular surgery
  - Postoperative intraocular hypertension
- Diplopia
  - Direct damage to the extraocular muscles from the following:
    - Retrobulbar anesthesia
    - Orbital surgery
    - Orbital hemorrhage after blepharoplasty
    - Scleral buckle placed for treatment of a retinal detachment
- Ptosis
  - Damage of the levator muscle from the ocular speculum

Visual loss during cranial surgery can result from compression, edema, ischemia, hemorrhage, or direct injury to the intracranial optic nerve, the chiasm, or the intracranial retrochiasmal visual pathways.

Visual loss during nonocular, noncranial surgery can result from the following:
- Anterior segment lesion
  - Corneal abrasion
  - Trauma (pressure on the eye during surgery)
  - Reversible retinal toxicity after prostate surgery (irrigating solution)
- Ocular ischemia
  - Central retinal artery occlusion
  - Ischemic optic neuropathy (anterior and posterior)
- Chiasmal lesion
  - Pituitary apoplexy
- Intracranial ischemia (homonymous hemianopia or cerebral blindness)

Ischemic optic neuropathies are particularly common after coronary artery bypass graft and after spinal surgery. Their mechanism remains debated.

Retinal and optic nerve ischemia may also occur during any procedure complicated by major bleeding with severe hypotension and after procedures involving the cervical vessels or dissection of the neck.

20.9 Phacomatoses

The phacomatoses are a group of disorders characterized by multiple hamartomas of the central and peripheral nervous systems, eye, skin, and viscera. The central nervous system lesions in phacomatoses have a very different natural history and prognosis than those found in other patients (e.g., the gliomas observed in the phacomatosis neurofibromatosis type 1 are often benign, whereas a glioma in a patient without neurofibromatosis may be a more aggressive tumor).

20.9.1 Neurofibromatosis Type 1

Neurofibromatosis type 1 (NF1; also known as von Recklinghausen disease) is the most common phacomatosis (1/5,000) and is autosomal dominant (NF1 gene localized on chromosome 17) with high penetrance and variable expressivity.

The diagnostic criteria for NF1 include two or more of the following:
- Café au lait macules (≥ 6) (▶ Fig. 20.49)
- Neurofibromas (≥ 2) (▶ Fig. 20.50 and ▶ Fig. 20.51)
- Freckling (axillary, inguinal)
- Lisch nodules (iris pigment epithelium hamartomas) (▶ Fig. 20.52)

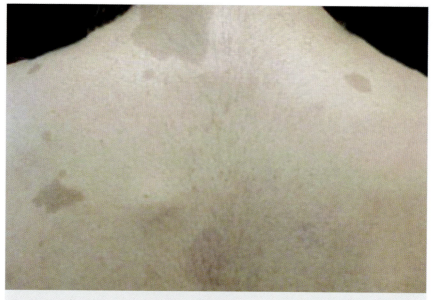

Fig. 20.49 Café au lait spots in neurofibromatosis type 1.

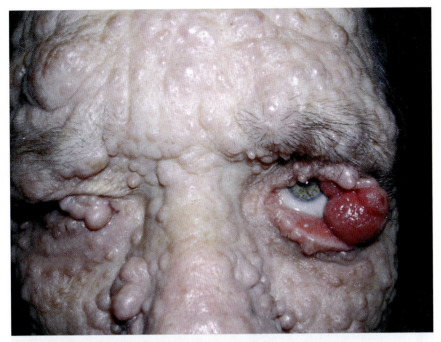

Fig. 20.50 Numerous cutaneous neurofibromas in neurofibromatosis type 1.

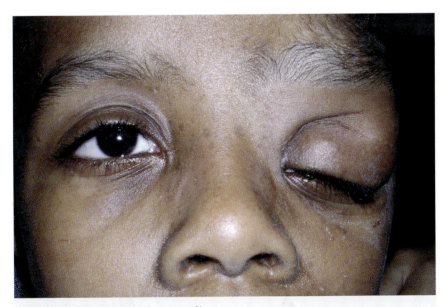

Fig. 20.51 Left upper lid plexiform neurofibroma.

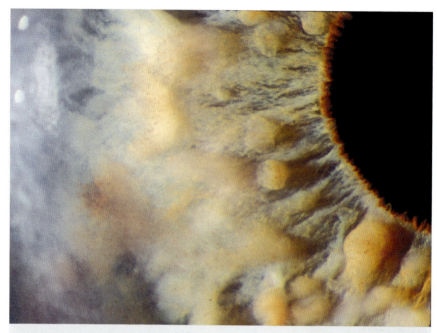

Fig. 20.52 Iris at the slit lamp with evidence of Lisch nodules. Lisch nodules appear during childhood.

- Optic nerve glioma (▶ Fig. 20.53)
- Sphenoid dysplasia (▶ Fig. 20.54)
- First-degree relative with NF1

The most prominent manifestation of NF1 is the involvement of cranial and peripheral nerves by two types of tumors:
- Schwannomas (neuromas, neurinomas, neurilemmomas)
  - Affect cranial nerves (fifth, third, fourth, and sixth nerves are most commonly affected)
- Neurofibromas
  - Plexiform neurofibromas
  - Localized neurofibromas

Central nervous system tumors (see ▶ Fig. 20.53) are common in NF1.
- Optic nerve or chiasmal gliomas (in 15–20% of NF1 patients)
  - Often asymptomatic
  - May produce progressive loss of vision
  - May improve spontaneously
  - Treatment (chemotherapy, radiation) is performed only in cases with documented worsening of visual function.
- Low-grade astrocytic tumors

Patients with NF1 may also have sphenoid dysplasia or absence of the sphenoid wing (see ▶ Fig. 20.54).

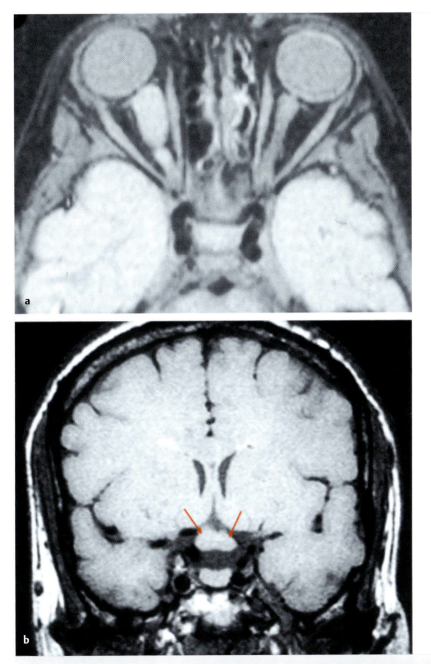

Fig. 20.53 (a) Axial T1-weighted magnetic resonance imaging (MRI) of the orbits without contrast showing bilaterally enlarged optic nerves consistent with optic nerve glioma. Note the kinking of the right optic nerve. (b) Coronal T1-weighted MRI of the orbits without contrast showing bilaterally enlarged optic nerves (*arrows*) consistent with optic nerve gliomas.

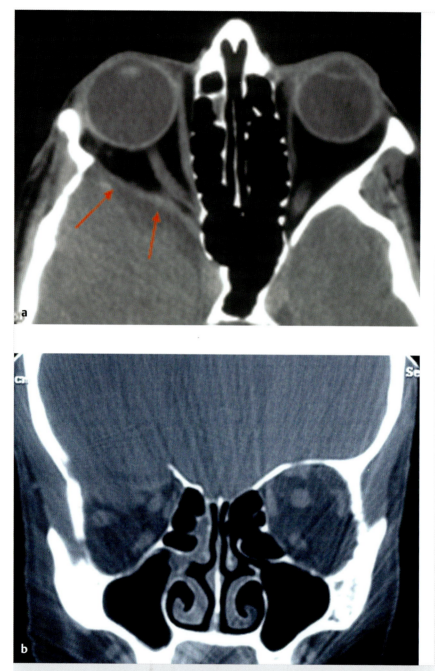

Fig. 20.54 (a) Axial and (b) coronal computed tomographic scan of the brain without contrast (bone window) showing the absence of the sphenoid wing on the right (the red arrows indicate where the sphenoid wing should be), with herniation of the brain into the orbit.

- Pulsatile exophthalmos or enophthalmos
- Herniation of dura, CSF, and brain into the orbit (encephalocele)
- May rarely result in compression of the extraocular muscles with diplopia and compression of the optic nerve with visual loss

20.9.2 Neurofibromatosis Type 2

Neurofibromatosis type 2 (NF2) is much less common than NF1 (1/50,000) and is an autosomal dominant disorder (NF2 gene localized on chromosome 22) with high penetrance.

The diagnostic criteria for NF2 include the following:
- Bilateral eighth cranial nerve mass identified on imaging *or* first degree relative with NF2 *and*
- Unilateral eighth nerve mass *or* two or more of the following:
  - Neurofibroma
  - Meningioma
  - Glioma
  - Schwannoma
  - Juvenile posterior subcapsular cataract
- Lisch nodules and skin lesions are less common in NF2 than in NF1.
- The most prominent manifestation of NF2 is bilateral acoustic neuromas (▶ Fig. 20.55).

20.9.3 Tuberous Sclerosis (Bourneville disease)

Tuberous sclerosis is an autosomal dominant disorder, with high penetrance, and variable expressivity.

Patients present with a classic triad including the following:
- Adenoma sebaceum
- Mental retardation
- Epilepsy

Diagnosis

Definite diagnosis requires one primary feature and two secondary features or one secondary feature and two tertiary features.
- Primary features
  - Facial angiofibromas (▶ Fig. 20.56)
  - Multiple ungual fibromas
  - Cerebral mass: cortical tubers, giant cell astrocytoma, calcified subependymal nodules protruding in the ventricle
  - Multiple retinal astrocytomas (▶ Fig. 20.57)
- Secondary features
  - Affected first-degree relative
  - Cardiac rhabdomyosarcoma
  - Retinal hamartoma or retinal achromatic patch
  - Shagreen patch
  - Forehead plaque
  - Pulmonary lymphangiomyomatosis
  - Renal angiomyolipoma, renal cysts

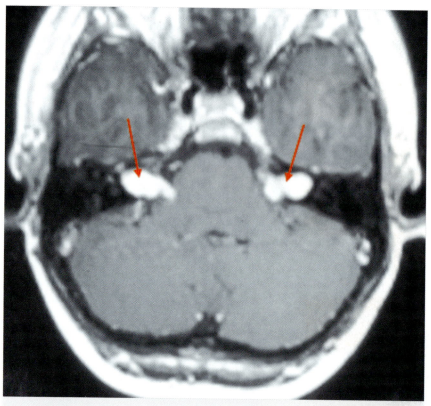

Fig. 20.55 Axial T1-weighted magnetic resonance imaging of the brain with contrast showing bilateral acoustic neuromas (*arrows*) in a patient with neurofibromatosis type 2.

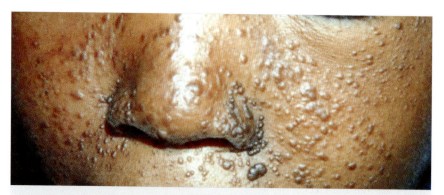

Fig. 20.56 Facial angiofibromas in tuberous sclerosis.

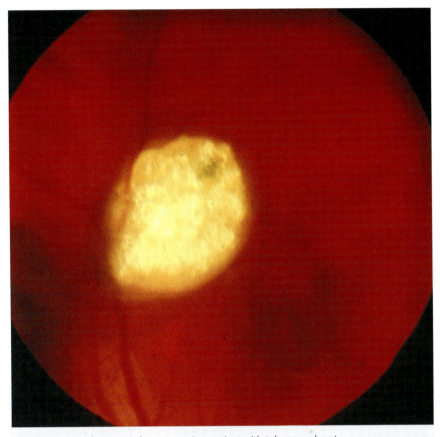

Fig. 20.57 Retinal astrocytic hamartoma in a patient with tuberous sclerosis.

- Tertiary features
  - Hypomelanotic macules
  - "Confetti" skin lesions
  - Renal, bone cysts
  - Nonrenal angiomyolipoma
  - Hamartomatous rectal polyps
  - Pulmonary lymphangiomyomatosis
  - Gingival lipomas
  - Infantile spasms
  - Cerebral white matter migration tracts or heterotopias

Seizures are the most common presenting symptom of tuberous sclerosis. Mental retardation occurs in > 50% of patients.

The most prominent ocular manifestation is hamartomas of the retina and optic nerve. They are observed in up to 50% of patients but rarely cause visual loss.

20.9.4 Von Hippel–Lindau Disease

Von Hippel–Lindau disease is an autosomal dominant disorder associating multiple, bilateral retinal angiomas and intracranial hemangioblastomas (most often in the cerebellum) (▶ Fig. 20.58). Twenty-five percent of patients will have a renal cell carcinoma. Five percent of patients will have a pheochromocytoma.

- Retinal angioma
  - Feeder vessel
  - Numerous exudates
  - Exudative retinal detachment

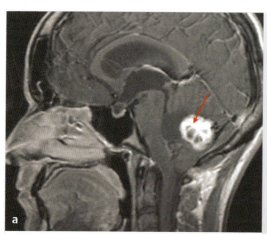

Fig. 20.58 (a) Sagittal T1-weighted magnetic resonance imaging of the brain with contrast showing a cerebellar hemangioblastoma (*arrow*). (b) Retinal angioma in the peripheral retina in a patient with von Hippel–Lindau disease. There are yellow exudates at the edge of the angioma.

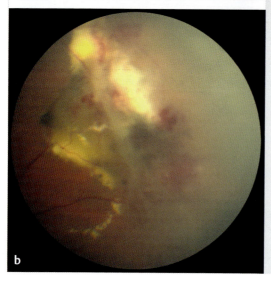

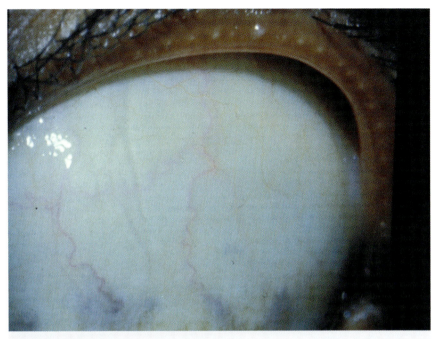

Fig. 20.59 Telangiectasias of conjunctival vessels.

20.9.5 Ataxia Telangiectasia (Louis-Bar Syndrome)

Ataxia telangiectasia is an autosomal recessive disorder associating cerebellar ataxia, telangiectasias, immune deficiency, and susceptibility to neoplasms.

Classic ophthalmologic manifestations include the following:
- Telangiectasias of the conjunctival vessels (▶ Fig. 20.59)
- Oculomotor apraxia

20.9.6 Sturge–Weber Syndrome (Encephalotrigeminal Angiomatosis)

- Characterized by cutaneous hemifacial hemangioma associated with hemangioma of the ipsilateral meninges and brain (▶ Fig. 20.60)
- Nonhereditary disorder
- Facial hemangioma present at birth (follows V1 and V2 innervation)
- Ocular manifestations ipsilateral to the hemangioma
  - Intraocular hypertension (increased episcleral venous pressure, immature angle, and neovascularization of the angle); glaucoma is particularly common when the hemangioma involves the upper eyelid.
  - Choroidal hemangioma

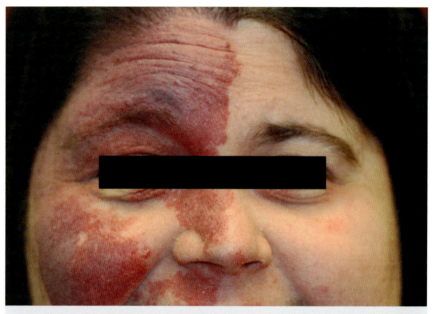

Fig. 20.60 Facial hemangioma involving the right side of the face in a woman with Sturge–Weber syndrome; she has a glaucomatous right optic neuropathy.

- Homonymous hemianopia contralateral to the meningeal hemangioma
- Seizures, headaches are common
- Raised intracranial pressure possible

20.9.7 Wyburn-Mason Syndrome

- Association of retinal arteriovenous malformations with an intracranial arteriovenous malformation, typically in the ipsilateral brainstem (see ▶ Fig. 20.17).
- Nonhereditary

20.9.8 Klippel–Trénaunay–Weber Syndrome

- Large cutaneous hemangiomas with hypertrophy of the related bones and soft tissues
- Retinal angiomas

20.10 Mitochondrial Disorders

The mitochondrial diseases are a heterogeneous group of disorders in which clinical presentation, inheritance, histopathology, or biochemical or genetic analysis suggest primary mitochondrial dysfunction. In many of these disorders, the central nervous system and the eye figure prominently. ▶ Table 20.4 lists the neuro-ophthalmic and systemic manifestations of several mitochondrial disorders.

Table 20.4 Neuro-ophthalmic manifestations of mitochondrial disorders

Disease	Ophthalmic manifestations	Systemic manifestations
LHON (Leber hereditary optic neuropathy)	Early: disc microangiopathy[a] Pseudo disc edema[a] Vascular tortuosity[a] Late: optic atrophy[a]	Cardiac conduction abnormalities Multiple sclerosis–like illness Minor neurologic/skeletal abnormalities Dystonia/basal ganglia lesions Encephalopathy
DOA (dominant optic atrophy)	Optic atrophy[a]	Hearing loss
CPEO (chronic progressive external ophthalmoplegia)/ KSS (Kearns–Sayre syndrome)	Ophthalmoplegia[a] Ptosis[a] Pigmentary retinopathy[a]	Myopathy/ragged red fibers[a] Peripheral neuropathy Deafness/vestibular dysfunction Dementia Ataxia Basal ganglia lesions Cardiac conduction abnormalities Short stature Gastrointestinal dysmotility Diabetes mellitus Delayed sexual maturation/ hypogonadism Hypomagnesemia Hypoparathyroidism Hypothyroidism
MNGIE (mitochondrial neuro-gastrointestinal encephalomyopathy)	Ophthalmoplegia[a] Ptosis[a] Pigmentary retinopathy	Gastrointestinal dysmotility[a] Cachexia[a] Sensorimotor peripheral neuropathy[a] Leukoencephalopathy
MELAS (mitochondrial myopathy, encephalopathy, lactic acidosis, and stroke-like episodes) syndrome	Homonymous hemianopia[a] Cerebral blindness[a] Pigmentary retinopathy[a] Ophthalmoplegia Optic atrophy	Headaches[a] Strokelike episodes[a] Seizures[a] Lactic acidosis[a] Psychiatric abnormalities Deafness Short stature Myopathy Basal ganglia lesions
NARP (neurogenic muscle weakness, ataxia, and retinitis pigmentosa)/Leigh syndrome	Pigmentary retinopathy[a] Optic atrophy	Neurogenic muscle weakness[a] Ataxia[a] Developmental delay[a] Sensory neuropathy Dementia Seizures Spongiform degeneration of basal ganglia and brainstem
MERRF (myoclonic epilepsy and ragged red fibers)	Optic atrophy	Myoclonus[a] Seizures[a] Myopathy[a] Ataxia[a] Dementia[a] Developmental delay
MIDD (maternally inherited diabetes mellitus and deafness)	Macular dystrophy[a]	Diabetes mellitus[a] Deafness[a]

[a]Commonly found.

The most common neuro-ophthalmic abnormalities seen in mitochondrial disorders include the following:
- Bilateral optic neuropathy (Leber hereditary optic neuropathy or dominant optic atrophy)
- Ophthalmoplegia with ptosis (chronic progressive external ophthalmoplegia)
- Pigmentary retinopathy
- Retrochiasmal visual loss (MELAS)

20.11 Chiari Malformations

Chiari malformations represent a continuum of hindbrain maldevelopments character-ized by downward herniation of the cerebellar tonsils. Chiari I malformation (Arnold–Chiari malformation) is defined as tonsillar herniation of at least 3 to 5 mm below the foramen magnum (▶ Fig. 20.61). It is sometimes associated with syringomyelia and other anomalies of the craniocervical junction.

There is overcrowding of the cerebellum within a small posterior cranial fossa leading to chronic tonsillar herniation. This overcrowding is believed to be responsible for the neurologic symptoms and signs that often develop during the second or third decade of life. Symptoms and signs may be related to changes in the CSF flow and to direct compression of the brainstem.

The clinical manifestations of Chiari I malformations are numerous, and it is often difficult to establish a direct relationship between nonspecific manifestations such as headache or dizziness and moderate tonsillar herniation.
- Often asymptomatic, discovered on a brain MRI obtained for another reason
- Headache (often with Valsalva or exercise)
- Dizziness, ataxia, vertigo
- Dysphagia, hoarseness
- Tinnitus

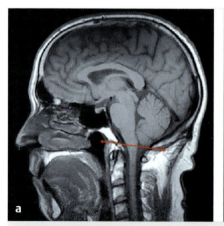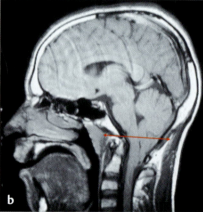

Fig. 20.61 (a) Sagittal magnetic resonance imaging (MRI) of the brain showing the normal position of the cerebellar tonsils in a healthy subject. The red arrow shows the line going through the foramen magnum (between the posterior part of the clivus and the lower level of the foramen magnum). (b) Sagittal MRI of the brain showing the herniation of the cerebellar tonsils in a patient with Chiari I malformation.

Neuro-ophthalmic manifestations of Chiari I malformations include the following:
- Downbeat nystagmus
- Diplopia
  ○ Unilateral or bilateral sixth nerve palsy
  ○ Divergence insufficiency

A specific MRI technique (Cine MRI) allows visualization of the CSF in the posterior fossa. The flow is abnormal in patients with symptomatic Chiari I malformation.

Treatment includes suboccipital decompression associated with C1 laminectomy and is performed only in patients with symptomatic Chiari I malformation.

Chiari II and Chiari III malformations are present at birth and consist of downward herniation of the lower cerebellum and medulla into the spinal canal, in association with complex anomalies of the brain.

20.12 Idiopathic Parkinson Disease

Although idiopathic Parkinson disease typically does not directly produce any clinically symptomatic ocular or neuro-ophthalmic complications, patients with idiopathic Parkinson disease have numerous ocular complaints, related either to the disease or to the medications used to treat the disease.

Neuro-ophthalmic manifestations of Parkinson disease include the following:
- Decreased vision during reading and ocular discomfort
  ○ Ocular surface irritation
    – Dry eyes
    – Blepharitis
  ○ Decreased blink rate (hypokinesia)
  ○ Convergence insufficiency
- Impaired visual function
  ○ Decreased color discrimination
  ○ Decreased contrast sensitivity
  ○ Visuospatial deficits
- Visual hallucinations
- Abnormal eyelid movements
  ○ Reduced spontaneous blink
  ○ Blepharospasm
  ○ Apraxia of lid opening
- Abnormal eye movements
  ○ Decreased saccade performance
  ○ Decreased adaptive modification of saccade amplitudes
  ○ Ocular microtremor
  ○ Convergence insufficiency
- Complications of pallidotomy or stimulation
  ○ Contralateral homonymous hemianopia
  ○ Square-wave jerks

Neuro-ophthalmic manifestations are also common with other Parkinson syndromes. For example, patients with Lewy body dementia often have terrifying visual hallucinations. Patients with supranuclear palsy have abnormal vertical eye movements early in the course of the disease.

Patients with Parkinson disease and similar syndromes may benefit from the following:

- Avoidance of medications that interact with tear secretion and accommodation
- Improved ambient light for reading to improve contrast
- Use of a music or cookbook stand to read if there is tremor or a downgaze deficit
- Treatment for ocular surface disease such as blepharitis
- Artificial tears
- Punctal occlusion for severe dry eye syndrome
- Avoidance of bifocals or progressive lenses
  - Increase the risk of fall
  - Not correctly used if head bent over
  - Cannot be used with a walker
  - Increase asthenopia and diplopia
- Separate pairs of glasses for distance vision (walking and watching TV) and reading (reading and close-up work or eating)
- Base-in prism in reading glasses if symptomatic of convergence insufficiency
- When prescribing spectacles, the spherical equivalent may be preferable to significant astigmatic correction because glasses tend not to be stable on patients with tremor, dyskinesias, or susceptibility to falling.
- Using a finger to lead the eyes across the page in the setting of decreased saccadic velocity
- Treatment of blepharospasm and apraxia of eyelid opening with botulinum toxin and/or surgery if not improved after treatment of ocular surface irritation

20.13 Wilson Disease (Hepatolenticular Degeneration)

- Hereditary disorder of copper metabolism (autosomal recessive); gene is on chromosome 13
- Reduced rate of incorporation of copper into ceruloplasmin and reduction in biliary excretion of copper resulting in deposition of copper in tissues
- Progressive degeneration of the central nervous system associated with liver cirrhosis (half of patients are symptomatic by age 15; early diagnosis is associated with a better prognosis)
- Neurologic syndrome
  - Extrapyramidal syndrome with tremor, motor dysfunction, and behavioral changes
- Ocular findings
  - Peripheral corneal ring of copper deposition involving the Descemet membrane (Kayser–Fleischer ring)
  - Copper pigment under lens capsule
  - Sunflower cataract
  - Various eye movement disorders
    - Paresis of accommodation
    - Jerky oscillations of the eyes, slow saccades

Screening for a Kayser–Fleischer ring is helpful in the diagnosis of Wilson disease. It is best performed with a slit-lamp examination and gonioscopy (▶ Fig. 20.62). The ring begins superiorly.

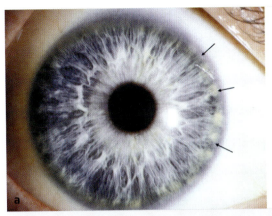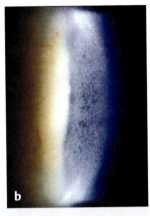

Fig. 20.62 (a) Kayser–Fleischer ring (slit lamp). Note the brown discoloration of the peripheral cornea (*arrows*). (**b**) Kayser–Fleischer ring is best seen on gonioscopy.

The ring may be absent at the initial stage of liver disease. The ring is always present once neurologic signs become manifest.

Other diagnostic tests include the following:

- Low serum ceruloplasmin level, low serum copper, increased urinary copper excretion
- Abnormal basal ganglia on brain imaging

Copper chelating agent (D-penicillamine) is used to treat Wilson disease, and the Kayser–Fleischer ring resolves with treatment.

21 The Visually Impaired Patient

Neuro-ophthalmic disorders often lead to some level of permanent visual impairment, and this needs to be addressed early in the course of the disease. Visual impairments may take many forms and be of varying degrees. Visual acuity alone is not always a good predictor of the degree of problems a person may have. Someone with relatively good acuity (e.g., 20/40) can have difficulty with daily functioning, while someone with worse acuity (e.g., 20/200) may function reasonably well (▶ Fig. 21.1).

Some people who fall into this category can use their residual to complete daily tasks without relying on alternative methods. The role of a low vision specialist is to maximize the functional level of a patient's vision by optical or nonoptical means.

21.1 Defining Visual Disability

The World Health Organization lists several categories of visual disability:
- Low vision is defined as follows:
  - Best corrected (with glasses) visual acuity between 20/60 and 20/200
  - Or corresponding visual field loss to < 20 degrees in the better eye
- Blindness is defined as follows:
  - Best corrected visual acuity of less than 20/400
  - Or corresponding visual field loss to < 10 degrees in the better eye

The Social Security Administration of the United States declares a taxpayer disabled for economic purposes and eligible for supplemental security income when
- the best corrected visual acuity is 20/200 or worse in the better eye, or
- the visual field is limited to 20 degrees or less in the better eye, or both.

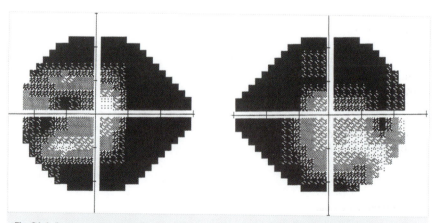

Fig. 21.1 Severe constriction of visual fields from chronic untreated papilledema, resulting in legal blindness. The patient's visual acuity is 20/30 in both eyes, but there is less than 10 degrees of residual central vision, resulting in severe visual impairment. Although the patient can read individual small letters and identify objects and people, reading sentences is very difficult, and ambulation without assistance is impossible. The patient is not legally allowed to drive.

21.2 Treatment of the Visually Impaired Patient

Aside from medical treatment of the cause of visual loss, information, rehabilitation, education, and work and social integration are essential for visually impaired patients. Such patients should be referred to specialized clinics dedicated to the management of visually impaired patients, such as low vision clinics or centers for the visually impaired.

Information is fundamental and must be offered by physicians, once a diagnosis of irreversible visual loss is made:

- Administrative aids are very important and range from help with applying for disability to where to find various resources,
- Adaptation to the disability and psychological help are priority issues and must be confronted from the start.
- Education of the patient and his or her family to confront the new situation is also essential and must be addressed early.
- Adaptation of the home is essential in maintaining autonomy and ensuring safety.
- Adaptation of the workplace is regulated by laws and must be considered before applying for disability.
- Information for the school is essential for visually impaired children and college students who can benefit from specific aids.
- Social integration aids facilitate adapted leisure and cultural activities. Information on such aids is most often obtained from low vision clinics or centers for the visually impaired, and from private foundations.

21.2.1 Optical Aids

The vast majority of patients with low vision can be helped to function at a higher level with the use of low vision devices. Low vision specialists recommend appropriate low vision devices (the general goal of which is to magnify the image) and counsel patients on how to better deal with their reduced vision in general. Many government and private organizations exist to aid the visually impaired.

Various aids and tools can improve distance vision, near vision, and sensitivity to contrast; others facilitate activities of daily life (alarms, talking watches, special phones, books in Braille, audiobooks, text-to-speech computer programs, etc.).

Computers are important tools of integration for the visually impaired person. They allow, using standard or specific programs, screen magnification and conversion of text into sound or touch (Braille line) and are useful for all levels of visual handicap. Scanners can, in conjunction with text-to-speech software, read the contents of books and documents aloud via computer. Vendors also build closed-circuit televisions that electronically magnify paper, and even change its contrast and color, for visually impaired users. The recent development of tablets and smartphones has revolutionized low vision aids; numerous applications allow magnification of objects or text (▶ Fig. 21.2), scanning of bar codes, dictation of messages or emails, and improved navigation with a Global Positioning System, among others.

21.2.2 Homonymous Hemianopia

Lesions involving the retrochiasmal visual pathways result in contralateral homonymous hemianopia. Often, associated neurologic deficits (such as hemiparesis, aphasia, neglect, cognitive impairment) predominate and make the visual loss a secondary issue

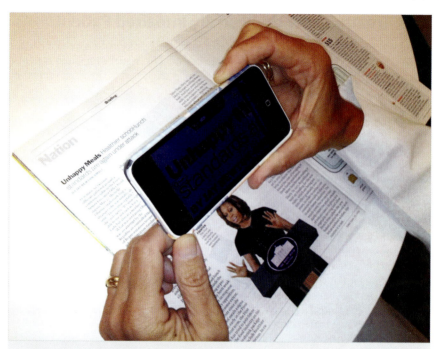

Fig. 21.2 Magnification of text using a smartphone. Most available applications use the light to illuminate the text, and a cursor allows easy control of the level of magnification. This type of application works particularly well on tablets that have a larger screen.

for the patient. However, isolated lesions of the visual pathways, particularly the occipital lobes, result in difficulty with ambulation, reading, and driving.

As for any neurologic deficit, rehabilitation can improve the outcome of patients with homonymous hemianopia. Treatment of associated cognitive deficits and neglect is essential.

Various strategies can be used to help hemianopic patients:
- Using a ruler to highlight the text when reading (avoids skipping lines) (▶ Fig. 21.3)
- Using a finger to follow the words when reading (helps making saccades into the blind field using proprioception) (▶ Fig. 21.3)
- Use of prisms on glasses to displace the seeing hemifield centrally (helpful for patients with mobility impairment)
- Computerized training with specific programs can enable the following:
  - Increased attention
  - Use of residual blindsight
  - Training to make saccades into the blind hemifield
  - Stimulation of cortical plasticity
- Driving rehabilitation with specific programs for use on the road or with driving simulators

Although none of these strategies is a "magic treatment," they all help improve the visual function of hemianopic patients. The choice of a specific strategy is based mostly on local availability as well as on a patient's specific complaints and needs. It is

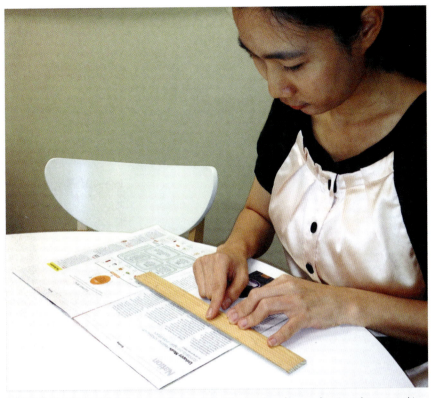

Fig. 21.3 Patient with homonymous hemianopia using a ruler when reading in order not to skip lines. Following each word with her finger allows her to read more easily.

important to emphasize that none of these strategies can truly enlarge the residual visual field; they are therefore usually not recommended in patients with a complete hemianopia whose only handicap is that they want to be legal to drive.

21.2.3 Driving with Visual Impairment

While there are strict federal vision standards in the United States for commercial licensing, there are no such international standards, and there are no federal standards for unrestricted noncommercial passenger vehicle drivers' licenses in the United States. Individual states and the District of Columbia have their own vision requirements for initial and renewal licensing. These requirements can vary widely and need to be verified individually with each state's Department of Motor Vehicles (DMV) (http://www.dmv.org/) prior to making recommendations.

Unrestricted Licenses

An unrestricted license allows its owner to drive without corrective lenses, in any location and for any distance, in all light conditions, both day and night, on any road, at

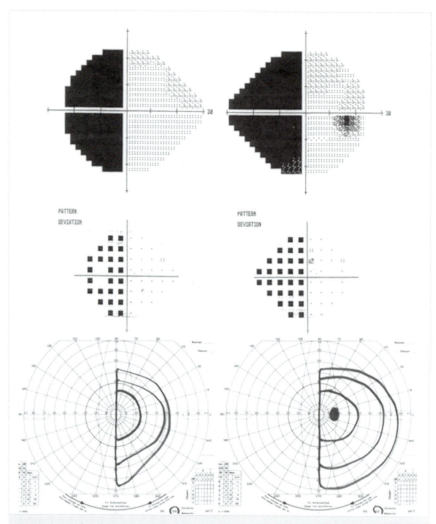

Fig. 21.4 Complete left homonymous hemianopia. Such a complete homonymous hemianopia would make it illegal for the patient to drive in most countries. The Humphrey visual field (top) tests the central visual field only, whereas the Goldmann visual field (bottom) tests the entire visual field. Both tests show a large deficit within the visual field.

any legal speed, and in any normally equipped vehicle, without additional or special mirrors.

Restricted Licenses

The most common restriction requires the use of corrective lenses when driving.

Restrictions based on vision testing vary from state to state and include mandated use of corrective lenses, limiting driving from sunrise to sunset only, prohibiting freeway driving, restricting the area in which driving is allowed, and requiring additional mirrors (left and right outside, wide-angle, panoramic, and fender-mounted). Most states have provisions that allow drivers to use telescopic lenses and to demonstrate competency with other visual assistance devices when necessary. The testing parameter that varies least from state to state is visual acuity. All states have visual acuity requirements for licensure, and most have set the minimum best corrected visual acuity (BCVA) requirement at 20/40 in the better eye. Horizontal visual field requirements are more varied. Although a few states have no required visual field most have a binocular horizontal visual field requirement, which ranges from 140 degrees to 105 degrees of contiguous visual field. Several states also list the horizontal dimension of the visual field of applicants with only one useful eye; this ranges from 55 degrees to 105 degrees. Most states will not issue any driver's license to a person with a homonymous hemianopia (▶ Fig. 21.4).

Index

A

Abducens nerve *306*, 328, *328*
Abducens nerve anatomy **383**, *385*
Abducens nerve palsies
– causes of *386*
– congenital **390**, *392*
– diplopia in *383*, *385*, *387–393*, *464*
– in children **393**
– microvascular *387–388*, *390*
– mimickers of *393*, **393**, *394*
– patient evaluation in **394**
Abnormal blinking **525**, *526*
Abnormal visual perceptions
– drugs in *279*
– in Anton syndrome **279**
– in blindsight *279*
– in Charles Bonnet syndrome **272**
– in dementia **273**
– in dysmetropsia *277*
– in maculopathy *271*, *272*
– in migraine *273*, **273**, *274*
– in narcolepsy **275**
– in occipital seizure *273*, **274**
– in oscillopsia *279*
– in palinopsia *275*, *276*
– in peduncular hallucinosis **274**, *275*
– in polyopia **276**
– in psychiatric disorders **271**
– in residual vision *279*
– in Riddoch phenomenon *278*
– in sensation of environment tilt phenomenon *277*, *278*
– in visual allesthesia *277*, **277**
– neurologic disorders in *273*, **273**, *274–276*, *278*
– ophthalmic disorders in **271**, *272*
– optic nerve disease in **272**
– optical causes of **271**
– toxins in *279*
Abuse, escape from **527**
Acalculia **269**
Acanthamoeba keratitis *116*
Accommodation paralysis, as nonorganic symptom **534**
Acoustic neuroma *499*, **556**
Acquired immunodeficiency syndrome (AIDS) **600**, *602–604*
– *See also* Human immunodeficiency virus (HIV)
Acute disseminated encephalomyelitis (ADEM) **196**

Acute idiopathic blind spot enlargement (AIBSE) syndrome **123**
Acute peripheral vestibulopathy **454**
Acute zonal occult outer retinopathy (AZOOR) **123**
ADEM, *see* Acute disseminated encephalomyelitis (ADEM)
Adenovirus **192**
Adie pupil **309**, *310–312*
Adipose body of orbit *467*
Adrenaline *282*, **308**
Agonist muscle **324**
Agraphia *267*, **269**
AIBSE, *see* Acute idiopathic blind spot enlargement (AIBSE) syndrome
AICA, *see* Anterior inferior cerebellar artery (AICA)
AIDS, *see* Acquired immunodeficiency syndrome (AIDS)
AION, *see* Anterior ischemic optic neuropathy (AION)
Akinetopsia *267*
Albinism **240**
Alcohol withdrawal **279**
Alexia, without graphica *267*
Alzheimer disease
– Balint syndrome in *266*
– in disorders of higher cortical function **270**
Amaurosis fugax **114**, 138
Amblyopia **120**, **124**, 285, 377, 415, 463, 493
Aminoglycosides **380**
Aminopyridines **501**
Amiodarone
– in toxic optic neuropathy **229**, *231*
– nystagmus with **495**
Amphetamines **282**
Amsler grid *6*, *7*, *28*, *46*, *47*
Ancillary testing
– electrophysiologic **77**, *78–79*
– indications for **77**
Aneurysm
– anterior communicating artery *573*
– anterior inferior cerebellar artery *573*
– basilar artery *573*
– carotid-cavernous **474**, *475–476*
– carotid-ophthalmic *573*
– cavernous sinus *423*, *426*, *573*

– in left posterior communicating artery *103*
– in oculomotor nerve palsy 415, *416*
– intracranial **572**, *573*, *575*
– ophthalmic artery *573*
– posterior communicating artery *103*, *108*, *111*, *573*
– posterior inferior cerebellar artery *573*
– superior cerebellar artery *573*
Angiofibroma, facial *616*
Angiography
– catheter **102**, *109–111*
– cerebral **546**
– computed tomographic **102**, *103–104*
– magnetic resonance **102**, *106–108*
– retinal fluorescein **81**, *83–85*
Angular artery *141*, *144*, *474*, *510*
Angular vein *144*, *255*, *473–474*, *510*
Aniridia **240**, 291
Anisocoria **14**, **15**, **287**, *290*
– causes of **288**
– diagnosis of **288**, *290–292*
– in Adie pupil **309**, *310–312*
– in Horner syndrome **297**, *298–307*
– in ipsilateral parasympathetic pathway dysfunction **309**
– in miosis **292**, *298–303*, *305–307*
– in mydriasis *293–295*, *308*, **308**, *309–315*
– in third nerve palsy *313*, **313**, *314–315*
– in tonic pupil **309**, *310–312*
– ocular causes of **291**, *293–297*, **308**
– patient approach in *315*
– pharmacologic *308*, **308**, *309*
– physiologic **288**, *293*
– traumatic **308**
Anterior cerebral artery **549**
Anterior communicating artery aneurysm *573*
Anterior ethmoidal artery *142*
Anterior inferior cerebellar artery (AICA) aneurysm *573*
Anterior intercavernous sinus *560*
Anterior ischemic optic neuropathy (AION) 204, *204–205*, **205**, *206–207*, *209–210*, **212**, *213*, 579, *579–580*
Anterior uveitis *18*, **595**

Index

Index